Student Workbook and Resource Guide for

Comprehensive Nursing Care

Roberta Pavy Ramont
Dee Maldonado Niedringhaus
Mary Ann Towle

Pearson

Boston   Columbus   Indianapolis   New York   San Francisco   Upper Saddle River
Amsterdam   Cape Town   Dubai   London   Madrid   Milan   Munich   Paris   Montreal   Toronto
Delhi   Mexico City   Sao Paulo   Sydney   Hong Kong   Seoul   Singapore   Taipei   Tokyo

Pearson® is a registered trademark of Pearson plc

Pearson Education LTD.
Pearson Education Australia PTY, Limited
Pearson Education Singapore, Pte. Ltd
Pearson Education North Asia Ltd
Pearson Education, Canada, Ltd

Pearson Educación de Mexico, S.A. de C.V.
Pearson Education—Japan
Pearson Education Malaysia, Pte. Ltd
Pearson Education, Upper Saddle River, New Jersey

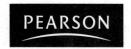

10 9 8 7 6 5 4 3 2 1
ISBN 10:   0-13-504100-7
ISBN 13: 978-0-13-504100-0

Contents

Preface

Students entering the field of nursing have a tremendous amount to learn in a short time. This Student Workbook and Resource Guide that accompanies *Comprehensive Nursing Care, Second Edition,* is designed to reinforce the knowledge that you—the student—have gained in each chapter and to help you master critical concepts.

At the beginning of each chapter, you will find a MyNursingKit box. Just as in the main textbook, this box identifies for you all the specific media resources and activities available for that chapter at www.mynursingkit.com. You will find references to animations as well as case studies and care plans to help you visualize and comprehend difficult concepts.

In addition, each chapter includes a variety of questions and activities to help you comprehend difficult concepts and reinforce basic knowledge gained from the textbook reading assignments.

Features Include:

- **Matching** exercises that contain key terms and definitions from each chapter.
- **Multiple Choice** questions that provide additional review on key topics.
- Thorough assessment of essential information in the text is provided through the **Learning Outcomes** activities.
- **Apply What You Learned** help you problem solve real nursing scenarios.
- **Answers** are included at the end of the book to provide immediate reinforcement and to permit you to check the accuracy of your work.

It is our hope that this Workbook will serve as a valuable learning tool and will contribute to your success in the nursing profession.

Debra S. McKinney, MSN, MBA/HCM, RN
Nursing Education Consultant

Chapter 1

Succeeding as a Nursing Student

EXPLORE PEARSON mynursingkit™

MyNursingKit is your one stop for online chapter review materials and resources. Prepare for success with additional NCLEX®-style practice questions, interactive assignments and activities, web links, animations and videos, and more!

Register your access code from the front of your book at www.mynursingkit.com

KEY TERMS

Match each of the following key terms to its proper definition.

_____ 1. Analysis

_____ 2. Application

_____ 3. Comprehension

_____ 4. Knowledge

A. The act of putting knowledge to use in a new situation

B. Understanding the meaning, translation, and interpretation of instructions and problems

C. The recall of information

D. The interpretation of a variety of data to recognize the commonalities, differences, and interrelationships among present ideas

LEARNING OUTCOMES

1. List essential nursing values concerning attitudes, personal qualities, and professional behaviors.

2. Explain ways to approach this textbook and plan your study time effectively.

3. What is the importance of time management for students in a nursing program?

4. Name the three important aspects of time management that support academic survival in nursing education.

1.

2.

3.

5. Name strategies for answering various types of test questions.

6. What are the responsibilities of the student nurse during the clinical experiences?

7. Explain the importance of prioritizing in the clinical setting.

APPLY WHAT YOU LEARNED

What concerns you regarding your success in completing the nursing program? List your concerns below.

Take this list of concerns to an upper level student and ask them how they overcame these concerns as they began the program. List their advice below.

MULTIPLE CHOICE QUESTIONS

Circle the answer that best completes each of the following statements.

1. The core characteristic of nursing is guided by the philosophy of:
   A. Good hygiene
   B. Critical thinking
   C. Precision
   D. Care

2. Which of the following approaches for planning your study time effectively is *least* helpful?
   A. Study questions at the end of the chapter.
   B. Use the MyNursingKit companion website provided with the textbook.
   C. Study with any group of people.
   D. Outline the chapter after reading it.

3. Which of the following would be used for documenting effective time management?
   A. A small tablet or notepad
   B. The rear section of your textbook
   C. Your cellphone
   D. A planning calendar

4. Which of the following *does not* support academic survival of the nurse in school?
   A. Maintaining current responsibilities
   B. Participating in group study sessions
   C. Maintaining a thorough planning calendar
   D. Securing financial aid

5. If asked to *contrast* a topic in an essay question, your response would contain information that would:
   A. Point out differences
   B. Describe in narrative form using "word pictures" to provide examples
   C. Present information in condensed form briefly giving main points
   D. Point out similarities and differences

6. Which of the following *is not* a responsibility of the student nurse during clinical experiences?
   A. Ensuring that you understand what you read and how to apply it to the care of real clients
   B. Taking advantage of all learning opportunities in the clinical setting
   C. Performing a task when you think you know what to do
   D. Practicing skills repeatedly so that you know exactly what to do

7. Prioritizing care in the clinical setting requires which of the following to be preformed first by the LPN/LVN?
   A. Review the pertinent client information prior to delivering care.
   B. Visit each of your clients and introduce yourself.
   C. Complete a head-to-toe examination.
   D. Prepare medications before seeing the client to maximize your time.

8. Which of the following would *not* be considered values and behavior that hallmark the professional nurse?
   A. Caring
   B. Perfection
   C. Precision
   D. Timeliness

9. A test question that requires you to understand information would be considered which of the following?
   A. An application question
   B. An analysis question
   C. A knowledge question
   D. A comprehension question

10. What should be foremost in the nurse's mind when working in the clinical setting pertaining to client care?
    A. Being flexible
    B. Having priorities correct
    C. Safety
    D. Attending post-conferences

Chapter 2

History of Nursing

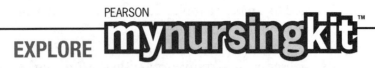

KEY TERMS

Match each of the following key terms to its proper definition.

_____ 1. Client

_____ 2. Consumer

_____ 3. Illness

_____ 4. NCLEX-PN®

_____ 5. Nurse practice acts

_____ 6. Patient

_____ 7. Profession

_____ 8. Wellness

A. The highly individualized response a person has to a disease

B. A person who is waiting for or undergoing medical treatment and care

C. A state of well-being; engaging in attitudes and behaviors that enhance the quality of life and maximize personal potential

D. A person who engages the advice or services of someone who is qualified to provide the service

E. A vocation requiring knowledge of some department of learning or science

F. An individual, a group of people, or a community that uses a service or commodity

G. Nurse must take in order to practice as an LPN or LVN

H. Laws in each state instrumental in defining the scope of nursing practice to protect public health, safety, and welfare

LEARNING OUTCOMES

1. Describe historical and contemporary factors that influence the development of nursing

Historical Factors	Contemporary Factors

2. Briefly describe the key figures in nursing history and their contribution to nursing.

Key Figures	Contribution

3. Outline the contribution made to the profession of nursing by males.

4. What are the four major areas within the LPN/LVN scope of practice?

    A.

    B.

    C.

    D.

5. Explain key contributions to the practical/vocational nursing history.

6. Summarize the customers, purpose, standards, and work settings of LPNs/LVNs.

Customers	Purpose	Standards	Work Settings

7. List professional organizations for the LPN/LVN and nursing students.

APPLY WHAT YOU LEARNED

Go to the State Board of Nursing website for your state and print the nurse practice act pertaining to the LPN/LVN practice. Read the act and then answer the following questions.

1. How is the "practice of practical nursing" defined in the nurse practice act?

2. What is required for you to call yourself a nurse?

3. What are grounds for discipline against your future license?

MULTIPLE CHOICE QUESTIONS

Circle the answer that best completes each of the following statements.

1. During the third and fourth centuries, several wealthy matrons of the Roman Empire converted to Christianity and used their wealth to provide houses of care and healing for the poor, the sick, and the homeless. Which of the following did this?
   A. Florence Nightingale
   B. Jean-Jacques Henner
   C. Marcella
   D. Mary Breckinridge

2. Which of the following key figures in nursing was noted for establishing the American Red Cross?
   A. Lillian Wald
   B. Clara Barton
   C. Margaret Higgins Sanger
   D. Mary Breckinridge

3. Which of these men is credited with starting the first ambulance service?
   A. James Derham
   B. Friar Juan de Mena
   C. St. Camillus de Lellis
   D. The Alexian Brothers

4. Which of the following would the nurse say was provided if giving a talk about drug and alcohol abuse?
   A. Restoring health
   B. Caring for the dying
   C. Preventing illness
   D. Promoting health and wellness

5. Which of the following organizations published a position paper clearly defining the two levels of nursing? (registered and technical)
   A. American Nurses Association
   B. The National League of Nursing
   C. The Association of Practical Nurse Schools
   D. Smith-Hughes Act

6. What is the common purpose of nurse practice acts regardless of jurisdiction?
   A. To protect the public
   B. To protect the nurse
   C. To protect the hospital or healthcare organization
   D. To protect the physician or doctor

7. Which of the following organizations serves as the central source of information on what is new and changing in practical/vocational nursing education and practice on the local, state, and national level?
   A. National Association for Practical Nurse Education and Service (NAPNES)
   B. National Federation of Licensed Practical Nurses (NFLPN)
   C. Health Occupation Students of America (HOSA)
   D. National League for Nursing (NLN)

8. The specific standards identified by the NFLPN state, "The LPN/LVN shall have at least _____ experience in nursing at the staff level" to be considered specialized in that field of nursing practice.
   A. Two years
   B. Six months
   C. One year
   D. Three years

9. Which state was first to require licensure for practical nurses?
   A. Pennsylvania
   B. Virginia
   C. New York
   D. California

10. Which woman devised a method for the treatment of poliomyelitis by stimulating and re-educating affected muscles?
    A. Mary Breckinridge
    B. Margaret Higgins Sanger
    C. Lavinia L. Dock
    D. Sister Elizabeth Kenny

Chapter 3

Promoting Culturally Proficient Care

KEY TERMS

Match each of the following key terms to its proper definition.

_____ 1. Prejudice

A. The modification of a group's or individual's culture as a result of contact with another group

_____ 2. Stereotypes

B. Interpretation of the beliefs and behaviors of others from the perspective of one's own cultural values and traditions

_____ 3. Ethnocentrism

C. Prejudgment or bias based on characteristics such as race, age, or gender

_____ 4. Discrimination

D. Oversimplified conceptions, opinions, or beliefs about some aspect of a group of people

_____ 5. Acculturation

E. Unfair and unequal treatment or access to services based on race, culture, or other bias

---

_____ 1. Cultural awareness

A. The intellectual identification with or vicarious experiencing of the feelings, thoughts, or attitudes of another culture

_____ 2. Cultural competence

B. An awareness of the needs and feelings of your own and others' cultures

_____ 3. Cultural empathy

C. Awareness of one's own cultural values

_____ 4. Cultural sensitivity

D. Knowledge about the similarities and differences among cultures

____	1.	Biocultural ecology	A.	The assessment of skin color and biologic variations
____	2.	Domains	B.	The exchange of messages by members of two or more cultures that is influenced by their different cultural perceptions
____	3.	Intercultural communication	C.	Physical separation of housing and services based on race
____	4.	Segregation	D.	Elements that describe a variable in scientific research

LEARNING OUTCOMES

1. What is the history of transcultural nursing?

2. List and define terminology of transcultural nursing.

3. List the 12 domains of culture and define each one.

Domain	Definition

4. What effect do healthcare disparities have on members of various cultural groups?

5. What is the role of communication in the delivery of culturally proficient care to hospitalized clients and their families?

6. What are the components of a cultural assessment?

7. What is the subculture of health care? Include cultural diversity among nurses in your answer.

APPLY WHAT YOU LEARNED

Using the Internet, research healthcare beliefs of different cultural groups and provide several culturally competent nursing actions you might use when caring for clients from the following cultures. Include common religious beliefs, communication style, decision maker in the family, or food preferences in your answer.

1. **African American –**

2. **Latino –**

3. **American Indian –**

4. **Middle Eastern –**

MULTIPLE CHOICE QUESTIONS

Circle the answer that best completes each of the following statements.

1. Which of the following person's work encouraged a broader awareness of cultural issues and led to the study of culture within the nursing curriculum?
   A. Dr. Madeleine Leininger
   B. Florence Nightingale
   C. Sojourner Truth
   D. Sister Elizabeth Kenny

2. Which word would be defined as interpreting the beliefs and behavior of others in terms of one's own cultural values and traditions?
   A. Stereotyping
   B. Cultural awareness
   C. Ethnocentrism
   D. Prejudice

3. Which of the following is not one of the 12 domains of culture?
   A. Communication
   B. Finances
   C. Workforce issues
   D. Death rituals

4. Cross-cultural education can be divided into three conceptual approaches that focus on:
   A. Stereotypes, bias, and clinical uncertainty
   B. Cultural awareness, sensitivity, and competence
   C. Mistrust, misunderstanding, and lack of knowledge
   D. Attitudes, knowledge, and skills

5. The nurse is assessing an infant client of Asian descent. During the assessment the mother of the infant becomes quiet and appears angry. She is verbalizing the word "curse" over and over. What might the nurse have done to cause this reaction?
   A. Smiled at infant
   B. Made eye contact with infant
   C. Dropped the infant's chart on the floor
   D. Touch the infant's head

6. What transcultural communication does the HIPAA regulation provide to the client?
   A. Prevents errors and noncompliance
   B. Ensures informed consent
   C. Provides customer satisfaction
   D. Reduces client stress and anxiety

7. The nurse, conducting a cultural assessment, asks the client, "What is your language preference?" The nurse is collecting what element of the assessment?
   A. The cultural elements of the relationship between the healthcare provider and the client
   B. The cultural explanation of the client's illness
   C. The cultural identity of the client
   D. The cultural factors related to the client's psychosocial environment

8. What term would be defined as the ability to experience *as* the client experiences rather than *how* they experience?
   A. Acculturation
   B. Cultural empathy
   C. Cultural diversity
   D. Cultural sensitivity

9. The nurse learns that a specific cultural group believes that an individual who brings shame on themselves brings shame on the entire family. Which cultural group holds this belief?
   A. Asian Pacific (or Pacific Rim) group
   B. Rasa-Latina group
   C. Caucasian group
   D. American Black group

10. Personal space is considered a factor in which of the 12 domains of culture?
    A. Family roles and organization
    B. Healthcare practices
    C. Spirituality
    D. Communication

Chapter 4

Legal and Ethical Issues of Nursing

KEY TERMS

Match each of the following key terms to its proper definition.

_____ 1. Credentialing

_____ 2. Bioethics

_____ 3. Malpractice

_____ 4. Defamation

_____ 5. Ethics

_____ 6. Libel

_____ 7. Assault

_____ 8. Negligence

A. Misconduct or practice that is below the standard expected of an ordinary, reasonable, and prudent practitioner that places another person at risk for harm.

B. The expected standards of moral behavior of a particular group as described in the group's formal code of professional ethics.

C. The way in which the nursing profession maintains standards of practice and accountability for the educational preparation of its members.

D. The ethics and philosophical implications of certain biological and medical procedures, technologies, and treatments.

E. Being legally responsible for one's acts and omissions.

F. Defamation by means of print, writing, or pictures.

G. Negligence that occurred while a person was performing as a professional.

H. The right and ability to make one's own decisions.

	9.	Slander	I.	Communication that is false or made with a careless disregard for the truth, resulting in injury to the reputation of a person.
	10.	Advocate	J.	Attempt or threat to touch another person unjustifiably.
	11.	Liability	K.	Defamation by the spoken word, stating information or false words that can cause damage to a person's reputation.
	12.	Autonomy	L.	One who expresses and defends the cause of another.
	13.	Battery	M.	Willful touching of a person that may or may not cause harm.

LEARNING OUTCOMES

1. What are the aspects of law that affect nursing practice? Include the difference between crimes and torts, and give nursing examples of each.

Aspects of Law	Crimes	Torts	Examples in Nursing

2. Define the following terms.

Unprofessional Conduct	Definition
Negligence	
Assault/battery	
False imprisonment	
Invasion of privacy	
Defamation	

3. What are the aspects of regulation of nursing practice, standards of care, agency policies, and nurse practice acts that affect the scope of nursing practice?

Regulation of nursing practice	
Standards of care	
Agency policies	
Nurse practice acts	

4. What legal protection is available for nurses?

5. What is the purpose of liability insurance?

6. How can nurses and nursing students minimize their chances of liability?

7. How does privileged communication impact the legal aspects of nursing practice?

8. What information needs to be included in an incident report?

9. What are the purposes and limitations of professional codes of ethics?

10. What is the advocacy role of the nurse?

11. What strategies could a nurse use to enhance ethical decision making?

12. Which common ethical issues are the healthcare professionals currently facing? Describe each issue briefly.

APPLY WHAT YOU LEARNED

The nurse, just beginning the shift, enters the client's room to check on the infusing intravenous line. The client's left forearm just above the wrist is red and swollen, the IV is no longer infusing, and there is fluid (most likely IV fluid) leaking from the insertion site. The skin of the arm is cool and pale. The nurse discontinues the IV, places a warm soak on the left arm, restarts the IV in the right hand, and notifies the physician of the IV infiltrate. The nurse documents the infiltrate in the client's medical record.

1. What other documentation must the nurse complete related to this event?

2. Document the event using objective terminology.

3. What is the nurse's legal liability related to this event?

MULTIPLE CHOICE QUESTIONS

Circle the answer that best completes each of the following statements.

1. What legal classification is given to a civil wrong committed against a person or a person's property?
   A. Negligence
   B. Tort
   C. Invasion of privacy
   D. Assault and battery

2. The nurse finds out a neighbor is admitted to the hospital where they work. After looking at their medical record on the computer, the nurse tells friends about the neighbor's admission and medical problems. The nurse is guilty of what?
   A. Invasion of privacy
   B. Slander
   C. Defamation
   D. Libel

3. Most locations require mandatory licensure for the nurse, but a few areas in Canada have a type of licensure allowing the nurse to practice without a license. What is this license called?
   A. Inclusive
   B. Accredited
   C. Permissive
   D. Selective

4. What legally protects any reasonably prudent individual, choosing to render emergency aid at an emergency scene, from being liable for their actions?
   A. Americans with Disabilities Act.
   B. Most auto insurance policy covers personal liability.
   C. Good Samaritan Act.
   D. There is no protection; an individual is responsible for their actions.

5. What legal term is defined as being legally responsible for one's acts and omissions?
   A. Liability
   B. Ethics
   C. Scope of practice
   D. Law

6. Which of the following strategies could minimize the risk of liability for the nurse?
   A. Being very pleasant and friendly with the client.
   B. Practicing procedures with which you are inexperienced on a willing client.
   C. Calling after end of your shift to add information to a client's chart.
   D. Asking for assistance with unfamiliar equipment.

7. The nurse is called to court to testify about a prior physician employer, and the lawyer asks for information about an uninvolved client. The nurse refuses to answer the question unless the client gives permission for the information to be shared in order to avoid what?
   A. Professional liability
   B. Privileged communication
   C. Collective bargaining
   D. Credentialing

8. Which of the following healthcare professionals is responsible for filling out an incident report on a client given an incorrect dosage of medication?
   A. RN or charge nurse on the floor.
   B. Pharmacist who prepared the dosage.
   C. The nurse who administered the medication.
   D. The nurse who discovered the error.

9. The nurse is caring for a client in a chronic vegetative state due to a recent injury. The family disagrees about how to proceed with the client's care. What resources could the nurse offer to help the family? (Select all that apply.)
   A. Local religious leader
   B. Ethics committee
   C. Social service referral
   D. Board of Nursing
   E. Healthcare team conference

10. The client tells the nurse he doesn't feel as though his doctor is hearing him when he voices preferences regarding his plan of care. The nurse calls the physician to discuss the client's concerns. What role is the nurse playing for this client?
    A. Advocate
    B. Care provider
    C. Nurturer
    D. Arbitrator

Chapter 5

Critical Thinking and Nursing Theory/Models

KEY TERMS

Match each of the following key terms to its proper definition.

_____ 1. Critical thinking

_____ 2. Deductive reasoning

_____ 3. Environment

_____ 4. Inductive reasoning

_____ 5. Objective data

_____ 6. Subjective data

_____ 7. Theories

A. Circumstances, objects, or conditions by which one is surrounded

B. Information detectable by an observer

C. Ways of looking at a discipline in clear, explicit terms that can be communicated to others

D. Information apparent only to the person being affected

E. The art of thinking about thinking

F. A process of forming generalizations from individual pieces of data

G. A process of moving logically from a general statement or concept to related specifics

1. What are the characteristics, skills, and attitudes of critical thinking?

Characteristics
Skills
Attitudes

2. What is the importance of critical thinking to the nursing process?

3. What is nursing theory?

4. How do different theories of nursing differ in terms of client, environment, health, and nursing?

5. How can the LPN/LVN incorporate critical thinking into their nursing practice?

6. Define evidence-based practice and explain how the LPN/LVN can participate in evidence-based practice.

APPLY WHAT YOU LEARNED

1. You go home from a long day at school, turn on your living room light switch, and nothing happens. Using critical thinking, how will you approach this problem?

2. What would happen if the nurse did not develop critical thinking skills?

3. Choose one nursing theory and one non-nursing theory, and describe how you will apply them to your nursing practice.

MULTIPLE CHOICE QUESTIONS

Circle the answer that best completes each of the following statements.

1. The nurse enters the client's room and finds her on the floor by her bed crying. The nurse assumes the client fell out of bed, is injured, and that is why she is crying. After helping the client back into bed, the nurse completes an incident report and notifies the supervisor of the client's fall. What one word in this scenario is incompatible with critical thinking?
   A. Helping
   B. Notifies
   C. Assumes
   D. Incident

2. Which of the following is *not* important to the critical thinking nursing process?
   A. Obtains information that clarifies the problem
   B. Evaluates all possible solutions
   C. Discards all other solutions after a specific solution is chosen
   D. Monitors the situation carefully to ensure effectiveness

3. Which of the following concepts are essential elements of nursing theory?
   A. Health, nursing, time, and environment
   B. Ethics, health, values, and nursing
   C. Environment, nursing, client, and health
   D. Nursing, training, bioethics, and attitude

4. Which theorist researched the individual's response to stressors?
   A. Florence Nightingale's environmental theory
   B. Dorothea Orem's general theory of nursing
   C. Betty Neuman's system model
   D. Sister Callista Roy's adaptation model

5. The LPN/LVN enters a client's room and notices blood on the bed. The LPN/LVN's priority action is to:
   A. Change the bed linens.
   B. Notify the physician.
   C. Ask the client where the blood came from.
   D. Examine the client.

6. The nurse reads a newspaper article about a new procedure for treating congestive heart failure. Which of the following would be an appropriate next step?
   A. Inform the physician that there is a better way of treating congestive heart failure the next time the nurse cares for a client with this diagnosis.
   B. Conduct a class for peers on the new treatment.
   C. Find other articles about the new treatment in other newspapers.
   D. Consult nursing and healthcare related articles to learn more about the study of the new procedure.

7. How can the LPN/LVN participate in evidence-based practice? Select all that apply.
   A. Read current literature
   B. Collect data
   C. Provide nursing care
   D. Collaborate with RN
   E. Participate in continuing education

8. Which of the following is an attribute of a critical thinker?
   A. We analyze other's thinking.
   B. We learn how to govern the thoughts that govern us.
   C. We subject the altruistic root of our thinking to close scrutiny.
   D. We embrace all standards.

9. Which type of statement is described as going beyond facts to make a statement about something currently known?
   A. Judgment
   B. Opinion
   C. Inference
   D. Fact

10. Have my assumptions affected my interpretation of the data? This question would be considered what part of the nursing process?
    A. Diagnosing
    B. Assessment
    C. Implementing
    D. Evaluating

Chapter 6

The LPN/LVN and the Nursing Process

KEY TERMS

Match each of the following key terms to its proper definition.

_____ 1. Assessment

_____ 2. Care plan

_____ 3. Diagnosing

_____ 4. Evaluation

_____ 5. Planning

A. A planned, ongoing, purposeful activity

B. The systematic collection, organization, validation, and documentation of data

C. The process of designing nursing activities required to prevent, reduce, or eliminate a client's health problems

D. Analyzing and synthesizing data to provide a statement of condition or need

E. Product of the planning phase of the nursing process

_____ 6. Collaborative interventions

_____ 7. Desired/expected outcomes

_____ 8. Manifestations

_____ 9. Objective data

_____ 10. Subjective data

A. The broader goals of a client in relation to a nursing diagnosis

B. Information apparent only to the person being affected

C. Nursing activities that reflect the overlapping responsibilities among healthcare personnel

D. Signs and symptoms

E. Information detectable by an observer

_____ 11.	Etiology	A.	A systematic, rational method of planning and providing individualized nursing care
_____ 12.	Goals	B.	Phase of the nursing process in which selected nursing interventions and activities occur
_____ 13.	Implementation	C.	The particular aspects of a desired outcome for a client
_____ 14.	Interventions	D.	Cause or origin
_____ 15.	Nursing process	E.	The actions initiated by the nurse to achieve client goals

LEARNING OUTCOMES

1. What are the essential characteristics of the nursing process?

2. What are the components of the nursing process?

3. What is the role of the LPN/LVN in the assessment process?

4. What is the purpose of collecting data? How will the data be used?

Purpose	How will it be used?

5. What differentiates objective from subjective data? What differentiates primary from secondary data?

Objective Data	Primary Data
Subjective Data	Secondary Data

6. What are three methods of data collection? How is each useful?

Methods of Data Collection	Use

7. What are the elements of the nursing diagnoses? What is the importance of each element?

8. What does the nurse do during the planning stage?

9. What activities occur during the implementing phase?

10. What is the value of the evaluation phase in the nursing process, and how does it relate to the other phases of the nursing process?

Value	Relationship to Other Phases

APPLY WHAT YOU LEARNED

While driving home from school, the car in front of you suddenly develops a flat front tire, skids and slides off the road, flips over the embankment, and lands on its roof. Using the nursing process, explain how you will respond to this emergency.

Assessment

Planning

Intervention

Evaluation

MULTIPLE CHOICE QUESTIONS

Circle the answer that best completes each of the following statements.

1. What component of the nursing process would the LPN/LVN use if they needed to determine how to prevent, reduce, or resolve the identified client problem?
   A. Diagnosing
   B. Assessing
   C. Planning
   D. Evaluating

2. Which component of the nursing process results in continuity of care?
   A. Diagnosis
   B. Planning
   C. Assessment
   D. Evaluation

3. How can the LPN/LVN contribute during the assessment phase of the nursing process?
   A. Performing the initial assessment
   B. Reviewing and revising the care plan
   C. Making observations of client status
   D. Identifying client strengths and health problems that can be prevented

4. During an assessment, the nurse documents that the client "Cried during the interview." This would be considered:
   A. Manifestation data
   B. Objective data
   C. Secondary data
   D. Subjective data

5. How is subjective data documented in the client's assessment?
   A. Paraphrased by nurse
   B. In red ink on the chart
   C. In as few words as possible to conserve space
   D. In the client's own words

6. While questioning the newly admitted obese client, he expresses a desire to lose weight. The type of data collection method is:
   A. An intervention
   B. An observation
   C. An interview
   D. An examination

7. Nursing diagnoses are created by what member of the healthcare team?
   A. The physician
   B. The nurse manager
   C. The LPN/LVN
   D. The RN

8. Setting priorities would happen in which phase of the nursing process?
   A. Planning
   B. Implementing
   C. Evaluating
   D. Diagnosing

9. The nurse enters the client's room and finds the client unresponsive. What is the first action of the nurse?
   A. Assess
   B. Plan
   C. Intervene
   D. Evaluate

10. The nurse learns in report that a client has been having a problem with urine retention and has required straight catheterization every six hours. The client is next due for catheterization at 9:00. Prior to performing the procedure, what will the nurse do first?
    A. Assess
    B. Plan
    C. Implement
    D. Evaluate

Chapter 7

Healthcare Delivery Systems

KEY TERMS

Match each of the following key terms to its proper definition.

_____ 1. Client-focused care

_____ 2. Managed care

_____ 3. Primary nursing

_____ 4. Team nursing

A. The delivery of individualized nursing care to clients led by a professional nurse.

B. A delivery model that brings all services and care providers to the client.

C. A healthcare system whose goals are to provide cost-effective, quality care that focuses on improved outcomes for groups of clients.

D. Total nursing responsibility for a group of clients 24 hours a day, 7 days a week.

_____ 5. Clinical pathways

_____ 6. Health maintenance organization

A. A system that limits the amount paid to hospitals that are reimbursed by Medicare.

B. A federal program to assist people age 65 and over with medical care.

_____ 7. Medicaid

C. A group healthcare agency that provides basic and supplemental health maintenance and treatment services to voluntary enrollees who pay a preset fee.

_____ 8. Medicare

D. An expected path of client needs, care, teaching, and progress for specific diagnosis.

_____ 9. Prospective payment system

E. A federal public assistance program paid out of general taxes to people who require financial assistance for medical care.

LEARNING OUTCOMES

1. List the three types of healthcare delivery services and provide examples of each.

Types of Healthcare Delivery Services	Examples

2. Describe the differences in providing nursing care in the outpatient versus the inpatient settings.

3. What are the purpose and functions of the following healthcare agencies?

Healthcare Agency	Purpose/Function
Public Health	
Home Healthcare Agencies	
Extended-Care Facilities	
Assisted Living Centers	
Hospice Services	

4. Why is health care considered a right, and what other rights do clients have?

5. List the members of the healthcare team and briefly explain what they do.

Member	Role

6. List and describe factors that affect healthcare delivery.

Factor	Effect on Healthcare Delivery

7. List the five models of care and explain the unique characteristics of each.

Model of Care	Unique Characteristics

8. List and describe the different reimbursement methods of payment for healthcare services.

APPLY WHAT YOU LEARNED

James Franklin, 26, is a famous professional basketball player. While running down the court, without any contact, his femur fractured. He was brought to the hospital, where they performed x-rays, bone scans, and a bone marrow biopsy, and diagnosed him with metastatic bone cancer with metastasis to the lungs, liver, bowel, and brain. His prognosis is extremely poor and he is not expected to live more than a few months. When the nurse enters the room he asks if the nurse thinks the physician may have made a mistake. The unit phone is ringing constantly with the news media trying to find out more about his condition.

1. Considering the client bill of rights, what does this client have the right to expect from you when you are caring for him?

MULTIPLE CHOICE QUESTIONS

Circle the answer that best completes each of the following statements.

1. Diagnosing and treating a complex illness is associated with what level of healthcare service?
   A. Primary
   B. Secondary
   C. Tertiary
   D. Ambulatory

2. A positive aspect of this type of healthcare setting is that cultural beliefs and practices are more visible to the nurse working independently. What healthcare setting is described?
   A. Home health care
   B. Day care center
   C. Retirement center
   D. Assisted living center

3. This type of healthcare agency can include skilled nursing facilities that provide personal care for those who are chronically ill or are unable to care for themselves without assistance:
   A. Hospitals
   B. Home healthcare agencies
   C. Retirement centers
   D. Extended-care facilities

4. A client refuses to participate in a research study examining the disease they are being treated for. The nurse's responsibility is to:
    A. Persuade the client to change her mind.
    B. Talk to the client's support group to have them try to change her mind.
    C. Respect the rights of the client not to participate.
    D. Get a court order to force the client to participate.

5. The member of the team responsible for finding placement in rehabilitation facilities for the client being discharged from the acute care facility is the:
    A. Hospitalist
    B. Social worker
    C. Nurse practitioner
    D. Paramedical technologists

6. The nurse works in a rural area where there are no doctors to treat clients. What factor is affecting healthcare in this situation?
    A. Access to health care
    B. Demographic changes
    C. Increasing number of elderly
    D. Uneven distribution of services

7. Which of the following models of care has cross-training of all members of the team as an essential element?
    A. Team nursing
    B. Functional method
    C. Client-focused care
    D. Primary nursing

8. Which system of payment would provide money to a blind client that could be used to cover costs of extended health care?
    A. Prospective payment system
    B. Medicaid
    C. Medicare
    D. Supplemental security income

9. A homeopath is considered what type of healthcare professional?
    A. Occupational therapist
    B. Alternative care provider
    C. Nutritionist
    D. Unlicensed assistive personnel

10. This was first adopted by the American Hospital Association (AHA) in 1973 to protect hospitalized clients.
    A. The Case Method Model of Nursing
    B. Medicaid
    C. The Patient's Bill of Rights
    D. Independent Practice Associations

Chapter 8

Complementary and Alternative Medicine in Health Care

KEY TERMS

Match each of the following key terms to its proper definition.

_____ 1. Alternative medicine

_____ 2. Complementary

_____ 3. Complementary and alternative medicine

_____ 4. Conventional medicine

_____ 5. Integrative medicine

_____ 6. Naturopathic medicine

A. Healing philosophies, approaches, and therapies that exist largely outside the main frame of conventional treatment.

B. A practice that integrates treatments and therapies from conventional medicine with complementary and alternative medicine that have been deemed safe and effective.

C. A medical treatment used in place of conventional medicine.

D. Alternative care system that uses a wide range of approaches to healing.

E. Medicine practiced by holders of a M.D., D.O., and by other healthcare professionals.

F. Used together with a standard approach to provide added benefit.

LEARNING OUTCOMES

1. What is the historical basis for complementary and alternative medical therapy?

2. List and define terminology used in complementary and alternative therapy.

3. Which nontraditional complementary and alternative medical therapies may be recommended to a client in addition to conventional therapy?

4. What complementary and alternative therapies should only be performed by a trained professional?

5. Why would it be important for the nurse to gather information about complimentary and alternative medicine being used by the client?

6. Apply the nursing process to a client using complementary and alternative medicine including interviewing the client during the admission process about their use of CAM therapy.

APPLY WHAT YOU LEARNED

The nurse is caring for a client who was admitted to the acute care facility yesterday. During the admission history the client denied taking any medications or supplements. While helping the client with morning hygiene needs the nurse notes several bottles of supplements in the client's bedside table.

1. Why might the client have failed to mention these supplements when questioned by the nurse yesterday?

2. What is the nurse's responsibility in this scenario?

3. How would you approach this client about the supplements found in the drawer?

MULTIPLE CHOICE QUESTIONS

Circle the answer that best completes each of the following statements.

1. The FDA requires which of the following in regards to herbal remedies?
   A. Submission of proof of the product's safety and efficacy.
   B. Proof of product purity and accuracy of amounts used in preparation.
   C. Side effects and potential interactions must be listed on the bottle or packaging.
   D. Recommended use of the product may be printed on the label.

2. What type of medicine would a doctor who practices internal medicine provide?
   A. Integrative
   B. Naturopathic
   C. Conventional
   D. Alternative

3. Which of the following CAM therapies uses hydrotherapy and exposure to the sun and air to promote energy-based healing?
   A. Naturopathy
   B. Reiki
   C. Ayurveda
   D. Homeopathy

4. Which of the following CAM therapies should only be performed by a trained professional?
   A. Massage therapy
   B. Chiropractic medicine
   C. Reiki
   D. Pilates

5. Why must the nurse have an understanding of CAM therapies? (Select all that apply.)
   A. The nurse may be asked to perform a religious healing practice.
   B. The nurse may be asked to administer herbal medication.
   C. The nurse needs to know of potential interference to prescription drugs.
   D. The nurse needs to know which herbal medications to recommend to the client.
   E. The nurse must understand the purpose and potential benefits of CAM therapies used by the client.

6. How long before surgery should a client stop taking the herbal supplement, *Angelica sinensis*, to prevent excessive bleeding intraoperatively?
    A. Two days
    B. Seven days
    C. Thirty days
    D. Fourteen days

7. Which of the following herbs may be useful for the client diagnosed with osteoarthritis?
    A. Harpagophytum procumbens
    B. Salix alba
    C. Melilotus officinalis
    D. Uncaria tomentosa

8. Which type of CAM therapy is believed to increase endorphins, promote blood flow, and relieve pain?
    A. Homeopathy
    B. Massage therapy
    C. Magnet therapy
    D. Acupuncture

9. What are the side effects of garlic?
    A. Headache, sweating, and hypoglycemia
    B. Insomnia, blood coagulation, and photosensitivity
    C. Diarrhea, low blood pressure, and GI discomfort
    D. Tinnitus, renal damage, and diarrhea

10. Which of the following is a common characteristic and philosophy of CAM therapists?
    A. They emphasize disease treatment instead of disease prevention.
    B. They treat a single pathology rather than the whole client.
    C. They individualize the diagnosis and treatment of clients.
    D. They believe in minimizing the body's inherent healing ability.

Chapter 9

Safety

KEY TERMS

Match each of the following key terms to its proper definition.

_____ 1. Body mechanics

_____ 2. External disasters

_____ 3. Internal disasters

_____ 4. Restraints

_____ 5. Triage

A. Protective devices used to limit the physical activity of the client or a part of the body.

B. Term used to describe safe, efficient use of one's body to move objects and carry out ADLs.

C. Events outside the hospital that produce a large number of victims.

D. System of prioritizing victims' care needs, from most severe to least injured or ill.

E. Events within the hospital that interrupt services and produce victims.

LEARNING OUTCOMES

1. What factors affect safety and people's ability to protect them from injury?

2. What would you teach a client to maintain safety at each stage of the life span?

Lifespan Stages	Safety Teaching Needs
Infant	
Toddler	
Preschool	
School age	
Adolescent	
Young adult	
Middle adult	
Elder	

3. What are common preventable injuries in the home and in healthcare settings?

Home	Healthcare Setting

4. What strategies do institutions use to maintain safety?

5. What emergency codes are commonly used in the healthcare setting?

Triage Codes	Emergency Codes

6. Why are restraints used? What are the legal implications?

7. What alternatives could you use to avoid use of restraints?

8. What strategies can you use to prevent self-injury?

9. Which strategies for self-protection would you use in violent or potentially violent situations?

APPLY WHAT YOU LEARNED

A three-year-old child was admitted to the pediatric unit after drinking a pine-scented cleaning solution. He is an only child and his mother reports he is "a real handful, getting into everything and never still." He lives with an extended family including an aging great-grandmother who has been diagnosed with Alzheimer's disease. His mother does not work outside the house and stays home to take care of the child and his great-grandmother, who has begun wandering and often does not recognize family members.

1. What strategies will you recommend to this mother to prevent the client from poisoning himself again?

2. What strategies can you teach this mother to maintain the safety of the client's great-grandmother?

3. What safety concerns do you have regarding the client's mother? How will you address them?

MULTIPLE CHOICE QUESTIONS

Circle the answer that best completes each of the following statements.

1. The client receiving narcotics could potentially be at risk for injury due to which factor?
   A. Sensory–perceptual alterations
   B. Cognitive alterations
   C. Mobility alterations
   D. Emotional alterations
   E. Environmental alterations

2. At what stage of the life span should a parent teach their child to obey traffic signs and wear reflective clothing at night?
   A. Preschoolers
   B. School-age children
   C. Adolescents
   D. Toddlers

3. The client experiencing orthostatic hypotension may be at risk for which of the following?
   A. Suffocation
   B. Radiation injury
   C. Falls
   D. Poisoning

4. The MSDS sheet is provided on all chemicals in the workplace to provide what information? Select all that apply.
   A. Relevant physical hazards
   B. Permissible exposure limits
   C. Treatment of overdose or overexposure
   D. CDC guidelines about the chemical
   E. Governmental regulations associated with the chemical

5. The nurse walks into a triage room and finds a bottle of sulfuric acid has been broken and fumes are emitted into the room. Which emergency code would the nurse use to report the incident?
   A. Code red
   B. Code yellow
   C. Code black
   D. Code orange

6. Which of the following would help the nurse tasked with applying restraints to a client avoid legal repercussions?
   A. Restraining a legally incompetent client without consent.
   B. Applying restraints for convenience to facilitate a procedure.
   C. Applying restraints only with a physician's order.
   D. Allowing a family member to sit with client in lieu of restraints.

7. Which of the following would be considered an alternative to restraints?
   A. Using a safety belt in a client's wheelchair
   B. Using full-length rails on the bed of a confused client
   C. Increasing a client's dosages of sedatives to relax them
   D. Assisting the confused client using a bedside commode

8. While performing an eye irrigation on an infant, the nurse determines that restraints are required. Which restraint may the nurse use?
   A. Mummy restraints
   B. Mitt or hand restraint
   C. Sleeveless jacket restraint
   D. Elbow restraint

9. What skills would assist the nurse confronted with a potentially violent situation?
   A. Social skills
   B. Cognitive skills
   C. Tai Chi training
   D. De-escalation techniques

10. Which of the following ethnic groups has twice the risk of death secondary to alcohol abuse in the 15–24 year age range?
    A. African American
    B. Native Americans
    C. Caucasian
    D. Latino

Chapter 10

Infection Control and Asepsis

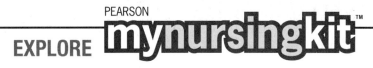

EXPLORE **mynursingkit™**

MyNursingKit is your one stop for online chapter review materials and resources. Prepare for success with additional NCLEX®-style practice questions, interactive assignments and activities, web links, animations and videos, and more!

Register your access code from the front of your book at
www.mynursingkit.com

KEY TERMS

Match each of the following key terms to its proper definition.

____ 1.	Antimicrobial	A.	Harmless micro-organisms found in and on the body
____ 2.	Pathogens	B.	The source of the microorganism
____ 3.	Resident flora	C.	Microbe-destroying
____ 4.	Vector	D.	An organism's ability to produce disease and survive both inside and outside the body
____ 5.	Virulence	E.	Microorganisms that cause disease
____ 6.	Reservoir	F.	A living means of transport for infection

____ 7.	Susceptibility of the host	A.	A potential source of infection for others
____ 8.	Transmission	B.	An inanimate object that can transmit infection from one area or person to another
____ 9.	Carrier	C.	The sixth link in the chain of infection
____ 10.	Fomite	D.	Spread or transmitted by direct or indirect contact
____ 11.	Communicable disease	E.	The manner in which a microorganism gets to the host

____ 12.	Disinfectants	A.	Guidelines for special care to be used with all body fluids
____ 13.	Antiseptics	B.	Fifth link in the chain of infection

_____ 14. Sterile field   C. Agents that destroy pathogens other than spores

_____ 15. Portal of entry   D. Agents that inhibit the growth of some microorganisms

_____ 16. Standard precautions E. A microorganism-free area

_____ 17. Bactericidal agent   A. Occurs after hospital admission and for which the client had no symptoms at the time of admission

_____ 18. Iatrogenic infection   B. Prevents growth and reproduction of only some bacteria

_____ 19. Systemic infection   C. Directly caused by any diagnostic or therapeutic source

_____ 20. Nosocomial infections D. State that exists when microorganisms spread from one area to other body areas

_____ 21. Bacteriostatic agent   E. Solution or chemical that destroys bacteria

_____ 22. Medical asepsis   A. Practice that keeps an object or an area completely free of microorganisms and spores

_____ 23. Portal of exit   B. The absence of disease-causing microorganisms

_____ 24. Surgical asepsis   C. The presence of infection

_____ 25. Sepsis   D. A way of leaving the reservoir

_____ 26. Asepsis   E. All practices used to confine a specific microorganism to a specific area

LEARNING OUTCOMES

1. What are the helpful and harmful actions of microorganisms?

Helpful Actions	Harmful Actions

2. Which agencies try to control the spread of infectious and communicable diseases?

3. List and define different types of infections.

4. What are the six links in the chain of infection? Describe strategies to break each link.

Link	Strategies to Break the Link

5. What are the factors that increase the client's risk of infection?

6. Describe the characteristics of specific and nonspecific defense systems of the body.

Specific	Nonspecific

7. What are common drug-resistant organisms? What nursing care and client teaching is indicated for each drug-resistant organism?

Drug-Resistant Organisms	Nursing Care	Client Teaching

8. What are the important means of controlling microorganisms in the environment?

9. How do standard precautions, transmission-based precautions, and CDC Guidelines relate to each other?

10. What equipment is used for infection control?

11. What are the nursing diagnoses and interventions for clients with an infection or who are at risk for developing an infection?

Diagnoses	Interventions

APPLY WHAT YOU LEARNED

What link in the chain of infection is broken by each of these nursing interventions?

A. Agent/Microorganism   B. Reservoir   C. Portal of exit
D. Method/Mode of transmission   E. Portal of entry   F. Susceptible host

_____ 1. Cleaning up a blood spill and following proper procedure

_____ 2. Use of antibacterial agents

_____ 3. Applying antiseptic spray to the over-bed table

_____ 4. Using proper cough hygiene

_____ 5. Wearing gloves when changing the dressing on a draining wound

_____ 6. Caring for the skin on the hands to prevent micro tears from dry skin

_____ 7. Providing adequate nutrition for clients

_____ 8. Cleaning the port of the IV tubing before inserting a needle

_____ 9. Disinfecting door handles

_____ 10. Hand washing

MULTIPLE CHOICE QUESTIONS

Circle the answer that best completes each of the following statements.

1. Which of the following statements about microorganisms is true?
   A. All microorganisms are harmful.
   B. Resident flora cannot cause disease.
   C. Pathogens are disease-causing microorganisms.
   D. Pathogens can be helpful as well as harmful.

2. While drawing blood to send to the lab, the nurse accidentally spills some onto the floor. What action should the nurse take to clean it up?
   A. Call housekeeping and ask them to come clean up the spill as soon as possible.
   B. Cover with a paper towel and spray bleach on the blood; wait for 20 minutes before cleaning it up.
   C. Call the hazardous material clean-up team to come and clean up the blood spill.
   D. Get some damp paper towels and clean up the spill as soon as possible.

3. What condition is created when bacteremia spreads through all the body systems?
   A. An iatrogenic infection
   B. Sepsis
   C. Septicemia
   D. A systemic infection

4. The client infected with the West Nile virus from exposure to bird feces would be the recipient of what type of transmission?
   A. Vector-borne
   B. Vehicle-borne
   C. Droplet or airborne
   D. Etiologic agent

5. Which of the following factors would elevate blood cortisol?
   A. Radiation treatments for cancer
   B. Stressors in life
   C. Genetic susceptibility
   D. Chronic pathologies that lessen the body's defense system

6. What type of defense system includes B cells?
   A. Cell-mediated defense
   B. Antibody-mediated defense
   C. Nonspecific defenses
   D. Immune defenses

7. Which of the following is considered to be the leading cause of healthcare-associated infections and recognized as a substantial contributor to outbreaks?
   A. Inappropriate hand hygiene
   B. Drug-resistant organisms
   C. Failure to complete a full course of prescribed antibiotics
   D. Physician's prescribing too many antibiotics

8. What type of technique would the nurse use when inserting a catheter into the bladder?
   A. Sepsis
   B. Asepsis
   C. Surgical asepsis
   D. Medical asepsis

9. Which of the following would be considered a component of Standard Precautions while disinfecting in a hospital setting?
   A. Know the type and number of infectious organisms present before disinfecting.
   B. Clean area with soap and water before applying disinfectant.
   C. Apply disinfectant directly on the blood present before cleaning.
   D. Mix extra disinfectant concentrate for heavily soiled surfaces.

10. Which of the following should be considered by the nurse while maintaining a sterile field?
    A. The edges of a sterile field are considered sterile.
    B. Reaching across a sterile field is sometimes necessary.
    C. It is acceptable for water to enter a sterile field.
    D. Objects below the waist of the nurse are considered unsterile.

Chapter 11

Client Communication

KEY TERMS

Match each of the following key terms to its proper definition.

_____ 1. Sender

_____ 2. Open-ended questions

_____ 3. Validation

_____ 4. Receiver

_____ 5. Closed-ended questions

A. A form of feedback that provides confirmation that both parties have the same basic understanding of the message and the feedback

B. The endpoint of the communication

C. Require only "yes" or "no" or short factual answers giving specific information

D. Invite clients to discover and explore their thoughts or feelings

E. Initiates the communication

_____ 6. Therapeutic communication

_____ 7. Interview

_____ 8. Personal space

_____ 9. Nonverbal communication

_____ 10. Verbal communication

A. A planned communication or a conversation with a purpose

B. Exchange of ideas using the spoken or written word

C. Exchange of ideas using gestures, facial expressions, or touch

D. The distance people prefer in interactions with others

E. Client-centered, goal-directed, and time-limited communication used by nurses to determine client concerns, problems, and feelings

LEARNING OUTCOMES

1. What are the essential aspects of communication and the communication process?

2. What are the factors that influence the communication process?

3. What is the difference between verbal and nonverbal communication?

4. What therapeutic techniques can be used to help clients express thoughts, feelings, and concerns?

5. What are the principles of communication used in the clinical setting?

6. What are the barriers to communication in a therapeutic setting?

7. What are the two approaches to interviewing a client?

8. What approaches can the nurse use for interviewing a client?

9. What are the different types of interview questions that could be used, and when would you use each type?

10. What factors affect client interviews?

11. What are the stages of an interview?

APPLY WHAT YOU LEARNED

You are working in a medical unit in an acute care facility. The nurse in the emergency room calls to give you the following report on a client being admitted to your unit: A 34-year-old woman brought to the emergency department by ambulance when her life partner found her unconscious on the living room floor. Toxicology studies indicated a high level of benzodiazepines in her gastric contents. A large-bore nasogastric tube was inserted, here stomach contents were removed, and the stomach was lavaged with sterile saline until clear. Activated charcoal was administered via the tube, an IV initiated in the left hand infusing normal saline solution at 125 mL/hour, and emergency hemodialysis was performed over three hours. The nasogastric tube has been removed and the client is currently awake, alert, and oriented. The life partner believes the client attempted suicide after losing custody of her two children and is in the process of a divorce from her husband. The client now admits to taking 24 Ativan 1 mg tablets because she just can't face life without her children. The client will stay on your unit until her medical condition stabilizes and then she will be admitted to a mental health facility to help her cope with her stressors.

1. When the client arrives on the unit, what questions will you ask her?

2. What therapeutic techniques can you use to help the client share her thoughts, feelings, and concerns?

3. What barriers could arise when caring for the client related to your own beliefs about homosexuality, suicide, or a mother who lost custody of her children?

MULTIPLE CHOICE QUESTIONS

Circle the answer that best completes each of the following statements.

1. What is the response from the receiver called?
   A. Content
   B. Interpretation
   C. Feedback
   D. Helpful communication

2. Territoriality can influence which of the following factors of communication?
   A. Personal space
   B. Development
   C. Family roles
   D. Environment

3. The nurse, while assessing ROMs on a client, notices the client grimaces when the left wrist is rotated. The nurse should:
   A. Continue with the assessment but document the expression in the clients chart.
   B. Repeat the previous procedure to see if they can get the same response.
   C. Ask the client if the left wrist is painful to validate their response.
   D. Tell the client you will not exercise the left wrist again.

4. What verbal technique involves verifying the meaning of specific words rather than the overall meaning of a message?
   A. Reflecting
   B. Checking perception
   C. Paraphrasing
   D. Summarizing

5. What form of communication does the nursing staff primarily use to provide continuity of care to the client?
   A. Looking up information on unassigned clients to remain current with plan of care
   B. Peer consultation
   C. Shift reports that may be taped or done as walking rounds
   D. Written report placed on the front of the client's medical record

6. What barrier to communication does the nurse create by responding in a way that fosters the client's dependence on them?
   A. Probing
   B. Using unwarranted reassurance
   C. Stereotyping
   D. Giving opinions

7. Rapport is built between client and nurse during which type of interview?
   A. Nondirective
   B. Closing
   C. Therapeutic
   D. Directive

8. Which of the following is an approach the nurse might use for interviewing a client?
   A. Use medical terminology to give complete information.
   B. Remain consistent, dependable, and honest in all communication.
   C. Use humor to avoid uncomfortable issues.
   D. Be rigid when communicating so there is no confusion in message.

9. Which type of question could create problems due to inaccurate responses by the client in order to please the nurse?
   A. Open-ended question
   B. Leading question
   C. Neutral question
   D. Closed-ended question

10. Where should the nurse sit while interviewing a client who is in bed?
    A. Sit on the edge of the bed.
    B. Sit on the other bed in the room.
    C. Place a chair at the end of the bed.
    D. Sit at a 45-degree angle to the bed.

Chapter 12

Client Teaching

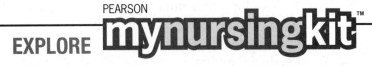
KEY TERMS

Match each of the following key terms to its proper definition.

_____ 1. Teaching

_____ 2. Feedback

_____ 3. Learning

_____ 4. Compliance

_____ 5. Retention

A. The extent to which a person's behavior aligns with medical or health advice

B. A lifelong process of acquiring knowledge or skills that cannot be solely accounted for by human growth

C. Ability to remember what is learned

D. The extent to which a person's behavior aligns with medical or health advice

E. A system of activities intended to produce specific learning

_____ 6. Motivation

_____ 7. Cognitivism

_____ 8. Readiness

_____ 9. Humanism

_____ 10. Relevance

A. Importance or applicability

B. Desire to act

C. System of thought that focuses on both cognitive and affective qualities of the learner

D. The belief that defines learning largely as a complex thinking process

E. Behaviors or cues that reflect the learner's motivation to learn at a specific time

_____ 11.	Psychomotor domain	A.	Area of learning that includes knowing, comprehending, and applying
_____ 12.	Behavior modification	B.	Area of learning that includes feelings, emotions, interests, attitudes, and appreciations
_____ 13.	Cognitive domain	C.	A system of positive reinforcement in which desirable behavior is rewarded and undesirable behavior is ignored
_____ 14.	Affective domain	D.	Area of learning that includes motor skills

LEARNING OUTCOMES

1. What are the key concepts of learning and topics for client education?

2. What are the three main theories of human learning?

3. What are the three domains of learning?

4. What are the factors that facilitate or inhibit learning?

5. Contrast the nursing process and the teaching process.

6. What role does the LPN/LVN have in client teaching?

7. Name effective teaching strategies.

8. What challenges are created when teaching clients from different cultures?

9. What methods can you use to evaluate learning in a client?

An 84-year-old Laotian woman, who speaks little English, has been experiencing black, tarry stools and is scheduled for a diagnostic workup that requires an extensive bowel prep. Realizing that she will not be able to understand the necessary teaching, you must decide how best to communicate with this client. Her family lives out of state, visits infrequently, and cannot provide you with help.

1. What cultural barriers and special considerations are present in this situation?

2. Where will you obtain the necessary information to assist you in understanding the Laotian culture?

3. Identify the necessary transcultural teaching guidelines for this situation.

4. How will you communicate clearly and effectively and evaluate the client's understanding?

MULTIPLE CHOICE QUESTIONS

Circle the answer that best completes each of the following statements.

1. The nurse teaching the mother about the need for an IV infusion for her child is educating about which of the following client areas?
   A. Promotion of health
   B. Prevention of illness/injury
   C. Restoration of health
   D. Adapting to altered health and function

2. What theory of learning involves imitating and modeling healthy behavior?
   A. Cognitivism
   B. Motivation
   C. Humanism
   D. Behaviorism

3. The nurse teaching a diabetic client about the safe storage of used needles is using what area of learning?
   A. Cognitive domain
   B. Affective domain
   C. Psychomotor domain
   D. Motivation

4. The client prescribed an inhaler to be used PRN is taught how to use it. Four weeks later the client calls the doctor for information on proper use of the inhaler. The client would be considered as having a problem with what?
   A. Relevance
   B. Retention
   C. Repetition
   D. Active learning

5. The nurse writing objectives for the client who is deficient in knowledge is following what type of process?
   A. Teaching
   B. Nursing
   C. Evaluation
   D. Fundamental

6. Which of the following roles in teaching might the LPN/LVN participate in? (Select all that apply.)
   A. Preceptor for new graduate LPNs/LVNs
   B. Teaching CPR for a community group
   C. Initiating discharge teaching
   D. Education for client transition from one level of care to another
   E. Contribute to the teaching plan

7. Which teaching strategy uses cognitive and affective theory as its major type of learning?
   A. Modeling
   B. Explanation
   C. Demonstration
   D. Role-playing

8. A guideline for transcultural teaching includes which of the following?
   A. Exclude the family in planning and teaching.
   B. Use medical terminology so meaning is not misinterpreted.
   C. Use humor to lighten the situation.
   D. Confirm the meaning of gestures and cues.

9. Which type of learning is the hardest to evaluate?
   A. Transcultural
   B. Affective
   C. Psychomotor
   D. Cognitive

10. Which of the following should be considered as a general teaching guideline?
    A. Teaching that limits the number of learner's senses often enhances learning.
    B. Rapport between teacher and physician is essential.
    C. Communication should not be vague or redundant.
    D. When the nurse is involved in planning, the desire to learn is increased.

Chapter 13

Documentation

KEY TERMS

Match each of the following key terms to its proper definition.

_____ 1. Database

_____ 2. Flow sheets

_____ 3. Charting

_____ 4. Record

_____ 5. Medication administration records

_____ 6. Report

A. Abbreviated progress notes

B. A written or computer-based collection of data

C. Used to gauge changes in client status

D. Making an entry on a client record

E. An oral, written, or computer-based communication intended to convey information to others

F. Record of the date of the medication order, the expiration date, the medication name and dose, the frequency of administration and route, and the nurse's signature

---

_____ 7. Objective data

_____ 8. Incident

A. Charting method in which the data are arranged according to the individual problems the client has rather than the source of the information

B. A widely used, concise method of organizing and recording data about a client

_____ 9. Subjective data

C. Charting method segmented into sections such as physician's orders, nurse's notes, radiology, and lab; each person or department makes notations in a separate section or sections of the client's chart

_____ 10. Kardex®

D. Information detectable by an observer

_____ 11. Source-oriented record

E. Any unexpected event

_____ 12. Problem-oriented medical record

F. Information apparent only to the person being affected

LEARNING OUTCOMES

1. Why is it important to keep client records?

2. What are the essential guidelines for reporting client data?

3. What abbreviations and symbols are commonly used for charting?

4. What are the effective guidelines for meeting ethical and legal standards when recording client data in the medical record?

5. How does the nurse maintain the confidentiality of records (both paper records and computerized records)?

6. What are the various systems for documenting in the medical record, and how is the nursing process utilized in each?

7. What role does the nurse have in reporting, conferring, and making referrals?

8. How does documentation differ for clients in acute care, home health care, and long-term care settings?

BP 140/86; P92; R18; T 99F; Alert and oriented ×3; grimacing; clenching jaw; dressing dry and intact; 20 mL light pink clear drainage in JP collection container; up in chair ×2 this shift; ambulated in hall ×1 with assist; stated, "I need something for pain"; rates pain at a 7 on a scale of 0–10. Drank 250 mL of various liquids for breakfast; tolerating fluids well; faint bowel sounds heard in all four quadrants; Indwelling urinary catheter draining clear amber urine; asks "How will I get over this in time for my daughter's graduation?" Demerol 75 mg IM given at 0800 and 1200; reports relief from pain meds; after receiving pain meds, rated pain at a 3 on a scale of 0–10.

1. Document the client's data in a SOAP format using the guidelines for recording found in this chapter of your text.

MULTIPLE CHOICE QUESTIONS

Circle the answer that best completes each of the following statements.

1. All of the following are purposes for nursing documentation *except*:
   - A. Communication
   - B. Planning client care
   - C. Nursing research
   - D. Preventing lawsuits

2. The nurse is caring for a client whose condition suddenly changes and becomes critical. When does the nurse document this change?
   - A. Immediately
   - B. After stabilizing the client
   - C. Before notifying the physician
   - D. When the incident report is completed

3. When reviewing the client's medical record the nurse finds an order for DAT. The nurse interprets this to mean:
   - A. Débride as tolerated
   - B. Demonstrate a technique
   - C. Diet as tolerated
   - D. Don't ambulate today

4. The nurse begins documenting in the client's record at the bottom of the last note. After starting the note the nurse realizes the page on which she was writing was from a week ago and the note should have been written several pages later. What does the nurse do?
   A. Discard the page she started to write on and start again.
   B. Continue the note where she began and write "out of sequence" at the end of the note.
   C. Call the nursing supervisor and complete an incident report.
   D. Put a line through the incorrectly placed note, write error, and begin the note again in the proper location.

5. While documenting in the client's computer record, the nurse turns to find a family member standing behind her. The priority nursing action is to:
   A. Minimize the screen with the client's information.
   B. Instruct the family member they are not to come into the nurse's station.
   C. Complete an incident report.
   D. Unplug the computer to make the screen go black immediately.

6. The nurse is documenting care using the focus charting method. Where is assessment data recorded?
   A. D
   B. A
   C. R
   D. Flow sheet

7. The nurse works in a facility where change of shift report is provided one-to-one with the off-going nurse reporting directly to the nurse who will assume care. When reporting to the on-coming nurse, how will the nurse provide a comprehensive report without forgetting something?
   A. Follow either a head-to-toe or system review order.
   B. Use the client's chart to review physician's orders.
   C. Obtain the client's Kardex to review all areas of care.
   D. Write everything down in advance so as not to forget anything.

8. The nurse begins a new job as a home care provider. When the nurse arrives at the client's home, where will the medical record be found?
   A. In a locked box next to the client's bed.
   B. The nurse brings the record from the agency.
   C. In the client's home.
   D. The nurse retrieves it from the physician's office.

9. The nurse has taught the newly diagnosed diabetic client how to care for the feet. Where does the nurse document this?
   A. On the nursing flow sheet
   B. In the nurse's progress notes
   C. On the teaching record
   D. On the medication administration record

10. The nurse's pen is empty and will no longer write. Which of the following available writing devices will the nurse substitute?
    A. A pencil
    B. A black gel pen
    C. A blue erasable ink pen
    D. A black marker

Chapter 14

Admission, Transfer, and Discharge

KEY TERMS

Match each of the following key terms to its proper definition.

_____ 1.	Coping behaviors	A.	Against the recommendation of the primary care provider
_____ 2.	Discharge	B.	Behaviors that people perform in times of crisis or stress in an attempt to deal with their feelings
_____ 3.	Transfer	C.	Introduction of clients to the people and the facility into which they have been admitted
_____ 4.	Admission	D.	Removal of unique human qualities
_____ 5.	Orientation	E.	Entry into the hospital
_____ 6.	Against medical advice	F.	A move
_____ 7.	Dehumanization	G.	The official procedure by which the client leaves the healthcare facility and returns home or goes to another setting

LEARNING OUTCOMES

1. What are the common reactions a client might have upon admission to a facility?

2. What are the steps to an admission of a client? What issues could be of importance when admitting a client?

3. What rules apply for distributing HIPAA information?

4. What are the interventions for orienting and caring for a newly admitted client?

5. Admitting a client involves what aspects of nursing care?

6. What are the reasons and guidelines for transferring a client?

7. What are the types of nursing care given a client who is being transferred?

8. What are the important factors to consider in discharging a client?

9. What are the nurse's responsibilities related to discharging a client?

APPLY WHAT YOU LEARNED

You are assigned to provide care for a 78-year-old Orthodox Jewish female client admitted to a long-term care facility after having a stroke. Prior to this admission, she lived in her own home, managed her own affairs, and took care of her own needs. For the past week, each time you pass medication to this client, she asks numerous questions about her medications, her diagnoses, and her physician, and complains vehemently about how much she dislikes being in the "nursing home." She angrily says, "I am a nonperson here. I can't make decisions for myself anymore. I hate being here. The aides call me 'sweetie' and 'honey.' I hate when they do that. I have always been known as Mrs. Levy. Who do they think they are?" You find yourself responding negatively to this client and are even hesitant to go into her room for any reason. When you speak to the client's son, he tells you that his mother was the family matriarch and made almost all the decisions for each family member. He says, "She was a strong woman with strong ideas about how the family should be, and we all pretty much did what she wanted us to."

1. Discuss what you think is going on with this client.

2. Discuss cultural considerations related to this client.

3. Describe nursing actions that would be appropriate in this situation.

4. Discuss how you might deal with your negative feelings toward this client.

MULTIPLE CHOICE QUESTIONS

Circle the answer that best completes each of the following statements.

1. The goal of nursing care during admission is to:
   A. Ensure the continuity of individualized client care
   B. Provide orientation to the family members
   C. Collect subjective and objective data
   D. Maintain a safe and effective nurse-client ratio

2. Because hospital admission is usually a very stressful time for a client and his or her family or significant others, it is most important for the nurse to:
   A. Make a good first impression and greet the client in a caring manner
   B. Delegate the initial assessment of vital signs to the nursing assistant
   C. Order a food tray for the client and each family member as soon as possible
   D. Show the family where the lounge, cafeteria, and vending machines are located

3. The client's response to hospitalization, although unique, is primarily influenced by:
   A. Level of knowledge, gender, and relationship with the primary physician
   B. Age, culture, religion, and lifelong, previously established coping behaviors
   C. Previous experiences, level of education, and psychological functioning
   D. Type of insurance, level of education, and support from family members

4. Which of the following is an example of dehumanization that occurs when a client is admitted to the hospital?
   A. Knocking on the door before entering the client's room
   B. Allowing the client to make food choices for each meal
   C. Asking the client personal and demographic data
   D. Having the client remove his clothing and put on a gown

5. The nurse hears the nursing assistant calling a newly admitted client "honey." The nurse decides to speak with the nursing assistant. The nurse's best response would be:
   A. "Why did you call the client 'honey'? That was very rude."
   B. "I heard you call the new client 'honey'—that needs to stop."
   C. "That new client is a real honey, isn't she?"
   D. "It is best to call the client by the name he or she prefers."

6. When preparing to transfer a client, the nurse must not only inform the client and family about the reason for the transfer, gather all of the client's belongings, and complete the required documentation, but, most importantly, the nurse must:
   A. Call admitting and indicate that the client will be transferred
   B. Ensure that there is a physician's order for the transfer
   C. Call the client's spiritual adviser and update about the transfer
   D. Remove all tubing, IVs, and urinary drainage collection bags

7. A client may require transfer to another unit in the hospital or to a different healthcare facility. The most likely reason for the transfer would be:
   A. The physician has only one other client at this facility
   B. The client does not like the day shift nursing staff
   C. The facility is too far for the family to drive every day
   D. The client's condition may require a different level of care

8. A client being discharged after undergoing a right total mastectomy asks if there are any support groups for women who have breast cancer. The nurse's most appropriate action would be to:
   A. Write a note to the physician requesting that she stop in to talk with the client
   B. Tell the client that she will contact the social worker and have her stop by
   C. Recommend that the client discuss this privately with her physician
   D. Provide the client with information on available community support groups

9. A common nursing diagnosis identified for a client being discharged is:
   A. Deficient knowledge
   B. Ineffective coping
   C. Impaired skin integrity
   D. Risk for injury

10. When reinforcing the discharge teaching plan with a client who is being discharged, the nurse's most important action would be to:
    A. Verify that the client has transportation to his home
    B. Provide the client with the opportunity to ask questions
    C. Remove all tubing, IVs, and unnecessary dressing
    D. Furnish necessary dressing change supplies

11. A child's most common reaction to being hospitalized is:
    A. Fear
    B. Denial
    C. Separation anxiety
    D. Loss of identity

12. When working with clients admitted to the hospital, the LPN/LVN must understand that:
    A. The client's feelings about admission help to determine the success of the hospital stay
    B. Discharge planning and teaching begin 24 hours prior to the anticipated discharge
    C. The nurse's primary responsibility at discharge is clear, concise documentation
    D. The LPN/LVN is required to complete the entire admission assessment

13. The initial assessment should be started once the client is settled into the room. The Joint Commission on Accreditation of Healthcare Organizations requires that:
    A. A registered nurse perform the admission assessment
    B. The admission assessment is completed by the admitting physician
    C. The social worker determine the client's psychosocial needs
    D. The RN delegate the entire assessment to the LPN/LVN

14. A client says, "I'm getting out of here. This place is awful! Nobody is doing a thing for me. Get me my clothes!" The physician has not been in to see the client today and there is no order for discharge. The LPN/LVN is aware that a client has the right to leave a facility against medical advice (AMA) as long as:
    A. The court has not issued an order to detain the client
    B. A family member signs appropriate release of liability form
    C. The nursing supervisor has been informed and given permission
    D. The client can walk and talk regardless of level of lucidity

15. The nurse is transporting a newly admitted client to the operating room for an emergency appendectomy. On the way, the patient says, "Oh my, gosh, I forgot to take off my engagement and wedding rings. What should we do?" The nurse's best action would be to:
    A. Take the ring from the client and tell her that she will give it to her husband after her lunch break as she makes your way back to the nursing unit
    B. Call the Loss Prevention department and request that security personnel come to the operating room to complete a property inventory, document the transfer of property, provide a receipt of the property, and secure the property
    C. Tell the client that she may continue to wear the ring and that the nurse will wrap some transparent tape around it for protection from microorganisms
    D. Whisper to the client that she should, "Just be quiet about it. Nobody will notice and it's no big deal anyway. We'll pretend it never happened."

Chapter 15

Theorists, Theories, and Therapies

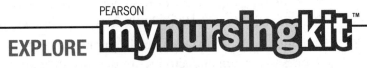

EXPLORE

MyNursingKit is your one stop for online chapter review materials and resources. Prepare for success with additional NCLEX®-style practice questions, interactive assignments and activities, web links, animations and videos, and more!

Register your access code from the front of your book at
www.mynursingkit.com

KEY TERMS

Match each of the following key terms to its proper definition.

_____ 1. Psychosocial needs   A. To turn an idea into fact or action

_____ 2. Superego   B. Doing things of one's choice, bringing ideas into action

_____ 3. Actualization   C. Needs having to do with physical processes in the human body

_____ 4. Physiologic needs   D. Concerned with moral behavior and takes into account the rules of society and the individual's personal values

_____ 5. Self-actualization   E. Needs having to do with relationships within oneself and others

_____ 6. Id   A. Internally includes self-respect, autonomy, and achievement; externally includes status, recognition, and attention

_____ 7. Esteem   B. Having to do with the divine or a higher power

_____ 8. Moral   C. Concept that connects the psyche with reality and promotes well-being and survival

_____ 9. Spiritual   D. Part of the unconscious concerned with immediate gratification

_____ 10. Ego   E. Relating to judgments of right or wrong

LEARNING OUTCOMES

1. What are the eight stages of Erikson's theory of psychosocial development? What are the negative and positive resolutions of each stage?

Stages of Theory	Positive Resolutions	Negative Resolutions

2. How do Freud and Erikson's theories differ? How are they similar?

3. What are Kohlberg's stages of moral development?

4. What is Piaget's theory of cognitive development?

5. What is Maslow's hierarchy of human needs?

6. What are the key points in the various developmental and psychological therapies?

7. What are the psychological therapies described in this chapter? How do they differ?

APPLY WHAT YOU LEARNED

As a student nurse, you are assigned to provide care to the following clients:

A 17-year-old high school senior admitted for an appendectomy. Her parents were killed in a motor vehicle crash, and she has been living on her own and trying to finish high school. She tells you that she lost her job last month and is being evicted from her apartment this week. She says, "I have exactly $2.36 in my pocket. I have no clue what I will do when I get out of here."

An 87-year-old widow who fell in her apartment and fractured her left hip. Up to this point, she has been managing on her own with some help from a neighbor. She says, "I don't think they'll let me go back to my house now. I don't want to go into a nursing home, but I don't know where I'll go."

A 56-year-old factory worker who was laid off from his job last week and was admitted for medically monitored detoxification from alcohol. He no longer has health insurance and is worried about how he will pay for this hospitalization.

A 34-year-old divorced bank executive, admitted for a right radical mastectomy after a routine mammogram showed a malignant lesion. She says, "This looks so awful. My boyfriend will leave me now, and I'll never find another person to share my life with."

1. Using Erikson's psychosocial developmental theory, identify the stage of development for each of your clients.

2. Applying Maslow's hierarchy of needs, identify the need level for each client.

3. Discuss how Rogers's person-centered therapies theory will help guide you through your interactions with these clients.

4. Identify how Peplau's theory is applicable to the nursing profession.

MULTIPLE CHOICE QUESTIONS

Circle the answer that best completes each of the following statements.

1. A baby cries when he or she is hungry, needs a diaper change, or wants to be held. According to Freud, this baby is operating out of which part of the psyche?
   A. Id
   B. Ego
   C. Superego
   D. Preconscious

2. The subconscious mind consists of an individual's:
   A. Moral behavior
   B. Reality and perceptions
   C. Memory
   D. Early experiences in infancy

3. A child being toilet trained is said to be in which of Freud's psychosexual developmental stages?
   A. Phallic stage
   B. Oral stage
   C. Latency stage
   D. Anal stage

4. The goal of Freud's genital psychosexual developmental stage is to:
   A. Develop awareness of the genital area and learn sexual identity
   B. Focus on pleasure of the mouth, lips, and tongue through various behaviors
   C. Develop satisfying relationships with the opposite sex
   D. Postpone gratification by controlling the sphincter muscles

5. According to Erikson, when a toddler is demonstrating autonomy as he explores the world around him and becomes frustrated during this period, he may develop:
   A. Initiative versus guilt
   B. Industry versus inferiority
   C. Shame versus doubt
   D. Identity versus role confusion

6. Kohlberg began working on his theory of moral development in the 1970s. He suggests that individuals progress through six stages in which they develop ethical behavior. Which of the following statements is true about Kohlberg's theory?
   A. Individuals must progress through these stages one stage at a time.
   B. Individuals who do not fully develop one stage may return at a later date and complete the necessary work.
   C. Individuals begin with a few inborn reflexes and progress to highly complex mental activities.
   D. When attachment behaviors are nurtured by the caregiver, the child develops a sense of security.

7. A client says, "I am scared to be alone in my house since it was vandalized." As the nurse planning care for this client, you will target your responses to the client using which level of Maslow's hierarchy of needs?
   A. Physiologic
   B. Safety
   C. Social
   D. Self-actualization

8. Your neighbor, a mother of a 3-year-old girl and an 11-year-old boy, asks you for help with parenting. She tells you that the children don't listen to her and tune her out when she tells them to do something. She says, "I just don't know what to do. They are driving me crazy." Using Skinner's behavior modification model, which of the following recommendations would be most appropriate?
   A. "You could set up a rewards program for good behaviors."
   B. "I think you should punish them when they don't listen."
   C. "Ignoring bad behavior is usually the best way to stop it."
   D. "You could send them to their respective rooms as punishment."

9. Cognitive theory focuses on distortion of thought as the cause of psychological distress. The aim or goal of cognitive therapy is to become aware of:
   A. Psychosocial issues or mental disorders present
   B. Feelings related to each situational life experience
   C. Thought distortions that are causing distress
   D. Early childhood experiences that impact relationships

10. Carl Rogers was the most influential psychologist in American history. Rogers believed that:
   A. Human beings have within themselves vast resources for self-understanding
   B. A person's behavior could be controlled by rewards
   C. It is important to present the client with moral dilemmas for discussion
   D. Involvement in religion often helps the older adult to resolve issues related to the meaning of life

11. Rogers's goal for therapy was to move the individual toward maturity. According to Rogers, which of the following characteristics is necessary for a supportive climate?
   A. Genuineness
   B. Unconditional positive regard
   C. Empathetic understanding
   D. All of the above

12. According to Piaget, a 10-year-old child is in which phase of child development and learning?
   A. Sensorimotor
   B. Preoperational
   C. Concrete operations
   D. Formal operations

Chapter 16

Life Span, Health Promotion, and Family Systems

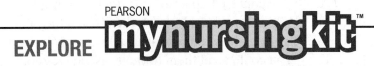

KEY TERMS

Match each of the following key terms to its proper definition.

_____ 1. Nuclear family

A. Treatment to a designated client with recognition that the family system or unit may also need intervention

_____ 2. Extended family

B. A family that includes adults and children who may or may not be related but where family decisions and responsibilities are shared

_____ 3. Family-centered care

C. Two or more individuals who come together for the purpose of nurturing

_____ 4. Communal family

D. A situation in which one or both spouses have had a previous marriage and children from that marriage

_____ 5. Family

E. An egocentric network of relatives

_____ 6. Blended family

F. A family consisting of parents and biological offspring

_____ 7. Development

A. Having to do with awareness of and interaction between oneself and the environment

_____ 8. Spiritual

B. Relating to judgments of right or wrong

_____ 9. Moral

C. An increase in the complexity of function and skill progression

© 2010 Pearson Education, Inc.

_____ 10. Cognitive

D. Having to do with the divine or a higher power

_____ 11. Puberty

E. Physical change and increase in size

_____ 12. Growth

F. Age when the reproductive organs become functional and secondary sex characteristics develop

LEARNING OUTCOMES

1. What is growth and what is development, how do they progress?

2. What are the components and principles of growth and development?

3. What are the normal development and characteristic milestones for each age group?

4. What are the types of families and stages in the family life cycle?

5. What are the roles, functions, and parenting styles in a family?

6. How does nursing care relate to lifespan differences?

APPLY WHAT YOU LEARNED

In today's world, one-half of first-time marriages and two-thirds of second marriages end in divorce. Single-parent households, blended families, and other nontraditional family structures are the norm. As a nurse practicing in health care today, it is important to be able to accept the client (family), identify the family's needs, plan for effective care, and provide support to these families.

1. Discuss the concept of family in the 21st century.

2. Identify and define four family types.

3. Identify the functions of the family.

4. Identify two important factors to consider when analyzing parenting styles.

MULTIPLE CHOICE QUESTIONS

Circle the answer that best completes each of the following statements.

1. Which of the following factors influences growth and development? Select all that apply.
   A. Physical stature
   B. Culture
   C. Religion
   D. Birth order
   E. Gender

2. Which of the following factors has the *most* negative impact on growth and development?
   A. Limited nutrition
   B. Single-parent household
   C. Cultural differences
   D. Gender

3. When assisting with a growth and development assessment of a child, the LPN/LVN should understand which of the following concepts?
   A. It is important to compare the progress of the growing child with the standards.
   B. Growth and development is totally individual and cannot be compared with that of others.
   C. Growth and development is totally dependent on race, culture, and genetics.
   D. It is not important to reflect on upbringing, parenting, or cultural customs.

4. At 4 months of age, the infant will be awake for two to three hours at a time during the day and then sleep through the night. During these hours of wakefulness, it is most important for the infant to:
   A. Explore his environment.
   B. Feed himself.
   C. Learn language skills.
   D. Develop fine motor skills.

5. Which of the following is true about a toddler's growth and development?
   A. His legs are short and his head large in relation to body size.
   B. He learns to make noise in response to voices and stores impulses for future reference.
   C. He is learning to obey rules and is becoming self-disciplined.
   D. He continues to grow about two inches and two pounds a year.

6. As a 10-year-old child moves through the school-age years, she will learn to:
   A. Examine hypothetical situations and apply the concepts to current issues.
   B. Adjust to life's crises, raise a family, and cope with changes in body function.
   C. Reason and understand cause and effect and reversibility.
   D. Obey rules and become increasingly self-disciplined.

7. Which of the following behaviors would you expect a preschool child to exhibit?
   A. Knows his name and age
   B. Has separation anxiety
   C. Cuts deciduous teeth
   D. Works independently

8. With a slowing of metabolism, adults may experience a(n)
   A. Increase in appetite.
   B. Decrease in energy.
   C. Increase in weight.
   D. Increase in sexual performance.

9. The nurse is caring for a 12-year-old pediatric client. The nurse promotes the family's life cycle by helping parents to recognize the importance of:
    A. Encouraging the child to explore his environment.
    B. Developing a stable family unit.
    C. Re-establishing the wife and husband roles.
    D. Promoting school achievement of child.

10. The nurse observes parents talking with a 13-year-old child who was admitted through the emergency department following a motor vehicle crash in which the child was driving a friend's car. The parents say, "I hope you will make better decisions in the future. You know we trust you to make good decisions because you are so smart and logical." The nurse assesses that, based on this parenting style, the child's attempt to drive prior to licensure was the result of:
    A. Authoritarian parents who value obedience resulting in children who have low internalization of parental values.
    B. Permissive parents who encourage children to make decisions they aren't mature enough to make.
    C. Authoritative parents who have clear expectations for their child's behavior resulting in children who have low ego development.
    D. Permissive parents who make few demands on their children and raise children who are mature, resilient and achievement oriented.

11. When planning care for a five-year-old the nurse considers the child's development before planning: (Select all that apply)
    A. Diet
    B. Teaching
    C. Medication dosage
    D. Diversional activities
    E. Performance of procedures

Chapter 17

Psychosocial Nursing of the Physically Ill Client

KEY TERMS

Match each of the following key terms to its proper definition.

_____ 1. Coping

A. Outward appearance of emotional state

_____ 2. Stressors

B. A state of mental uneasiness, apprehension, dread, or foreboding

_____ 3. Anxiety

C. Dealing with problems and situations

_____ 4. Counseling

D. Sources of stress

_____ 5. Crisis

E. A form of therapy in which trained professionals help people think about the problems they are experiencing in their lives and find new ways of coping

_____ 6. Affect

F. A sudden change of events of a pyrexic condition

_____ 7. ICU psychosis

A. Unconscious attempts to manage anxiety

_____ 8. Defense mechanisms

B. Presence of substance abuse along with a concurrent psychiatric disorder

_____ 9. Posttraumatic stress disorder

C. A specific type of anxiety, defined as out-of-proportion fear

_____ 10. Obsessive-compulsive disorder

D. A form of delirium or acute brain failure that may result from alcohol withdrawal

_____ 11. Phobias

E. An anxiety disorder characterized by patterned behaviors that are focused on some topic of fixation and that are repeated in order to relieve the anxiety

_____ 12. Dual diagnosis

F. An anxiety disorder that can develop after exposure to one or more terrifying events in which grave physical harm occurred or was threatened

LEARNING OUTCOMES

1. What types of data are collected for a psychosocial assessment?

2. What are the components of a mental status exam?

3. What are the common psychological responses to a serious medical illness?

4. What are the types of depression? How do their manifestations differ by age group? Which therapies are used to treat depression?

5. What are the conditions associated with an increased risk of suicide? What emotional or behavioral changes may be seen?

6. What is the difference between stress and anxiety? How can clients cope with each?

7. What ways do clients cope? Include defense mechanisms.

8. What are the psychosocial factors in medical illness?

9. How can the LPN/LVN meet the psychosocial needs of the medically ill adult or child?

10. How does the nursing process meet the psychosocial needs of the client?

APPLY WHAT YOU LEARNED

A 49-year-old African American male client is admitted to your unit. Together with the RN, you conduct a psychosocial assessment. During this assessment the client says, "I drink every day after work. I usually have at least six beers and a couple of shots. It helps me to relax after a long, hard day." When asked if the drinking has caused any problems in his life, he replies, "Oh, I've been picked up once or twice for drunk driving. But it's not a problem, really. I can stop anytime I want."

1. Identify one ineffective coping behavior that this client is exhibiting.

2. Identify the primary defense mechanisms the client is using to defend his drinking habits.

3. Identify cultural considerations that may need to be incorporated into the care plan.

MULTIPLE CHOICE QUESTIONS

Circle the answer that best completes each of the following statements.

1. A common response to a physical illness is:
    A. Anxiety
    B. Grief
    C. Fear of dependency
    D. All of the above

2. Which skill is crucial in helping clients share important information with the nurse?
   A. Clear, accurate documentation
   B. Good listening ability
   C. Multitasking organization
   D. Sharing relevant personal stories

3. Symptoms of depression:
   A. Vary by age group
   B. Are the same for everyone
   C. Are time-limited
   D. Are normal in the elderly

4. Though most new antidepressants have fewer side effects, the client must still be monitored for unpredictable reactions, also known as:
   A. Idiosyncratic reactions
   B. Drug toxicity
   C. Drug tolerance
   D. Iatrogenic disease

5. Crying, the client tells you that the physician, as a last effort, plans to order electroconvulsive therapy for her. "I'm so scared. I don't know much about this type of therapy except what I've seen in the movies. What exactly is it, and how does it work?" Which of the following responses would be most appropriate?
   A. "Electroconvulsive therapy, or ECT, may be used for people with severe depression who have not responded well to medication or other treatment. A small electrical 'shock' is applied to the brain. Let me get more information for you, and we can talk about what will happen."
   B. "ECT was used years ago and wasn't very helpful. Doctors today don't use it much. It does nothing to help people with depression."
   C. "You know, I don't know much about it either. I have seen it in the movies and think it is scary, don't you? If I were you, I'd tell my doctor I don't want it."
   D. "Actually, you need to speak to your doctor about that. He should have explained everything to you and had you sign a consent."

6. Which of the following individuals are most likely to experience posttraumatic stress disorder (PTSD)?
   A. A young mother who just gave birth
   B. An elderly woman who fell down and broke her hip
   C. A young man just returning from a military assignment in a war zone
   D. A toddler who became separated from his mother at the shopping mall

7. An elderly woman yells at you every time you answer her call light. "Where have you been? I've waited for hours for you to come to help me to the bathroom. Oh, I just wish I could do these things for myself again!" Which of the following statements best explains the client's reactions and responses?
   A. The client is in denial about the amount of care she requires.
   B. The client is projecting her anger at becoming increasingly dependent.
   C. The client doesn't like you and is trying to make your life miserable.
   D. The client is just an angry old lady who needs to be put in her place.

8. When an individual experiences stress, the body produces increased chemicals in preparation for an emergency. Which of the following statements correctly identifies the changes that take place in the body when it is under stress?
   A. Adrenaline and noradrenaline raise the blood pressure and increase the heart rate.
   B. Adrenaline and noradrenaline increase blood flow to your skin and speed up stomach activity.
   C. Cortisol releases fat and sugar into the system and increases the efficiency of the immune system.
   D. Cortisol decreases respirations and the rate of perspiration.

9. You have been feeling sad and irritable and experiencing frequent headaches for the past month or two. It is difficult to get out of bed in the morning and go to work. Each shift you have more and more clients to care for and just can't take it any more. You have a hard time identifying anything that gives you pleasure and you are drinking one or two alcoholic beverages daily. What should you do?
   A. Tell yourself that you don't have time to feel sorry for yourself and go on with life.
   B. Do not tell anyone because, as a nurse, you should know better.
   C. Contact the Employee Assistance Program where you work and arrange for counseling.
   D. Increase your alcohol consumption because this seems to relieve some stress, at least temporarily.

10. Which of the following combinations is an example of a dual diagnosis?
    A. Hypertension and depression
    B. Alcohol abuse and bipolar affective disorder
    C. Diabetes and schizophrenia
    D. Opiate abuse and heart disease

11. Which of the following activities is an example of an ineffective coping behavior?
    A. Meditating
    B. Smoking a cigarette
    C. Keeping a journal
    D. Taking a walk

12. A client admitted to the intensive care unit after extensive surgery begins to hear voices and becomes paranoid and delirious. Which of the following nursing interventions would be most appropriate for this client?
    A. Place the client in restraints until the psychosis diminishes.
    B. Coordinate the lighting with the normal day–night cycle.
    C. Seclude the client in a corner room.
    D. Encourage visitors to provide stimulation.

13. A 15-year-old client has been giving her favorite DVDs and pictures to friends, saying, "I want you to have a remembrance of me when I'm gone." She has been undergoing treatment for depression. Which of the following statements by the nurse would be most appropriate in this situation?
    A. "Why are you giving away your favorite things? You'll probably want them next week."
    B. "You need to stop talking so foolishly. You are a smart girl and have everything to live for."
    C. "Anyone who tries to kill herself must be crazy."
    D. "I'm very concerned about you. Are you thinking of killing yourself?"

14. Which of the following statements is considered a myth associated with suicide?
    A. Most individuals who commit suicide have given some clue or warning.
    B. Individuals who are suicidal are not psychotic or insane.
    C. Clients who commit suicide do not want death; they want the pain to stop.
    D. People who talk about suicide won't really do it.

Chapter 18

Loss, Grief, and Death

KEY TERMS

Match each of the following key terms to its proper definition.

_____ 1. Loss

A. An attempt to ignore unacceptable realities by refusing to acknowledge them

_____ 2. Distancing

B. The process and rituals through which grief is eventually resolved

_____ 3. Grief

C. Third stage of grief

_____ 4. Mourning

D. An unconscious response of professionals in which they hold back emotionally, especially from dying clients

_____ 5. Bargaining

E. A real or potential situation in which something that is valued is gone, is unavailable, or is changed

_____ 6. Denial

F. The whole range of feelings, thoughts, and behaviors related to loss and signifying emotional responses, especially overwhelming distress and sorrow

____	7.	Medical power of attorney	A. An order to prevent interventions the client does not wish to have performed when death approaches
____	8.	Bereavement	B. Energy directed through the hands of the practitioner to activate the healing response of the recipient
____	9.	Do-not-resuscitate	C. The normal grieving period experienced by the surviving loved ones
____	10.	Therapeutic touch	D. Fourth stage of grief
____	11.	Acceptance	E. A written statement appointing someone else to manage healthcare treatment decisions when the client is unable to do so
____	12.	Depression	F. Last stage of grief in which the client comes to terms with loss

LEARNING OUTCOMES

1. How do loss, grief, and death relate to each other?

2. What factors affect a loss or grief response?

3. What are the common myths about grief as related to children?

4. What are the stages and manifestations of grieving?

Stages	Manifestations

5. What are the "four tasks" of William Worden's grief model?

6. What is the mourner's bill of rights and the six reconciliation needs?

7. What are the three legal issues that arise when a client is dying?

8. What nursing strategies can be used to assist clients and families at times of grief, loss, and death?

9. Why is self-care important for the nurse working with dying clients?

APPLY WHAT YOU LEARNED

You are talking with a 72-year-old client whose husband died in a motor vehicle crash two weeks ago. She says, "I cannot believe that he is gone! I can hardly breathe sometimes when I think about how he died. I miss him so much and I don't know how I can go on without him. We just celebrated our 50th wedding anniversary last month. Part of me died with him. We didn't have any kids, so I really have no one to help me. Will I ever be okay again? Why did God take him from me?"

1. Identify the Kübler-Ross stage(s) of grieving this client is currently demonstrating.

2. Identify factors that may be affecting this client's grieving response.

3. Identify four important questions you will need to ask this client in order to determine her current physical and emotional status.

4. Discuss various nursing interventions that could be used to help this client work through her grief. Provide rationales for each intervention.

MULTIPLE CHOICE QUESTIONS

Circle the answer that best completes each of the following statements.

1. A 70-year-old woman is exhibiting signs of unresolved grief following the death of her husband a year ago. The nurse knows that unresolved grief can lead to:
   A. Resolution of death and dying issues.
   B. Acceptance of the loss of a loved one.
   C. Development of new coping strategies.
   D. Significant physical and emotional problems.

2. Crying, a client who recently lost her husband of 32 years, says, "Oh, I am so lost these days. I miss my husband so much. I feel so guilty sometimes because he really wanted me to quit smoking. I never listened and kept right on. I'd stop in a heartbeat now if I could have him back again!" According to Kübler-Ross, this client's statement is reflective of which stage of the grieving process?
   A. Denial
   B. Bargaining
   C. Depression
   D. Acceptance

3. Which statement made by a client represents acceptance of the death of a loved one?
   A. "Why did he have to leave me? How could he do that to me?"
   B. "I don't know what to do. I'm never going to be the same again."
   C. "I miss him terribly, but we had a great, long life together."
   D. "I still don't believe he is gone. It just doesn't seem possible."

4. When caring for a client whose death is imminent, the nurse would expect to see which physiological change?
   A. Increased respirations
   B. Stiffening of the extremities
   C. Heightened sense of hearing
   D. Dusky or bluish nail beds

5. The nurse admits a client scheduled for a bowel resection and ostomy creation in the morning. The surgeon has informed the client that the ostomy will be permanent. The client tells the nurse, "I can't believe I'm going to be walking around with a bag filled with stool for the rest of my life." The nurse recognizes the client is experiencing:
   A. Dysfunctional grief.
   B. Anticipatory grief.
   C. Disenfranchised grief.
   D. Maturational loss.

6. Mrs. Dyson has died and her granddaughter is talking with the nurse about ways to tell her children that their great-grandmother has died. The children are 3, 5 and 6 years of age. Which of the following strategies suggested by the nurse would be helpful?
   A. "It would be best not to tell the children but just let them forget about her naturally."
   B. "Tell them she has gone to sleep and will never wake up again."
   C. "Tell them simply and then assess what their understanding of the situation is."
   D. "Take them to church and have the spiritual leader explain it to them."

7. The husband of a client who died 30 minutes ago is met in the hallway by family members who hug and console him and then the man's father reaches over and tears a corner of his pocket away from his shirt. The nurse, observing this behavior, will:
   A. Call security and describe the violent behavior witnessed.
   B. Interpret the behavior as part of Orthodox Jewish beliefs.
   C. Gather several staff members to restrain the man's father.
   D. Inform the man's father he will need to leave the hospital if he can't behave properly.

8. While admitting the elderly client the nurse learns that she goes to church every day and lights a candle in memory of her dead husband. The client says she has been depressed and withdrawn ever since he died three months ago. The nurse documents the client's process of grieving as including:
   A. Going to church every day.
   B. Lighting a candle in memory of her husband.
   C. Going to church and lighting a candle.
   D. Depression.

9. After a client at the long-term care facility died, a few of the staff decided to attend his funeral because they had cared for him for many years. At the viewing the client's daughter tells the nurse that she's worried about her mother because she has no energy, she has been emotionally labile (changing from one emotion to another in a short period of time), and she's suddenly been spending hours reading the Bible. The daughter is afraid these behaviors indicate the mother has impaired cognition. The nurse correctly tells the daughter:
    A. "Your mother would benefit from seeing a psychiatrist because her behavior is irrational."
    B. "Your mother's behavior is normal and could last for 4 to 5 years. I wouldn't worry about her."
    C. "Your mother's behavior is to be expected. Call her doctor if she shows signs of illness or confusion.'
    D. "Your mother's behavior is normal."

10. A client is brought to the emergency department and later determined to be in a chronic vegetative state, permanently dependent on mechanical ventilation and tube feedings. The family was notified of the client's injuries at the time of admission and cannot agree about discontinuing life support, with the client's spouse wanting life support continued and the parents wanting it discontinued. The family doctor shows the family the client's advanced directive asking that no artificial measures be used to continue life. The nurse recognizes the legal thing to do is to respect:
    A. The parent's wishes.
    B. The husband's wishes.
    C. The client's wishes.
    D. The physician's wishes.

11. The nurse works in a long-term care facility and becomes close to one of the residents, often stopping by her room on her way home at the end of the day to talk and share a cup of tea. When the resident dies the nurse finds herself feeling sad, lacking energy, and sleeping longer than usual. The nurse needs to:
    A. Maintain a distance between herself and clients.
    B. Recognize she is grieving and allow herself time to mourn the client's loss.
    C. Quit the long-term care facility and work in a place where clients are short-term.
    D. Talk with a counselor to help recover from depression.

12. The nurse, working in a provider's office, admits a 52-year-old female client who has smoked for 36 years and was recently diagnosed with lung cancer. Which of the following statements made by the client would indicate denial?
    A. "I don't want to be in pain."
    B. "I don't want to die and plan to fight this disease."
    C. "I don't think my husband understands how I'm feeling."
    D. "The type of cancer I have is the slow-growing type so I'm not worried."

13. The nurse, caring for a client who is dying of cancer, prepares to administer an analgesic for pain when the client's family member says, "Don't give that now. You're going to turn him into a drug addict." How would the nurse best reply?
    A. "The doctor has ordered it so it must be given."
    B. "The client is in pain and that's more important than worrying about addiction."
    C. "Dependence may occur but we can treat that when he's no longer in pain."
    D. "If the client doesn't mind becoming addicted then I will give the medications."

14. The nurse is caring for a client admitted for testing to determine the cause of a lump found in the abdomen following chemotherapy for breast cancer. The nurse reviews the client's record and sees the lab results as well as a note in the progress notes written by the provider saying the client is terminal with metastases to the brain, bone, and bowel. The provider plans to inform the client of the diagnosis this evening. The client's awareness of approaching loss is:
    A. Closed awareness.
    B. Mutual pretense.
    C. Open awareness.
    D. Partial awareness.

15. The nurse is asked by the client to witness a consent to donate organs. The nurse will:
    A. Assist the client in obtaining a notary public.
    B. Ask the facility legal department to assist the client.
    C. Witness the consent.
    D. Inform the client the nurse is not legally allowed to act as a witness.

Chapter 19

Health Assessment/Head-to-Toe Data Collection

KEY TERMS

Match each of the following key terms to its proper definition.

_____ 1.	Accommodation	A.	Alternating change in pupil size
_____ 2.	Inferior	B.	Farther from the origin of a structure
_____ 3.	Palpation	C.	Toward the front of the body or the belly
_____ 4.	Superior	D.	Reduced ability or inability to speak or understand verbal or written language
_____ 5.	Distal	E.	A point lower than or below a reference point
_____ 6.	Ventral	F.	The presence of excess interstitial fluid
_____ 7.	Edema	G.	Examination of the body using the sense of touch
_____ 8.	Capillary	H.	The refill time the nail bed takes to return to its usual color after being pressed
_____ 9.	Aphasia	I.	Above or in a higher position than a point of reference
_____ 10.	Lateral	J.	Toward the side; the opposite of medial

1. What are the three types of physical health assessments, and what role does the LPN/LVN have in each?

Type of Physical Health Assessment	LPN/LVN Role

2. What are the elements to check by body systems?

3. What preparations of the client and the environment are needed before an examination?

4. What are the potential variables in data by age or condition?

5. What are the four methods of examination and which are commonly used by the LPN/LVN?

Method of Examination	LPN/LVN Uses

6. What are the common terms used during an examination to identify body parts or locations?

7. What nursing care is involved in a client undergoing an assessment?

8. What terms are used in the physical assessment of the lungs?

9. What is the suggested sequencing to conduct a physical health assessment in an orderly fashion?

APPLY WHAT YOU LEARNED

A client was admitted after being involved in a serious motor vehicle crash. She is semicomatose but responds to deep pain stimuli. There is an order for a focused assessment with neurologic checks every hour.

1. Describe neurologic status related to level of consciousness.

2. Describe the elements of a focused assessment.

3. Identify the components of a neurologic check and describe each one.

4. Describe the Glasgow Coma Scale, what it measures, and how it would be used to assess LOC for this client.

MULTIPLE CHOICE QUESTIONS

Circle the answer that best completes each of the following statements.

1. When determining a client's level of consciousness (LOC), which question would be most helpful in obtaining appropriate data?
   A. "How are you doing today?"
   B. "Are you having any pain this morning?"
   C. "Where are you now?"
   D. "What do you do for a living?"

2. To auscultate the anterior chest, the nurse would begin by placing the stethoscope:
   A. Just above the clavicle starting on the client's right side.
   B. On the posterior chest wall starting distal to the clavicle.
   C. At the fifth intercostal space to the left of midline.
   D. Inferior to the thorax and proximal to the dorsal cavity.

3. The physician has written an order for a daily weight on the client. The nurse plans to delegate this task to the nursing assistant and, because accuracy is essential, she must instruct the certified nurse assistant (CNA) to:
   A. Take the weight whenever possible and time allows.
   B. Weigh the client immediately after breakfast.
   C. Use the bed scale today since is readily available.
   D. Weigh the client at the same time each day.

4. Pallor usually occurs when:
   A. There is too little circulating blood or hemoglobin.
   B. Bruised areas blanch when pressure is applied.
   C. There is excess interstitial fluid or third spacing.
   D. The nail beds look bluish or purplish.

5. During the assessment of a 3-year-old child, the mother asks why her child has such a "pot belly." The nurse's best response would be:
   A. She is eating too many snack foods.
   B. It could be an early sign of malnutrition.
   C. It is normal for a child her age.
   D. Her liver may be enlarged.

6. In infants or children, asymmetric gluteal folds may suggest which circumstance or condition?
   A. Lordosis, or swayback
   B. Genu varum, or bowleggedness
   C. Normal growth and development
   D. Developmental dysplasia of the hip

7. As part of a focused assessment the nurse lightly palpates the client's abdomen. Which client response would be the best indicator that the client is experiencing pain or tenderness?
   A. Client asks, "How much longer?"
   B. Client grimaces and clenches his jaw.
   C. Client states, "I'm fine, really."
   D. Client grabs and moves nurse's hand.

8. Skin turgor of a 90-year-old male client should be assessed in which location?
   A. Over the sternum
   B. Inside the wrist
   C. Under the chin
   D. Top of the hand

9. When inspecting the gums and oral mucous membranes, which finding would be considered a deviation from normal?
   A. Bluish hue in dark-skinned clients
   B. Freckled brown pigmentation in dark-skinned clients
   C. Uniform pink color in light-skinned clients
   D. Yellowish discoloration in light-skinned clients

10. During an abdominal assessment, the nurse observes purple striae on the skin. This finding may indicate:
    A. Malnutrition
    B. Hernia or tumor
    C. Ascites or edema
    D. Cushing's disease

11. The nurse is listening for bowel sounds in a 70-year-old client who has an order for bed rest with bathroom privileges. After using the flat-disk diaphragm of the stethoscope to auscultate the four quadrants of the abdomen for 5 to 20 seconds, the nurse is unable to hear any bowel sounds.

    The nurse's next best action would be to:
    A. Document that bowel sounds are absent.
    B. Call the physician to report the finding.
    C. Continue to listen for an additional 3 to 5 minutes.
    D. Ask the RN to listen and verify the absence of sounds.

12. The father of a 15-month-old toddler says, "My kid seems to be bowlegged and pigeon-toed. He looks goofy. Is he always going to be like that?" The nurse's best response would be:
    A. "Yeah, I can see that. Does he trip and fall down a lot? He should probably have x-rays done and may need corrective surgery in the near future."
    B. "He certainly does look goofy, doesn't he? I wouldn't worry too much about it, though. He'll adapt and will probably grow out of it once his bones develop."
    C. "I would suggest talking with the doctor about both of those conditions. Sometimes the child needs to be placed in a corrective cast."
    D. "Actually, it is quite common for a child his age to have some in-turning of the feet and bowleggedness. It should go away within 6 to 12 months."

13. An older adult client says, "Nothing tastes very good any more. I really don't enjoy food like I used to." The most likely reason for this change is:
    A. Age-related atrophy of the taste buds
    B. Underlying pathology or systemic disease
    C. Increased use of preservatives in food processing
    D. Presence of periodontal or gum disease

Chapter 20

Hygiene

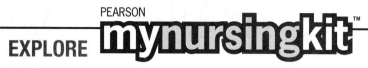

KEY TERMS

Match each of the following key terms to its proper definition.

_____ 1. Pediculosis   A. Bad breath

_____ 2. Gingiva   B. Ear wax

_____ 3. Cerumen   C. An infestation with lice

_____ 4. Hirsutism   D. Gums of the mouth

_____ 5. Halitosis   E. Condition of excessive hair growth

_____ 6. Cleaning baths   A. A device designed to keep the top bed-clothes off the feet, legs, and even abdomen of a client

_____ 7. Hygiene   B. Hygienic care given for physical effects

_____ 8. Bed cradle   C. Baths given chiefly for hygiene purposes to remove accumulated oil, perspiration, dead skin cells, and some bacteria

_____ 9. Therapeutic baths   D. The science of health and its maintenance

LEARNING OUTCOMES

1. What kinds of hygienic care does the nurse provide to the client?

2. What factors influence personal hygiene?

3. What are the normal and abnormal findings and interventions for nursing care of the skin, feet, and nails?

Body Section	Normal Findings	Abnormal Findings	Interventions
Skin			
Feet			
Nails			

4. What are the different types of baths and what is the purpose of each?

Type of Bath	Purpose

5. What are the teaching points for client foot care?

6. What are the normal and abnormal findings and interventions for nursing care of the hair?

Body Section	Normal Findings	Abnormal Findings	Interventions
Hair			

7. What are the normal and abnormal findings and interventions for nursing care of the mouth, eyes, ears, and nose?

Body Section	Normal	Abnormal	Interventions
Mouth			
Eyes			
Ears			
Nose			

8. How can the nurse support a hygienic environment?

9. What are the methods for making an unoccupied and an occupied bed?

10. What infection control measures are part of bed-making procedures?

APPLY WHAT YOU LEARNED

You are caring for a 48-year-old woman admitted for treatment of bacterial pneumonia. She is currently menstruating. As you enter her room, you detect a mild body odor. For her morning care, you suggest that she take a shower and freshen up. She replies, "I am menstruating, and I may not bathe until the bleeding stops. In my religion, women are considered to be in a fragile condition during menstruation, and we restrict showers and strenuous exercise." During the morning report, the other nurses comment on this client's hygiene practices, saying, "How can anyone believe such stuff? She needs to take a bath regardless of what her religion says. She smells and we shouldn't put up with that."

1. Identify factors that influence individual hygiene.

2. How do culture and religion influence hygiene practices for this client?

3. Discuss how the dominant North American culture may influence competent cultural care.

4. Discuss how the cultural and religious beliefs of this client can be factored into the nursing care plan.

MULTIPLE CHOICE QUESTIONS

Circle the answer that best completes each of the following statements.

1. For a dependent, debilitated, or unconscious client, the LPN/LVN must provide frequent and often special mouth care. Which solution would be most appropriate to use when cleaning the teeth and oral mucous membranes?
   A. Normal saline
   B. Mineral oil
   C. Mouthwash containing alcohol
   D. Hydrogen peroxide

2. While inspecting the skin of a debilitated, immobile client, the nurse notices slight plantar flexion of both feet. As a preventative measure, the nurse orders a:
   A. Bed cradle
   B. Footboard
   C. Egg-crate mattress
   D. Sheepskin pad

3. While giving a client a complete bath, the nurse notices a significant amount of cerumen in both ears. The nurse's best action is to:
   A. Contact the client's primary physician for an order.
   B. Push a corner of the washcloth into the ear as far as it will go.
   C. Retract the auricle downward to loosen and remove visible wax.
   D. Use a cotton-tipped applicator to remove the wax buildup.

4. In older adults, the hair generally:
   A. Becomes thicker
   B. Grows more quickly
   C. Becomes oilier
   D. Loses its color

5. When teaching nail care to a client with diabetes, which recommendation should the nurse include?
   A. File the nail straight across beyond the end of the finger or toe.
   B. Cut the nails with a scissors rather than using a nail file.
   C. Use a very sharp scissors to prevent tissue injury.
   D. Dig into the lateral corners to prevent ingrown toenails.

6. During an initial assessment, the client says, "I really itch, especially during the night." The nurse observes short, wavy brown or black threadlike lesions between the webs of the fingers and the folds of his wrists and elbows. Based on the subjective and objective data, the nurse suspects that the client has:
   A. Hirsutism
   B. Pediculus capitis
   C. Tularemia
   D. Scabies

7. Clients' hygiene practices are influenced to a large degree by their:
   A. Sociocultural background
   B. Religious beliefs
   C. Educational background
   D. Age and functional ability

8. Which action by the nurse will help to provide a comfortable environment for the client?
   A. Lowering the room temperature to 65°F.
   B. Spraying room deodorizer every 2 hours.
   C. Disposing of soiled materials in a timely manner.
   D. Watering the plants and flowers daily.

9. A client has an artificial eye that must be removed regularly for cleaning. To remove the artificial eye, the nurse should:
   A. Separate the eyelid with the nondominant hand, moving the eye down to the inferior part of the sclera, using the pad of the dominant index finger.
   B. Use clean gloves and the dominant thumb to pull the client's lower eyelid down over the infraorbital bone, exerting slight pressure below the eyelid.
   C. Soften dried secretions by placing a sterile cotton ball moistened with sterile water or normal saline over the lid margins.
   D. Ask the client to look straight ahead, and gently exert pressure on the upper and lower lids, gently pushing the eye forward.

10. A homeless person faces numerous difficulties that influence his or her hygiene. The factor(s) posing the greatest challenge would most likely be:
    A. Personal preferences
    B. Cultural aspects
    C. Limited resources
    D. Religious beliefs

11. A 60-year-old client says that his skin becomes so dry and itchy during the winter that he sometimes scratches his skin until it bleeds. The best recommendation for this client would be to:
    A. Take more frequent baths rather than showers during the colder months.
    B. Bathe less frequently when environmental temperature and humidity are low.
    C. Wear only clothes that contain natural fibers such as wool and cotton.
    D. Contact his physician for an order for a prescription for hydrocortisone cream.

12. Before using a safety razor to shave a client, the most important client-centered action by the nurse would be to:
    A. Wipe the client's face with a wet washcloth to remove any debris and to soften the bristles.
    B. Hold the skin taut, particularly around creases, in order to prevent cutting or damaging the skin.
    C. Don gloves in order to reduce exposure to blood from open facial nicks, blemishes, or lesions.
    D. Check the client's medication record to determine whether he is receiving any anticoagulants.

13. An older adult client receiving all nourishment via tube feedings has significant cheilosis. Which nursing intervention would be most appropriate for this client?
    A. Check the oral cavity for ill-fitting dentures.
    B. Increase fluid intake as health status permits.
    C. Lubricate the lips with antimicrobial ointment.
    D. Advise the client to seek oral care from a dentist.

Chapter 21

Vital Signs

KEY TERMS

Match each of the following key terms to its proper definition.

_____ 1. Dysrhythmia

_____ 2. Tachycardia

_____ 3. Afebrile

_____ 4. Korotkoff's sounds

_____ 5. Pulse pressure

_____ 6. Cardiac output

A. Condition that occurs when the heartbeats become irregular and abnormally fast

B. Without fever

C. Sounds heard through the stethoscope when measuring blood pressure

D. The amount of blood pumped by the ventricles in 1 minute; stroke volume X pulse rate

E. Pulse with an irregular rhythm

F. The difference between the diastolic and the systolic pressures

_____ 7. Orthopnea

_____ 8. Cheyne-Stokes respirations

_____ 9. Eupnea

_____ 10. Radiation

A. Rapid respiration marked by quick, shallow breaths

B. Cessation of breathing

C. Ability to breathe only in upright sitting or standing positions

D. Normal respirations

_____ 11. Tachypnea

E. Rhythmic waxing and waning of breath, from very deep to very shallow breathing and temporary apnea

_____ 12. Apnea

F. Heat lost by transfer to cooler objects that are nearby but not in direct contact

_____ 13. Evaporation

A. The resistance supplied by the blood vessels as a result of compliance

_____ 14. Arrhythmia

B. A blood pressure that drops when the client sits or stands

_____ 15. Orthostatic hypotension

C. Pulse with an irregular rhythm

_____ 16. Conduction

D. A blood pressure cuff

_____ 17. Peripheral vascular resistance

E. Transfer of heat by direct contact with a cooler object

_____ 18. Sphygmomanometer

F. Change of water to a gas or vapor, which causes cooling

_____ 19. Bradycardia

A. Indrawing beneath the breastbone

_____ 20. Point of maximal impulse

B. The dispersion of heat by air currents

_____ 21. Vaporization

C. A very high fever

_____ 22. Convection

D. Condition in which heartbeats become irregular and abnormally slow

_____ 23. Substernal retractions

E. The area where the pulse is heard the loudest and strongest

_____ 24. Hyperpyrexia

F. A continuous change into vapor of moisture from the respiratory tract, mucosa of the mouth, and perspiration on the skin

_____ 25. Suprasternal retractions

A. Difficult and labored breathing during which the individual has a persistent, unsatisfied need for air and feels distressed

_____ 26. Dyspnea

B. Indrawing above the clavicles

_____ 27. Insensible water loss

C. Any difference between the apical pulse rate and the radial pulse

_____ 28. Pulse deficit

D. Abnormally slow breathing

_____ 29. Bradypnea

E. A continuous and unnoticed loss of water from the body

LEARNING OUTCOMES

1. At what times should vital signs be measured?

2. What are the normal ranges of each vital sign by age group?

3. What factors affect temperature and the accurate measurement of it?

4. What factors affect pulse rate and the accurate measurement of it?

5. What are the sites commonly used to assess the pulse and why might each site be used?

6. What are the normal ranges for pulse rate? What effect does quality of pulse rate have on the assessment?

7. What factors affect respirations and the accurate measurement of it?

8. What are the mechanics of breathing? What are the components of the respiratory assessment?

9. What factors affect blood pressure and the accurate measurement of it?

10. What is the difference between systolic and diastolic blood pressure? What are the five phases of Korotkoff's sounds?

APPLY WHAT YOU LEARNED

In report you learn that one of the clients you are assigned to has been intermittently febrile. When you make your initial contact with the client, she tells you she is very cold, has begun shivering, and needs an extra blanket, which you provide. You check on her thirty minutes later and she says, "I am so hot and all sweaty now."

1. Identify factors that affect body temperature.

2. What three physiological processes are taking place when the client is shivering and requests an additional blanket?

3. When you check her an hour later, she complains about being hot and diaphoretic. What two physiological processes are now at work?

4. Describe what happens when a client experiences an intermittent fever.

MULTIPLE CHOICE QUESTIONS

Circle the answer that best completes each of the following statements.

1. A 76-year-old male client is shivering and says, "I need another blanket. I am so cold." Which statement would best explain the client's need for additional warmth?
   A. Body temperatures normally change throughout the day, reaching the lowest point between 1600 and 2000 hours.
   B. Progesterone secretion at the time of ovulation lowers body temperature by about 0.3 to 0.6°C (0.5 to 1.0°F).
   C. Because of decreased muscle activity in older adults, body temperatures fluctuate significantly.
   D. Older adults (over 75 years old) lose subcutaneous body fat and are sensitive to extremes of temperature.

2. The adult client is experiencing rapid respirations marked by quick, shallow breaths. The nurse counts the rate of respiration at 23 breaths per minute. This would be documented as:
   A. Bradypnea
   B. Apnea
   C. Tachypnea
   D. Orthopnea

3. The doctor in the emergency department has diagnosed a 17-year-old female client with hyperventilation. Which statement best describes hyperventilation?
   A. An increase in the amount of air in the lungs characterized by prolonged, deep breaths that may be associated with anxiety
   B. Gurgling sounds heard as air passes through moist secretions in the respiratory tract and bronchial tree
   C. A reduction in the amount of air in the lungs, characterized by shallow respirations, diaphoresis, and dusky nail beds
   D. Difficult and labored breathing during which the individual has a persistent, unsatisfied need for air and feels distressed

4. The doctor has diagnosed hypothermia for a homeless person who spent the night outside in frigid temperatures. Which manifestations of hypothermia would the nurse expect to observe?
   A. Diaphoresis; red, ruddy complexion; fever
   B. Alert, oriented; flushed, dry skin; subnormal temperature
   C. Hypertension; decreased pulse and respirations
   D. Pale, cool, waxy skin; disorientation; shivering

5. An adult client has a temperature of 102.3°F. Which intervention would be most appropriate for this client?
   A. Encourage frequent, rapidly paced walks in the halls.
   B. Provide at least 2500–3000 mL of fluids per day.
   C. Monitor vital signs, including temperature, every eight hours.
   D. Offer extra blankets for warmth and to "break" the fever.

6. A client has moderately severe burns over most of his neck, trunk, and upper and lower extremities. Which pulse site would it be most appropriate to use to assess his pulse?
   A. Radial
   B. Femoral
   C. Carotid
   D. Temporal

7. A client's initial blood pressure at a blood pressure screening clinic was 146/92. What follow-up recommendation should the nurse make?
   A. Confirm within two months
   B. Refer to a physician within one week
   C. Recheck in two years
   D. Recheck in one year

8. A client with pneumonia has a persistent cough and expectorates large amounts of rust-tinged sputum. When the nurse documents the findings, which statement would be most appropriate?
   A. Coughing and spitting up large amounts of brown-tinged stuff
   B. Persistent, productive cough; blood in sputum; probable bronchitis
   C. Nonproductive cough; large amounts of red-looking sticky phlegm
   D. Productive cough; expectorates large amounts of rust-tinged sputum

9. As a student, you are working with the RN in caring for a 77-year-old client admitted after falling down and hitting his head on a concrete floor. The RN tells you that the physician suspects that there is increasing intracranial pressure. As you look through the previous shift's documentation, you read, "The client's breathing is rhythmically waxing and waning from very deep to very shallow with periods of temporary apnea." You have just completed studying the respiratory system in one of your nursing classes and know that this type of breathing is called:
   A. Intercostal retraction
   B. Orthopnea
   C. Cheyne-Stokes
   D. Hypoventilation

10. The physician has ordered a blood pressure for a client with orthostatic hypotension. The nurse's first action would be to:
    A. Assist the client to sit or stand slowly; support the client in case of faintness.
    B. Place the client in a supine position for two to three minutes to allow for stabilization of the blood pressure and pulse.
    C. Encourage the client to ambulate in the halls for approximately five minutes and then rest for another five minutes.
    D. After one minute in the upright position, check the client's pulse and blood pressure in the other upper arm.

11. Although the thermometer must be left in place a long time to obtain an accurate measurement, this site is the safest and most noninvasive.
    A. Oral
    B. Rectal
    C. Tympanic
    D. Axillary

12. A 51-year-old client is in her second postoperative day after undergoing a total joint replacement of the left knee. To determine circulation to her foot, the nurse would palpate which pulse site?
    A. Femoral
    B. Brachial
    C. Popliteal
    D. Pedal

13. A client rides his bicycle to the clinic to have his blood pressure rechecked. To obtain an accurate reading, the nurse asks the client to:
    A. Drink a large glass of water.
    B. Rest 20 to 30 minutes.
    C. Do 10 cool-down exercises.
    D. Drive to the clinic tomorrow.

14. The physician has ordered a digitalis preparation for the client. This medication would be expected to:
    A. Decrease the client's heart rate.
    B. Increase the client's heart rate.
    C. Make no change in the client's heart rate.
    D. Initially decrease the client's heart rate, then increase it.

Chapter 22

Pain: The Fifth Vital Sign

KEY TERMS

Match each of the following key terms to its proper definition.

_____ 1. Gate control theory

A. The amount of pain stimulation a person requires in order to feel pain

_____ 2. Exogenous opioid analgesics

B. The maximum amount and duration of pain that an individual is willing to endure

_____ 3. Pain threshold

C. Pain relievers

_____ 4. Pain tolerance

D. The autonomic nervous system and behavioral responses to pain

_____ 5. Analgesia

E. Peripheral nerve fibers carrying pain to the spinal cord can have their message modified at the spinal cord level before transmission to the brain

_____ 6. Pain reaction

F. Bind to receptor sites to provide pain relief

_____ 7. Visceral pain

A. Chronic discomfort that persists despite therapeutic interventions

_____ 8. Radiating pain

B. Discomfort that results from stimulation of pain receptors in the abdominal cavity, cranium, and thorax

_____ 9. Intractable pain

C. Discomfort felt in a part of the body that is considerably removed from the tissues causing the pain

_____ 10.   Somatic pain

D.   Discomfort that is the result of a disturbance of the nerve pathways either from
past or continuing tissue damage

_____ 11.   Neuropathic pain

E.   Diffuse discomfort that arises from ligaments, tendons, bones, blood vessels, and
nerves

_____ 12.   Referred pain

F.   Discomfort that is perceived at the source
of the pain and extends to nearby tissues

LEARNING OUTCOMES

1.   What are the types and categories of pain according to location, etiology, and
duration?

Pain	Types	Categories
Location		
Etiology		
Duration		

2.   What are pain threshold, pain tolerance, and other concepts associated with
pain? How do they differ?

3.   What is the physiology of pain and what are the types of pain stimuli?

4.   What application does the gate control theory have to nursing care?

5.   Which factors affect the experience of pain?

6.   What is the three-step ladder approach to cancer pain endorsed by the
World Health Organization?

7. What are the pharmacologic interventions for pain and their nursing implications?

Pharmacologic Interventions	Nursing Implications

8. What are nonpharmacologic pain interventions?

9. What are the key factors in providing effective pain management?

10. What are the rationales for various analgesic delivery routes?

11. What are the barriers to effective pain management?

12. What data needs to be collected and what important interventions of the nursing care for the client in pain need to be accomplished?

Data Collected	Important Interventions

13. What are the adaptations by developmental level that need to be considered in the care of client with pain?

14. What criteria are used by the nurse to evaluate a client's response to interventions for pain?

APPLY WHAT YOU LEARNED

You are caring for an 85-year-old woman who, up until this hospitalization, has been living in her own home. You speak with the client's daughter, who says, "My mom has really bad arthritis and on some days, she can hardly get around. She's in constant severe pain. But she's stubborn, won't take her medications and refuses help." When you talk with the client, she says she doesn't like to take pain medication but refuses to elaborate on why. She goes on to say, "I'm old and I'm supposed to hurt some. I don't dwell on it because that doesn't make it any better." To obtain baseline information, you and the RN decide to conduct a pain assessment. You begin by thinking about:

1. Why might this client be reluctant to report the extent of her pain?

2. What possible misconceptions about pain and pain management might the client and her daughter have?

3. Is this client's pain acute or chronic? What rationale from your textbook readings do you have for your answer?

4. What one question you might ask the client to determine the impact of the pain on her life?

5. What nursing actions would be appropriate for individualizing this client's care?

MULTIPLE CHOICE QUESTIONS

Circle the answer that best completes each of the following statements.

1. If the physician orders a nonopioid analgesic for a client who is rating her pain at a 3 on a pain scale of 1 to 10, the client would most likely receive which medication?
   A. Darvocet
   B. Percocet
   C. Tylenol
   D. Tegretol

2. A client is experiencing chronic back pain and moderate anxiety. From readings on the impact of anxiety on a client's perception of pain, the nurse knows that:
   A. Anxiety, depression, and hopelessness often accompany chronic pain.
   B. Expressing concerns to an attentive listener does nothing to reduce pain.
   C. Fatigue has no impact on a person's perception of pain and ability to cope.
   D. Chronic pain is self-limiting and responds to the usual therapeutic interventions.

3. The burning sensation felt when a finger is burnt on a hot pan can be classified as:
   A. Neuropathic pain
   B. Somatic pain
   C. Visceral pain
   D. Cutaneous pain

4. A postoperative client is experiencing a significant level of acute pain. The nurse would expect to see:
   A. Dry, warm skin
   B. Normal pupillary response
   C. Diaphoresis
   D. BP 120/80; P 80; R 16

5. Before administering an opioid analgesic such as morphine, it is most important for the nurse to assess for:
   A. Muscle spasms
   B. Bradypnea
   C. Indigestion
   D. Drowsiness

6. Pharmacologic management of mild to moderate pain should begin with which class of medications?
   A. Opioids
   B. NSAIDs
   C. Anticonvulsants
   D. Anxiolytics

7. When taking a pain history on a newly admitted client, it is important to understand what the pain means to the client and how the client copes with it. To determine this, the nurse's best first response would be:
    A. "Since everyone has pain from time to time, can I assume that you are no different from the rest of the population?"
    B. "After your surgery, most nurses will try to keep you as comfortable as possible, though we can't over-medicate you."
    C. "I read in your chart that you have been having pain for quite some time. Is that correct? I'm assuming you're having a hard time now."
    D. "I'm interested in hearing from you about your pain, how it impacts on your life, and what you do to manage it."

8. The most reliable indicator of the presence or intensity of pain is the:
    A. Client's self-report
    B. Family's interpretation
    C. Nurse's judgment
    D. Physician's exam

9. A client receiving Demerol for pain management is complaining of constipation. Which preventive measure would be most appropriate?
    A. Place a call to the physician.
    B. Monitor intake and output.
    C. Stop administration of Demerol.
    D. Increase fluid intake to 2000 mL/day.

10. A postoperative client has been receiving morphine sulfate every three hours for pain management. The client's rate of respiration has gradually dropped from 18 breaths per minute to 10 breaths per minutes over the past one to two hours. The nurse contacts the physician and expects that he will order which medication?
    A. Methylphenidate hydrochloride (Ritalin)
    B. Diphenhydramine hydrochloride (Benadryl)
    C. Naloxone hydrochloride (Narcan)
    D. Prochlorperazine maleate (Compazine)

11. A client is reluctant to take the Percocet ordered by the physician. She says, "I'm afraid I'll get hooked on it. I'm trying to get by without taking anything." The nurse's best response would be:
    A. "Yes, that is a definite possibility, but wouldn't you rather be more comfortable now and worry about that later?"
    B. "You really need to take that medication. I've been a nurse for 10 years and I know what is best for my clients."
    C. "Actually, individuals are unlikely to become addicted to the medication when it is being used to treat pain."
    D. "You really shouldn't even need the Percocet since you only had minor surgery rather than major surgery."

12. Which route is the least desirable for opioid pain medication administration?
    A. Oral
    B. Transdermal
    C. Subcutaneous
    D. Intramuscular

13. When performing an assessment to determine the quality of a client's pain, which question would provide the most appropriate response by the client?
    A. What causes you pain?
    B. What does your pain feel like?
    C. When did the pain start?
    D. What relieves your pain?

14. A client recovering from a left leg above-the-knee amputation two days ago tells the nurse, "The toes on my left foot tingle and burn like fire. Can I have something for pain?" This client is likely experiencing:
    A. Referred pain
    B. Phantom pain
    C. Radiating pain
    D. Somatic pain

15. A client with an advanced malignancy is experiencing intractable pain. Although the physician has ordered PCA for self-administration of an analgesic for the client, the nurse recognizes that in order to help relieve the client's pain and promote client comfort, she must also:
    A. Use a number of nonpharmacologic pain intervention methods such as guided imagery and massage.
    B. Limit opioid use because of fears of addiction, despite its great value in relieving the severe and chronic pain in clients.
    C. Quantify each person's pain threshold and pain tolerance before medicating with an opioid analgesic.
    D. Explain the gate control theory to the client and stress the importance of the power of positive thinking.

Chapter 23

Activity, Rest, and Sleep

KEY TERMS

Match each of the following key terms to its proper definition.

_____ 1. Equilibrium

_____ 2. Pétrissage

_____ 3. Sleep apnea

_____ 4. Range of motion

_____ 5. Atrophy

A. Periodic cessation of breathing during sleep

B. Decrease in size

C. The maximum movement possible for a joint

D. Kneading or making large quick pinches of the skin, subcutaneous tissue, and muscle

E. The sense of balance

_____ 6. Hypersomnia

_____ 7. Ambulation

_____ 8. Parasomnia

_____ 9. Effleurage

_____ 10. Insomnia

A. Stroking of the body

B. The inability to obtain an adequate amount or quality of sleep

C. The act of walking

D. Excessive daytime sleep

E. Behavior that may interfere with sleep

LEARNING OUTCOMES

1. What are the basic elements of normal movement?

2. What factors affect body alignment and mobility?

3. What are the effects of immobility on body systems?

4. What assistive devices are used to support mobility?

5. How does the nursing process relate to a client with immobility?

6. What are the different body positions and how do they compare?

7. What actions will the nurse perform to support client mobility?

8. What are the proper procedures for assisting a client with mobility issues?

9. What are the stages and functions of sleep?

Stages of Sleep	Function

10. What factors affect sleep, and how does age or development affect sleep?

11. What are the common sleep disorders listed in this chapter, and what interventions are applied to promote normal sleep?

Sleep Disorder	Intervention

12. What tests are used to diagnose sleep disorders?

APPLY WHAT YOU LEARNED

You are caring for an immobile elderly client. Collaborating with the RN, you plan to implement nursing strategies to maintain or promote body alignment and mobility.

1. Discuss the importance of proper body alignment.

2. Discuss the effects of immobility.

3. Identify specific nursing strategies you will implement to maintain or promote body alignment and mobility.

4. Identify proper body mechanics the nurse must use to avoid personal injury when moving or transferring a client.

MULTIPLE CHOICE QUESTIONS

Circle the answer that best completes each of the following statements.

1. The primary purpose of conducting passive range of motion (ROM) exercises on an immobile client is to:
   A. Maintain joint flexibility.
   B. Strengthen tendons and ligaments.
   C. Build new muscle mass.
   D. Maintain cardiorespiratory function.

2. A client underwent an abdominal hysterectomy yesterday. The doctor has written an order that reads, "Ambulate every shift." When the nurse approaches the client, she says, "I'm not moving from this bed. I'm not ready to walk yet." The nurse's best response would be:
   A. "I'll leave for 10 minutes, and when I get back, you will get up!"
   B. "The doctor has ordered you to walk, and walk you must."
   C. "Getting up and moving about is critical to your recovery."
   D. "That's fine. You have the right to refuse treatment."

3. Poor oxygenation and buildup of carbon dioxide in the blood can result in:
   A. Respiratory acidosis
   B. Respiratory alkalosis
   C. Metabolic acidosis
   D. Metabolic alkalosis

4. Which of the following are considered weightbearing joints?
   A. Umbilicus and symphysis pubis
   B. Ankles and feet
   C. Sacrum and pelvis
   D. Hips and knees

5. An immobile client, without the stress of weightbearing activity, will likely experience osteoporosis, which is caused by depletion of which mineral?
   A. Iron
   B. Calcium
   C. Magnesium
   D. Potassium

6. A client reports having difficulty sleeping. He says he feels tired when he goes to bed but cannot fall asleep. Which recommendation would be most helpful for this client?
   A. Drink several alcoholic beverages.
   B. Raise the room temperature.
   C. Wear loose-fitting nightwear.
   D. Exercise immediately before going to bed.

7. As the nurse conducts passive range of motion (ROM) exercises for a client on bed rest, she adducts each limb. Which statement best describes this action?
   A. The nurse is moving the limb (bone) away from the midline of the body.
   B. The nurse is turning the sole of the foot outward by moving the ankle joint.
   C. The nurse is moving the bones of the forearm with the palm of the hand facing upward.
   D. The nurse is moving the limb (bone) toward the midline of the body.

8. The nurse is repositioning a client in a low-Fowler's position. To prevent external rotation of the hips, the most effective action would be to:
   A. Order a footboard for lower body support.
   B. Roll a small pillow under the lumbar curvature.
   C. Place a trochanter roll lateral to each femur.
   D. Place a pillow under the lower legs at the knees.

9. A client is experiencing rapid eye movement (REM) sleep deprivation. Which clinical sign would the nurse expect this client to exhibit?
   A. Apathy
   B. Irritability
   C. Withdrawal
   D. Hyporesponsiveness

10. The nurse is helping a client from the bed to the bathroom. Before helping the client to sit up on the edge of the bed, the nurse will:
   A. Move the mattress to the edge of the bed frame.
   B. Assist the client to a supine position.
   C. Lower the head of the bed slowly as low as it will go.
   D. Raise the head of the bed slowly as high as it will go.

11. Which physiologic change is characteristic during non-rapid eye movement (NREM) sleep?
   A. Irregular muscle movement
   B. Fall in arterial blood pressure
   C. Depressed muscle tone
   D. Active, vivid dreaming

12. A client has chronic obstructive pulmonary disease (COPD), which limits the supply of oxygen to vital organs. When planning care, which nursing consideration would be most appropriate for this client?
   A. Complete ADLs as rapidly as possible to conserve energy.
   B. Omit ADLs until the client regains his strength.
   C. Have the client do the ADLs himself.
   D. Pace activities based on the client's tolerance.

13. To facilitate drainage from the mouth and prevent aspiration, the nurse positions an unconscious client halfway between the lateral and prone positions. At the end of the shift, the nurse reports this position as:
   A. Dorsal recumbent
   B. Sims'
   C. Fowler's
   D. Supine

14. Proper body alignment provides the client with:
   A. Little strain on the joints, muscles, tendons, or ligaments.
   B. Greater stability and balance when sitting or in a supine position.
   C. An offset to the constant pull of gravity, which enhances self-esteem.
   D. An imaginary vertical line drawn through the body's center of gravity.

15. A client has been experiencing a significant drop in blood pressure when she changes positions. She says, "Boy, I sure get dizzy when I get up. I feel like I'm going to pass out." Which action would be most effective for this client as she experiences these episodes?
   A. Take a hot bath.
   B. Hold her breath and bear down.
   C. Become active first thing in the morning.
   D. Wear elastic stockings at night.

Chapter 24

Wound Care and Skin Integrity

KEY TERMS

Match each of the following key terms to its proper definition.

_____ 1. Maceration	A. Wound caused by a blow from a blunt instrument
_____ 2. Contusion	B. Surface scrape, either unintentional or intentional
_____ 3. Laceration	C. Penetration of the skin and often the underlying tissues by a sharp instrument, either intentional or unintentional
_____ 4. Abrasion	D. Softening of tissue by prolonged wetting
_____ 5. Puncture	E. Tissues torn apart, often from accidents

_____ 6. Phagocytosis	A. Lesions caused by unrelieved pressure resulting in damage to underlying tissue
_____ 7. Shearing force	B. A process by white blood cells to ingest and digest bacteria and cellular debris
_____ 8. Decubitus ulcers	C. Production of pus
_____ 9. Pressure ulcers	D. A combination of friction and pressure
_____ 10. Suppuration	E. Lesions caused by unrelieved pressure resulting in damage to underlying tissue

_____ 11.	Fistula	A.	Dead matter that is sloughed off the surface of the skin
_____ 12.	Eschar	B.	A deficiency in the blood supply to the tissue
_____ 13.	Ischemia	C.	Pus-filled
_____ 14.	Exudate	D.	An abnormal passage from a body cavity or tube to another cavity or surface
_____ 15.	Purulent	E.	Material that has escaped from blood vessels during the inflammatory process and is deposited in tissue or on tissue surfaces

_____ 16.	Granulation tissue	A.	Type of discharge consisting of serum
_____ 17.	Keloid	B.	A discharge of large amounts of red blood cells frequently seen in open wounds
_____ 18.	Serous exudate	C.	Washing or flushing out of an area
_____ 19.	Irrigation	D.	Translucent red tissue that grows in a wound
_____ 20.	Sanguineous exudate	E.	Watery, blood-tinged
_____ 21.	Serosanguineous	F.	A progressively enlarging scar

LEARNING OUTCOMES

1. What are the factors that affect skin integrity?

2. What terms are used to describe or classify wounds?

3. How do wounds heal? What are the phases of wound healing? What are the types of wound drainage?

4. What factors affect wound healing and what complications can occur?

5. What is involved in nursing care of wounds?

6. What are the different types of dressings used in wound care and what are the methods of application?

7. What are methods of applying dry and moist heat and cold to aid in wound healing?

8. What are the interventions for nursing care of clients with wounds?

9. How do pressure ulcers form and what are the risks factors involved and the preventive measures of them?

10. What are the stages of pressure ulcer formation and how is the data collected to assess status of a pressure ulcer?

11. How does the nursing process relate to clients with pressure ulcers?

APPLY WHAT YOU LEARNED

You are giving a report to the nursing assistant who will be providing care for an elderly immobile client. You must provide her with instructions on care for this client. Before you begin, the nursing assistant says, "I know what to do. I'll turn her when I get to it, do a two-person transfer to the chair, try to feed her breakfast and lunch, order a doughnut cushion for her to sit on when she is up, and massage those areas that look red." After listening to the nursing assistant, you realize that you must provide specific instructions and a rationale for each action, as well as an explanation for those statements on tasks that would be inappropriate or contraindicated for this client. Your goal for this client is the maintenance of skin integrity.

1. Identify specific approaches to be used when assessing common pressure sites.

2. Identify specific tasks targeting prevention of the formation of pressure ulcers to be completed for this client.

3. Provide a rationale for each of the delegated tasks.

4. Review the nursing assistant's comments and provide an explanation for those statements on tasks that would be inappropriate or contraindicated for the client.

MULTIPLE CHOICE QUESTIONS

Circle the answer that best completes each of the following statements.

1. The nurse observes a bright, sanguineous exudate on the abdominal dressing of a postoperative client. This finding indicates:
   A. Old blood
   B. Fresh bleeding
   C. Pus
   D. Dehiscence

2. A closed surgical incision is an example of which type of healing?
   A. Primary intention
   B. Secondary intention
   C. Tertiary intention
   D. Deliberate intention

3. A keloid can be defined as a:
   A. Hypertropic scar or an abnormal amount of collagen formation.
   B. Black, leathery formation of dried plasma proteins and dead cells.
   C. Fluid that has escaped from blood vessels during the inflammatory process.
   D. Combination of clots and dead or dying tissue on the surface of a wound.

4. Secondary intention healing differs from primary intention in which way?
   A. The repair time is shorter.
   B. The scarring is less.
   C. The risk of infection is greater.
   D. Depends on the size of the wound.

5. Wound healing requires a diet rich in protein, carbohydrates, lipids, minerals, and which vitamins?
   A. A and C
   B. D and E
   C. A and D
   D. C and E

6. A postoperative client who is obese has an increased risk of wound infection because:
   A. Fibroblast activity is decreased with increased adipose tissue.
   B. Obese clients heal by secondary intention.
   C. Obesity reduces the number of available macrophages.
   D. Adipose tissue usually has a minimal blood supply.

7. The physician writes an order for wound care that includes packing the client's wound with moistened gauze. Which statement provides the best rationale for this action?
   A. The gauze packing acts as a temporary skin and provides thermal insulation.
   B. Gauze packing decreases pain and thus reduces the need for analgesics.
   C. Packing a wound provides the client with psychologic comfort.
   D. Gauze packing facilitates the formation of granulation tissue and healing.

8. Hydrocolloid dressings are frequently used over venous stasis leg and pressure ulcers. One disadvantage of using this type of dressing is that it:
   A. Facilitates anaerobic bacterial growth.
   B. Needs to be changed every day.
   C. Causes maceration of surrounding skin.
   D. Must be covered with a dry sterile dressing.

9. You have learned in class that laboratory data often support the nurse's clinical assessment of the wound's progress in healing. So as you prepare and plan care for a client who has several stage IV pressure ulcers, you check the client's lab results and notice that his leukocyte count has steadily decreased over the past three to four days. From this data, you conclude the client may be at increased risk for:
   A. Delayed healing and the possibility of infection.
   B. Blood clots that may impede blood flow to the wounds.
   C. Decreased oxygen supply to new granulation tissue.
   D. Vitamin A and K deficiency and malnourishment.

10. When repositioning a client, the nurse observes a reddened area over the left greater trochanter. When light pressure is applied to this erythematous area, it does not blanch and the skin integrity remains intact. When documenting these findings, the nurse notes this stage of pressure ulcer formation to be:
    A. Stage I
    B. Stage II
    C. Stage III
    D. Stage IV

11. To ensure that an elderly immobile client who is at risk for impaired skin integrity will be repositioned at least every two hours, the nurse will:
    A. Delegate this task in writing to the nursing assistant assigned to the client.
    B. Establish a written schedule for turning and repositioning and post above the bed.
    C. Encourage the client to move at least every 15 to 30 minutes or as much as possible.
    D. Try to get into the client's room as often as possible to do this.

12. In an attempt to prevent pressure ulcer formation, the nurse should:
    A. Keep the skin clean, dry, and free of urine, feces, and perspiration.
    B. Transfer the immobile client without the use of a lifting device.
    C. Massage areas over bony prominences to stimulate circulation.
    D. Order an inflatable doughnut-like cushion for use when the client is sitting.

13. To reduce shearing force in clients on bed rest, the head of the bed should be elevated no more than:
    A. 90 degrees
    B. 60 degrees
    C. 30 degrees
    D. 15 degrees

14. A client with a Stage III pressure ulcer has been given the nursing diagnoses of *Impaired Skin Integrity* and *Risk for Infection*. Which expected outcome would be most appropriate for this client?
    A. The client and family will learn wound care by discharge.
    B. The wound will heal by primary intention by discharge.
    C. The wound will be maintained without evidence of infection.
    D. The client will consume 100% of meals and drink 2500 mL of water.

15. Wound healing in the older adult is most likely to be inhibited or delayed by:
    A. Enhanced flexibility of collagen tissue.
    B. Increased formation of antibodies.
    C. Diminished respiratory capacity.
    D. Atrophy of capillaries in the skin.

Chapter 25

Nutrition and Diet Therapy

KEY TERMS

Match each of the following key terms to its proper definition.

_____ 1. Obesity

_____ 2. Lipids

_____ 3. Protein–calorie malnutrition

_____ 4. Amino acids

_____ 5. Parenteral nutrition

A. Organic substances that are greasy and insoluble in water but soluble in alcohol or ether

B. Weight loss and visible muscle and fat wasting

C. The building blocks of proteins

D. Provided when the client is unable to ingest or absorb foods

E. Body weight that exceeds ideal body weight by more than 20%

_____ 6. Glycogenesis

_____ 7. Basal metabolic rate

_____ 8. Enteral nutrition

_____ 9. Undernutrition

_____ 10. Calories

A. Units of heat energy

B. Condition occurring when nutrient intake is insufficient to meet daily energy requirements

C. Process of glycogen formation

D. The pace at which the body utilizes food to maintain the energy requirements of a person who is awake and at rest

E. Nourishment given through a tube or stoma directly into the small intestine, thus bypassing the upper digestive tract

1. What are the essential nutrients, dietary sources, and elements of metabolism?

2. What are the essential aspects of energy balance? What tools are there for individualizing food choices?

3. What are the requirements of nutrition throughout a person's life span?

4. Define the following diets:

Type of Diet	Definition
Therapeutic Diets	
Diet Modifications For Disease	
Elective Diets	
Dietary Changes Related To Food Allergies	

5.   What are nursing interventions to promote nutrition?

APPLY WHAT YOU LEARNED

You are administering 0900 medications. A client with an enteral tube is to receive seven different medications. Three of the medications are available as liquids, three are in tablet form, and one is a capsule. After looking up each medication in your drug handbook, you determine that all but one of the tablets may be crushed.

1.   Identify essential data that you must gather prior to administering any medications to this client.

2.   Discuss which medications may be given through the tube and which ones may not. Provide rationales for your choices.

3.   Discuss how you will administer the crushable medications through the tube.

4.   Discuss what action(s) you will need to take related to the medication that may not be crushed.

MULTIPLE CHOICE QUESTIONS

Circle the answer that best completes each of the following statements.

1.   A client who was recently diagnosed with diabetes mellitus has been instructed to restrict or eliminate processed or refined sugars from her diet. Which foods should she avoid?
      A.   Apples
      B.   Soft drinks
      C.   Whole milk products
      D.   Whole grain breads

2. Glucose that cannot be stored by the body as glycogen is converted to:
   A. Protein
   B. Nitrogen
   C. Fat
   D. Starch

3. Which foods or beverages could be included for a client receiving a clear liquid diet?
   A. Skim milk and tea
   B. Ginger ale and pudding
   C. Clear broth and plain Jell-O
   D. Ice cream and coffee

4. When caring for a client receiving continuous tube feedings, the placement of the tube should be checked:
   A. Every hour and when administering water or other liquids through the tube.
   B. At least once per shift and prior to administering medications through the tube.
   C. Every four hours regardless of when medications are administered.
   D. Each time a new bag of feeding solution is hung and the tubing is changed.

5. An intermittent enteral feeding of 400 mL should be administered over at least:
   A. 5 minutes
   B. 15 minutes
   C. 30 minutes
   D. 60 minutes

6. When working with a client with a nutritional imbalance, the nurse must first:
   A. Set the goals for the client and insist that the client follow all directions.
   B. Involve the client in the determination of short- and long-term goals.
   C. Show a video and provide follow-up printed materials for use at home.
   D. Arrange for the registered dietician or nutritionist to meet with the client.

7. Prior to insertion of a nasogastric tube, the client should be placed into which position?
   A. Side-lying
   B. Supine
   C. Semi-Fowler's
   D. High-Fowler's

8. A coworker asks the nurse to help her place a nasogastric tube into a client who has not been eating. As she prepares the tube for insertion, the nurse notices that the coworker is lubricating the tip of the tube with Vaseline. The nurse's best response in this situation is to:
   A. Say nothing, since she knows that Vaseline is an acceptable lubricant for use when inserting a nasogastric tube through the nasopharynx.
   B. Volunteer to get a water-based lubricant since an oil-based lubricant could cause respiratory complications if it enters the lungs.
   C. Pretend not to see that the coworker is using Vaseline since the nurse is not her supervisor and she has not asked for the nurse's opinions or ideas.
   D. Leave the room and report this coworker's actions to the RN supervisor, who is the person ultimately responsible for this client.

9. The nurse is assessing placement of a feeding tube by aspirating alimentary secretions. After withdrawing the stomach contents, the nurse measures the amount and finds it to be approximately 125 mL. After recording the amount, the nurse should:
   A. Discard the aspirated contents.
   B. Send the contents to the lab for analysis.
   C. Check the pH to make sure it is 6 or above.
   D. Reinstill the gastric contents into the stomach.

10. To prevent peristomal skin excoriation and breakdown in a client with a percutaneous endoscopic gastrostomy (PEG) tube, the nurse should:
    A. Cleanse the area with mild soap and water and leave the site open to air.
    B. Cleanse with a 50% hydrogen peroxide solution and cover with a 4 × 4 gauze.
    C. Remove the old dressing and spray with tincture of benzoin before washing.
    D. Wash the site with sterile water and apply an antibacterial ointment.

11. The physician has ordered an enteric-coated medication for a client with an enteral feeding tube. After looking up the medication in the drug handbook, the nurse realizes that this medication may not be crushed. What is the nurse's next best action?
    A. Call the pharmacist to discuss the situation.
    B. Dissolve the medication in a small amount of warm water.
    C. Crush the medication anyway since the physician ordered it.
    D. Try to give the medication orally with a small amount of juice.

12. The client at most risk for *Nutrition, Less than Body Requirements*, or undernutrition, would be a(n):
    A. 17-year-old high school athlete
    B. 20-year-old aspiring model
    C. 87-year-old widower living alone
    D. 2-year-old active toddler

13. Based on the client's body mass index (BMI), a 27-year-old male who is 6 foot 3 inches tall and weighs 230 pounds would be considered:
    A. Underweight
    B. Normal
    C. Overweight
    D. Obese

14. During an admission interview, a client who adheres to a strict vegetarian diet says, "I'm always a little worried about not getting enough complete protein in my diet." The nurse's best response would be:
    A. "You probably should consult a dietician. Protein is essential for building and maintaining our body's tissue."
    B. "Eating complementary proteins, such as beans and rice, is a good way to ensure adequate protein intake."
    C. "Why don't you just include a couple of eggs, some cheese, and a glass of milk in your diet on a daily basis?"
    D. "Does your doctor know that you don't eat any meat, chicken, or fish? I'd think he'd be upset about that."

15. A client says, "My doctor told me that my triglycerides are way too high and that I have to cut down on certain foods with a lot of saturated fat. My question is, how do I know which fats are high in saturated fats and which are not?" The nurse's best response would be:
    A. "Actually, all fats are very high in saturated fat. You'll just have to eliminate most of them from your diet."
    B. "That's a good question. It kind of takes the fun out of life and eating, doesn't it? I'm supposed to cut back as well."
    C. "The hardness of the fat at room temperature is a good indicator. The harder the fat, the more saturated it is."
    D. "Most fats that are liquid at room temperature and found in plant products are generally considered the most harmful."

Chapter 26

Fluids, Electrolytes, and Acid-Base Balance

KEY TERMS

Match each of the following key terms to its proper definition.

_____ 1. Passive transport

A. Less than normal acid within the plasma

_____ 2. Metabolic alkalosis

B. Drop in blood ph from carbonic acid buildup

_____ 3. Respiratory acidosis

C. Greater than normal acid within the plasma

_____ 4. Active transport

D. An elevated pH due to a decrease in $PaCO_2$

_____ 5. Metabolic acidosis

E. Movement of solutes through membranes without energy expenditure

_____ 6. Respiratory alkalosis

F. Movement that occurs when it is necessary for electrolytes to move from an area of low concentration to an area of high concentration

_____ 7. Osmosis

A. Force that develops as solute particles collide against one another, causing movement of fluid

_____ 8. Filtration

B. Extracellular fluid that surrounds the cells and includes lymph

_____ 9. Intravascular fluid

C. Only that fluid which is found within the blood

_____ 10. Interstitial fluid

D. Body water found within cells

_____ 11. Osmotic pressure

E. The transfer of water and dissolved substances from a region of high pressure to a region of low pressure

_____ 12. Intracellular fluid

F. The passage of water from an area of lower particle concentration toward an area of higher concentration of particles

_____ 13. Isotonic

A. Chemicals that prevent marked changes in hydrogen ion concentration

_____ 14. Buffers

B. pH above 7 on a scale of 0 to 14

_____ 15. Alkaline

C. Electrolytes with positive charge

_____ 16. Anions

D. Having the same concentration of solutes as blood plasma

_____ 17. Cations

E. Electrolytes with negative charge

LEARNING OUTCOMES

1. What are the definitions, compositions, and distribution of fluids in the body?

2. What are the mechanisms for regulation of body fluids and electrolytes?

3. What is the normal range of acid-base balance? What are the important regulators of pH in the blood?

4. Name the important electrolytes, their normal ranges, and manifestations of imbalances.

Electrolytes		
Normal Ranges		
Manifestations of Imbalances		

5. List four acid-based imbalances, and explain how they are treated.

Acid-based Imbalances	Treatment

6. What substances are considered part of fluid intake?

7. Define the nursing care for clients with fluid or acid-based disorders:

APPLY WHAT YOU LEARNED

With the RN, you are preparing a discharge teaching plan for an African American client admitted with pneumonia, uncontrolled diabetes mellitus, dehydration, hyperkalemia, fluid and electrolyte imbalance, and metabolic acidosis.

1. Identify common strategies for prevention of fluid and electrolyte imbalance you will include in the teaching plan.

2. Provide the client with an explanation of the relationship between uncontrolled diabetes and metabolic acidosis.

3. Describe how the client can prevent metabolic acidosis from occurring in the future.

4. Discuss cultural considerations that may influence this client's health status.

MULTIPLE CHOICE QUESTIONS

Circle the answer that best completes each of the following statements.

1. Which electrolyte is an example of a cation?
   A. Chloride
   B. Potassium
   C. Phosphate
   D. Fluoride

2. Which of the following foods would provide the best source of dietary calcium?
   A. Split pea soup
   B. Nonfat yogurt
   C. Cantaloupe
   D. Macaroni and cheese

3. Which arterial blood pH is considered basic and may result in alkalosis?
   A. 7.35
   B. 7.45
   C. 7.15
   D. 7.55

4. This regulatory system is the body's first line of defense against acid-base balance changes in the body.
   A. Buffer regulation
   B. Respiratory system regulation
   C. Renal system regulation
   D. Carbonic regulation

5. When the level of carbon dioxide rises, the arterial blood pH subsequently falls, causing the respiratory system regulators to respond. During this process, the nurse would observe which change in the vital signs of the client?
   A. Decreased rate and depth of respirations
   B. Increased rate and depth of respirations
   C. Decreased rate and strength of the pulse
   D. Increased rate and strength of the pulse

6. A client's (ABG) arterial blood gas results are as follows: $pH = 7.29$; $PCO_2 = 49$ mm Hg; $HCO_3^- = 24$ mEq/L. This client is experiencing:
   A. Respiratory acidosis
   B. Respiratory alkalosis
   C. Metabolic acidosis
   D. Metabolic alkalosis

7. A client's (ABG) arterial blood gas results are as follows: pH = 7.51; PCO_2 = 39 mm Hg; HCO_3^- = 31 mEq/L. This client is experiencing:
    A. Respiratory acidosis
    B. Respiratory alkalosis
    C. Metabolic acidosis
    D. Metabolic alkalosis

8. A client with a high fever may be at increased risk for which acid–base imbalance?
    A. Respiratory acidosis
    B. Respiratory alkalosis
    C. Metabolic acidosis
    D. Metabolic alkalosis

9. A client who has a nasogastric tube attached to low suction is at risk for:
    A. Respiratory acidosis
    B. Respiratory alkalosis
    C. Metabolic acidosis
    D. Metabolic alkalosis

10. A client reports taking "numerous" antacid pills per day for "heartburn" or "indigestion." Because of the excessive intake of the antacid, the client may be at risk for:
    A. Respiratory acidosis
    B. Respiratory alkalosis
    C. Metabolic acidosis
    D. Metabolic alkalosis

11. A client with poorly controlled diabetes mellitus is experiencing Kussmaul's respirations. The physician has ordered ABGs drawn. The nurse would expect the uncompensated results to be similar to which of the following?
    A. pH 7.20; PCO_2 30 mm Hg; HCO_3^- 20 mEq/L
    B. pH 7.35; PCO_2 35 mm Hg; HCO_3^- 24 mEq/L
    C. pH 7.45; PCO_2 30 mm Hg; HCO_3^- 30 mEq/L
    D. pH 7.65; PCO_2 50 mm Hg; HCO_3^- 26 mEq/L

12. A client has been admitted with acute renal failure. For the past several months, he has been taking a loop diuretic and a potassium supplement. The client is complaining of weakness in his legs and arms, and an ECG reveals a significant dysrhythmia and altered T-waves that were not present on past tracings. Based on this data, the nurse concludes the client is most likely experiencing:
    A. Hypocalcemia
    B. Hypernatremia
    C. Hyperkalemia
    D. Hypomagnesmia

13. The kidneys provide the primary long-term regulation of acid-base balance by:
    A. Selectively excreting or conserving bicarbonate and hydrogen ions.
    B. Altering the hemoglobin to make it give up its oxygen and carbonic acid.
    C. Neutralizing excess acids or bases with bicarbonate and carbonic acid.
    D. Eliminating or retaining carbon dioxide, thereby altering the pH.

14. A client with severe anxiety who hyperventilates is at increased risk for:
    A. Respiratory acidosis
    B. Respiratory alkalosis
    C. Metabolic acidosis
    D. Metabolic alkalosis

15. A 15-year-old female client has been diagnosed with anorexia nervosa. She has lost 60 pounds over the past two months. She presents with weakness and complains of a constant headache. This client must be monitored for signs and symptoms of which acid-base imbalance?
    A. Respiratory acidosis
    B. Respiratory alkalosis
    C. Metabolic acidosis
    D. Metabolic alkalosis

Chapter 27

Medications

KEY TERMS

Match each of the following key terms to its proper definition.

_____ 1. Metabolism   A. Unintended drug actions

_____ 2. Generic   B. The process by which the drug is sent to various body tissues

_____ 3. Absorption   C. The desired result

_____ 4. Therapeutic effect   D. Family name of a drug

_____ 5. Distribution   E. The process by which some drugs are converted in the liver to inactive compounds

_____ 6. Side effects   F. The process by which a drug passes into the bloodstream

---

_____ 7. Suppository   A. Into the muscle

_____ 8. Intravenous   B. Under the tongue

_____ 9. Subcutaneous   C. Into the dermis or skin

_____ 10. Intradermal   D. Below the skin

_____ 11. Intramuscular   E. One or several drugs mixed with a firm base and shaped for insertion into the body

_____ 12. Sublingual   F. Into the vein

_____ 13.	Meniscus	A.	Part of the needle that fits into the syringe
_____ 14.	Bevel	B.	Injectable
_____ 15.	Syrup	C.	Pertaining to the cheek
_____ 16.	Parenteral	D.	The slanted part of the tip of needle of a syringe
_____ 17.	Hub	E.	An aqueous solution of sugar
_____ 18.	Buccal	F.	Crescent-shaped upper surface of a column of liquid

_____ 19.	Drug interaction	A.	Occurs when a person requires increases in dosage to maintain the therapeutic effect
_____ 20.	Adverse effects	B.	Deleterious effects of a drug on an organism or tissue
_____ 21.	Drug toxicity	C.	Problem that occurs when the administration of one drug alters the effect of another drug
_____ 22.	Drug allergy	D.	Severe side effects or drug reactions
_____ 23.	Drug tolerance	E.	An immunologic reaction to a drug

LEARNING OUTCOMES

1. What are the terms related to the administration of medication?

2. What are drug standards and what are the legal aspects of administering drugs?

Drug Standards	Legal Aspects

3. What are the physiologic actions and effects of drugs and what are the factors affecting medication action?

4. What are the essential parts of a medication order? How are they communicated and how can the nurse avoid common errors?

Essential Parts	Communicated How?	Avoiding Errors

5. What systems of measurement and formulas are commonly used in medication orders?

6. What equipment is required for administrating parenteral medications?

7. What are the routes of medication administration and drug dispensing systems?

Routes	Drug Dispensing Systems

8. What are the nursing interventions in relation to oral medication administration?

9. What are the required steps for administering nasogastric and gastrostomy tube medications?

10. How would the nurse mix selected drugs from vials and ampules?

11. What are the essential steps for safely administering parenteral medications by intradermal, subcutaneous, and intramuscular routes?

Intradermal	Subcutaneous	Intramuscular

12. What are the essential steps in safely administering topical medications?

APPLY WHAT YOU LEARNED

You are preparing morning medications for a client receiving the following:
- Haloperidol 1 mg IM for agitation now
  - On hand: The vial labeled *Haloperidol* reads *5 mg/mL*.
  - How many milliliters will you give?
  - ANSWER: _____
- Xanax 0.25 gm PO t.i.d. for acute anxiety
  - On hand: The bottle of oral solution labeled *Xanax* reads *500 mg/mL*.
  - How many milliliters will you give per dose?
  - ANSWER: _____

- KCL 40 mEq PO. Daily
  - On hand: The bottle of oral solution labeled *Potassium chloride (KCL)* reads *30 mEq/15mL.*
  - How many milliliters will you give per dose?
  - ANSWER: _____

1. Begin this exercise by briefly describing the nurse's legal responsibilities when administering drugs.

2. Determine if each order above contains the essential parts of a medication order.

3. Define each abbreviation contained in the orders.

4. For each of the above medications, using the information provided, calculate the appropriate dosage.

5. List the essential steps to follow when preparing and administering medications.

6. Identify one nursing action to determine the effectiveness of medications.

MULTIPLE CHOICE QUESTIONS

Circle the answer that best completes each of the following statements.

1. The nurse enters a client's room with the morning medications. After looking at the pills, the client says, "What is that yellow pill for? I've never had that one before." What is the nurse's best response?
   A. "I checked them all very carefully and I believe they are correct."
   B. "Let's wait with that one, and I'll go back and check the original order."
   C. "It's probably the same but just manufactured by a different company."
   D. "It's what your doctor ordered, so you will need to take it."

2. The rate of absorption of a medication is determined by the:
   A. Administration route
   B. Prescribed amount
   C. Type of medication
   D. Time of day it is administered

3. Before administering a dermatologic preparation, the nurse must:
   A. Use sterile technique when filling the syringe.
   B. Instruct the client to place the medication under the tongue.
   C. Hold the bevel of the needle upward.
   D. Clean the area with mild soap and water and pat it dry.

4. The client has an order for Demerol 50 mg IM every four hours for pain. Which route will the nurse choose when administering this medication?
   A. Intravenous
   B. Subcutaneous
   C. Intramuscular
   D. Intradermal

5. The nurse is withdrawing a solution for a subcutaneous injection from the vial, and notices white sediment at the bottom of the bottle. What is the nurse's next best action?
   A. Proceed without taking any action.
   B. Rotate the vial between the palms of her hands.
   C. Shake the bottle vigorously.
   D. Call the pharmacy and request a new vial.

6. The physician has written an order for Prozac 20 mg daily. This is an example of a:
   A. PRN order
   B. Standing order
   C. Single order
   D. Stat order

7. An insulin order reads U-100 NPH insulin 15 units and U-100 regular insulin 4 units. It is imperative to choose the correct specially calibrated scale syringe. There are two insulin syringes to choose from: a low-dose syringe (50 units) and a 100-unit syringe. Based on the above order, select the appropriate syringe.
   A. U-100; low-dose syringe
   B. U-50; low-dose syringe
   C. U-100; 100-unit syringe
   D. U-50; 100-unit syringe

8. The physician prescribes Benadryl, an antihistamine, for a client with seasonal allergies. Because it is impossible to memorize pertinent information about every drug, the nurse refers to a current drug reference and sees that the medication can cause drowsiness. When teaching the client about the medication, the nurse refers to this response as a(n):
   A. Desired effect
   B. Adverse effect
   C. Idiosyncratic effect
   D. Side effect

9. Which class of medications can produce drug tolerance?
   A. Insulin
   B. Barbiturates
   C. Antihypertensives
   D. Cholesterol-lowering drugs

10. A sweetened and aromatic solution of alcohol used as a vehicle for medicinal agents is known as a(n):
    A. Elixir
    B. Aqueous solution
    C. Liniment
    D. Syrup

11. When evaluating the effects of any medication, the LPN/LVN should:
    A. Return to the client when the medication is expected to take effect.
    B. Tell the client to report any unusual effects to the RN.
    C. Wait for the client to say something because the LPN/LVN is busy with other clients.
    D. Send the nursing assistant into the client's room to ask him how he is feeling.

12. A client is receiving ASA (aspirin) every six hours for arthritic pain. This medication has which therapeutic action?
    A. Palliative
    B. Curative
    C. Restorative
    D. Supportive

13. When injecting a medication using a Z-track technique, the nurse must:
    A. Use the nondominant hand to pull the skin laterally and downward approximately 2.5 cm (1 in.) at the site.
    B. Grasp the syringe in the dominant hand and quickly insert the needle at a 45-degree angle.
    C. Hold the syringe between the thumb and forefinger and pierce the skin quickly at a 90-degree angle.
    D. Use a surgical marker to draw a 2.5-cm-long "Z" at the landmark injection site.

14. A physician has written a new order for Lasix. When attempting to determine the dosage, the nurse realizes that the writing is unclear and she cannot determine whether it reads 40.0 mg or 400 mg. The drug reference indicates that 400 mg is beyond the usual adult dosage. What is the nurse's next best action?

    A. Have the unit clerk/secretary try to decipher the writing and determine the dosage.

    B. Decide that if the order is wrong, the physician is ultimately responsible.

    C. Give the 40 mg because the drug reference indicates 400 mg is far too much.

    D. Discuss the order with the RN and contact the physician for clarification of the order.

15. After preparing oral medications for a client and taking them to the client's room, the nurse realizes that the client is unable to hold the pill cup. What is the nurse's next best action?

    A. Ask the nursing assistant to put the pills into the client's hot breakfast cereal.

    B. Take each pill with his fingers and place it in the client's mouth.

    C. Take the pills back to the medication room and chart that the client could not take them.

    D. Using the pill cup, introduce the medication into the client's mouth, giving only one at a time.

Chapter 28

IV Therapy

KEY TERMS

Match each of the following key terms to its proper definition.

_____ 1. Extravasation

_____ 2. Phlebitis

_____ 3. Drip factors

_____ 4. Osmolarity

_____ 5. Thrombosis

_____ 6. Infiltration

A. Clot formation in the vein

B. Passage of the IV solution out of the vein and into the surrounding tissue

C. Inflammation of the vein

D. Severe infiltration of a solution into surrounding tissue

E. Rates at which IV solution passes through the drip chamber and into the tubing

F. The concentration of a solute in a volume of solution

_____ 7. Hypotonic

_____ 8. Septicemia

_____ 9. Isotonic

_____ 10. Hypertonic

_____ 11. Venospasm

_____ 12. Bacteremia

A. Virulent microorganisms in the bloodstream from a localized source of infection

B. Having the same concentration of solutes as blood plasma

C. Constriction of the inner lining of the vein

D. Spread of bacteria from a local infection into the bloodstream

E. Having greater concentration of solutes than plasma

F. Having lesser concentration of solutes than blood plasma

LEARNING OUTCOMES

1. What are the nurse's responsibilities and concerns in administering IV therapy?

2. What is the purpose of IV therapy and what types of solutions are used?

3. What equipment is used in providing parenteral therapy?

4. How are IV rates accurately calculated?

5. What are the peripheral veins appropriate for use in IV therapy?

6. What are the factors that influence IV site and needle selection?

IV Site	Needle Selection

7. What is the technique for venipuncture, and what are the responsibilities of the LPN/LVN in monitoring an IV drip rate?

8. What are the complications associated with infusion therapy?

9. What is the procedure for administering blood products and what nursing measures prevent potential complications?

APPLY WHAT YOU LEARNED

One of the clients you are caring for puts on her call light to report that the IV pump alarm is sounding. She has a 22-gauge ONC (inserted 48 hours ago) attached to a primary line of D_5W 0.45% NS running at 125 mL per hour into a peripheral metacarpal vein on the dorsal surface of her right hand. The physician has written orders for the client to be up as tolerated.

1. Discuss the appropriateness of the selected gauge of the ONC.

2. Given the data provided in the case study, discuss the appropriateness of the chosen IV site.

3. Describe what you will look for when assessing the IV insertion site.

4. Identify those areas you will check when troubleshooting the source of the pump alarm.

MULTIPLE CHOICE QUESTIONS

Circle the answer that best completes each of the following statements.

1. The physician has ordered a potassium supplement to be given to a client receiving a daily diuretic. The order reads: KCL 20 mEq once daily PO. The nurse knows that this medication is expressed in millequivalents rather than milligrams because:
   A. Millequivalents measure the chemical activity of the positively charged ion (K^+) and a negatively charged ion (Cl^-).
   B. Millequivalents measure the weight of the potassium supplement KCL, making it easier to administer.
   C. Millequivalents ensure that the client receives an equal balance of cations and anions in any solution of KCL.
   D. Actually, the unit secretary made an error in transcription. The order should be written as: KCL 20 mg once daily PO.

2. A 90-year-old client admitted with a medical diagnosis of congestive heart failure (CHF) is experiencing shortness of breath, has a productive cough, and shows 3$^+$ pitting edema in both feet and ankles. Upon auscultation of her lungs, the nurse hears moist-sounding rales over all lung fields. The client has a peripheral IV running at 50 mL/hr. The nurse plans to monitor this client's IV closely since she is at risk for:
   A. Fluid Volume, Overload
   B. Fluid Volume, Deficient
   C. Fluid Volume, Imbalance
   D. Nutrition, Imbalanced

3. You are caring for a client who will be receiving blood. Though you will not be inserting the over-the-needle catheter (ONC), you tell the RN you will gather the needed supplies. When selecting the cannula, you decide on a(n):
   A. 24 gauge
   B. 22 gauge
   C. 18 gauge
   D. 14 gauge

4. When preparing to hang blood or blood products, the nurse must select an administration set that includes a(n):
   A. Burrette
   B. Inline filter
   C. Microdrip
   D. Rubber bung

5. The RN asks you to get a bag of IV solution to be used with a blood transfusion. Because you are in a hurry, you quickly select a bag of 0.45% sodium chloride. When you recheck the bag, you realize your mistake. You know that if this solution were to be hung with blood, the blood cells would:
   A. Hemolyze or burst
   B. Dilute and shrink
   C. Remain stable
   D. Adjust accordingly

6. A client at risk for respiratory alkalosis would most likely be asked to:
   A. Breathe slowly into a paper bag.
   B. Place her head between her legs.
   C. Drink additional fluids of her choice.
   D. Eat foods high in potassium and sodium.

7. After blood has been checked out of the blood bank, it should be initiated within:
   A. 2 hours
   B. 1 hour
   C. 30 minutes
   D. 20 minutes

8. According to INS standard, a peripheral short catheter should be removed every:
   A. 24 hours
   B. 36 hours
   C. 48 hours
   D. 72 hours

9. Which signs would the nurse expect to observe when assessing a client with possible dehydration and fluid and electrolyte imbalance?
   A. Weight gain; sunken eyes; cool extremities
   B. Weight loss; low BP; increased hematocrit
   C. Bounding pulse; dyspnea; low body temperature
   D. Puffy eyelids; low serum osmolarity; dry, cracked lips

10. You are working the day shift on an acute care medical unit. The night nurse reports that a client's IV pump malfunctioned and she received an additional 800 mL of IV solution. As you assess this client, you will observe for:
    A. Increased respiratory rate
    B. Decreased respiratory rate
    C. Low blood pressure
    D. Low body temperature

11. A client admitted with gastrointestinal bleeding has a nasogastric tube attached to intermittent low suction. The nurse knows it is important to monitor this client for signs and symptoms of:
    A. Respiratory acidosis
    B. Respiratory alkalosis
    C. Metabolic acidosis
    D. Metabolic alkalosis

12. A client who was admitted through the emergency department with diabetic ketoacidosis (DKA) would most likely be given which medication as treatment?
    A. Lidocaine HCL
    B. Theophylline bromide
    C. Sodium bicarbonate
    D. Potassium chloride

13. A 17-year-old female comes to the emergency department complaining of anxiety, lightheadedness, palpitations, chest tightness, and numbness and tingling of her hands and feet. Upon examination, her vital signs are: BP 180/90, T 99°F, P 130, R 38. This client is at risk for which acid–base imbalance?
    A. Respiratory acidosis
    B. Respiratory alkalosis
    C. Metabolic acidosis
    D. Metabolic alkalosis

14. The best place to insert an over-the-needle catheter (ONC) to begin IV therapy would be:
    A. Antecubital cephalic vein
    B. Digital veins
    C. Metacarpal veins
    D. Great saphenous vein

15. Which IV solution is considered isotonic?
    A. Lactated Ringer's
    B. D_5 W 0.45% NS
    C. 0.45% NS
    D. D_5% 0.9% NS

Chapter 29

Nursing Care of Clients Having Surgery

KEY TERMS

Match each of the following key terms to its proper definition.

_____ 1. Dehiscence

_____ 2. Atelectasis

_____ 3. Paralytic ileus

_____ 4. Embolus

_____ 5. Anesthesia

A. The collapse of a lobe or of an entire lung

B. Clots moved from their place of origin, causing circulatory obstruction elsewhere

C. The alteration in the level of sensation and consciousness

D. Intestinal obstruction characterized by lack of peristaltic activity

E. The partial or total rupturing of a sutured wound

_____ 6. Evisceration

_____ 7. Thrombophlebitis

_____ 8. Ablative

_____ 9. Sutures

_____ 10. Palliative

A. Threads used to sew body tissues together

B. Relieving or reducing pain or symptoms of a disease

C. Condition with inflammation and clot formation in a vein

D. Describing a procedure involving removal of a tissue or body part, or destruction of its function

E. The protrusion of the internal viscera through an incision

LEARNING OUTCOMES

1. What are the phases of the perioperative period?

2. What are the various types of surgery according to the purpose, degree of urgency, and degree of risk?

Purpose	Degree of Urgency	Degree of Risk

3. What are the types of wounds and their complications?

Types of Wounds	Complications

4. What are the tests that may occur and what are the overall nursing responsibilities in the perioperative period?

5. What is essential preoperative teaching?

6. What are the essential aspects of nursing care when preparing a client for surgery?

7. What are the types of anesthesia that may be used intraoperatively?

8. What is the nurse's role in the care of the postoperative client?

9. What are the potential postoperative problems? How can they be prevented?

10. What is the ongoing care of the surgical client, including suture and staple removal and discharge considerations?

11. In what ways can the LPNs/LVNs provide wound care and support healing?

APPLY WHAT YOU LEARNED

Together with the RN, you are conducting a preoperative assessment on a 76-year-old male scheduled to undergo a total replacement of the right knee. When asked how he feels about this surgery, he replies, "Well, I'm not looking forward to it. And actually, I'm pretty darn scared." The client indicates that he is in "pretty good shape" and denies having significant health problems. However, when you look at his old records from previous admissions, you find that he is diabetic and has a diagnosis of hypertension. When asked whether he adheres to a therapeutic diet, he states, "No, not since my wife died last year. I live alone and eat what I want. In fact, I usually go out to eat since I don't really know how to cook. I don't really know how to do any of the stuff my wife used to do. The house is too big and has lots of steps. I just can't keep up." He admits to smoking a pack of unfiltered cigarettes per day, and to drinking "several" alcoholic beverages every evening.

1. Discuss factors that will influence the client's degree of risk when having this surgery.

2. Which risk factors must the nurse consider when planning care for this client?

3. Identify all possible nursing problem areas that require a nursing diagnosis and care plan.

4. Identify at least three areas requiring client teaching prior to discharge.

MULTIPLE CHOICE QUESTIONS

Circle the answer that best completes each of the following statements.

1. Histamine-receptor antihistamines such as cimetidine (Tagamet) and ranitidine (Zantac) may be given preoperatively to:
   A. Reduce oral secretions
   B. Induce general calmness
   C. Reduce gastric fluid volume
   D. Reduce anxiety

2. A sequential compression device is used to:
   A. Promote venous return from the legs
   B. Aid in wound healing
   C. Secure abdominal dressings
   D. Prevent hemorrhage postoperatively

3. An approximated surgical incision is an example of which type of healing?
   A. Secondary intention
   B. Tertiary intention
   C. Primary intention
   D. Deliberate intention

4. You observe a bright, sanguineous exudate on the abdominal dressing of a postoperative client. This finding indicates:
   A. Fresh bleeding
   B. Older bleeding
   C. Hemorrhage
   D. Dehiscence

5. After surgery, infection will most likely become apparent within:
   A. 24 hours
   B. 2 to 4 hours
   C. 2 to 11 days
   D. 14 days

6. Wound healing requires a diet rich in protein, carbohydrates, lipids, minerals, and which vitamins?
   A. A and C
   B. D and E
   C. A and D
   D. C and E

7. Which of the following statements best explains why obese clients have an increased risk of wound infection?
   A. Adipose tissue usually has a minimal blood supply.
   B. Obesity reduces the number of available macrophages.
   C. Obese clients heal by secondary intention.
   D. Fibroblast activity is decreased with increased adipose tissue.

8. The nurse reviews the clients laboratory data and interprets a decreased leukocyte count as indicating:
   A. Prolonged Clotting Time
   B. The body's nutritional reserves
   C. Potential delay in healing with increased risk of infection
   D. The need for initiation of antibiotic therapy

9. Hydrocolloid dressings are frequently used over venous stasis leg and pressure ulcers. Which of the following is one advantage of using this type of dressing?
   A. It can be molded to uneven body surfaces.
   B. It contains wound odor.
   C. It is easy to remove.
   D. A and B.

10. Laboratory data often support the nurse's clinical assessment of the wound's progress in healing. A decreased leukocyte count:
    A. Indicates prolonged clot absorption.
    B. Provides an indication of the body's nutritional reserves.
    C. Can delay healing and increase the risk of infection.
    D. Identifies the sensitivity of specific antibiotic therapy.

11. Postoperative pain is usually greatest after:
    A. 12 to 36 hours
    B. 1 to 2 hours
    C. 6 to 8 hours
    D. 48 to 72 hours

12. Because general anesthetics and analgesics depress the action of both the cilia of the mucous membranes lining the respiratory tract and the respiratory center in the brain, the nurse must encourage the postoperative client to:
    A. Limit the amount of pain medication used.
    B. Drink large quantities of fluid.
    C. Cooperate with the physical and respiratory therapists.
    D. Do deep breathing and coughing exercises hourly.

Chapter 30

Clients with Integumentary System Disorders

KEY TERMS

Match each of the following key terms to its proper definition.

_____ 1. Alopecia

A. Superficial loss of tissue, usually with inflammation, on the surface of the skin or mucous membrane

_____ 2. Wheal

B. A circumscribed, slightly reddened, papule or irregular plaque of edema of the skin

_____ 3. Jaundice

C. A condition caused by excess bilirubin in the blood

_____ 4. Atrophy

D. Decrease in size

_____ 5. Petechiae

E. Absence of hair on the head and/or body

_____ 6. Ulcer

F. Condition of excessive hair growth

_____ 7. Hirsutism

G. Pinpoint hemorrhages

_____ 1. Cerumen

A. A deep furrow or slit extending into the dermis

_____ 2. Purpura

B. Ear wax

_____ 3. Fissure

C. Pus in the blood

_____ 4. Hematoma

D. Condition characterized by hemorrhaging into the skin

_____ 5. Pyemia

E. A small, circumscribed elevation of the skin containing purulent matter

_____ 6. Ecchymosis

F. Purplish patch caused by extravasation of blood into the skin

_____ 7. Pustule

G. Accumulation of blood in the soft tissue under the skin that may appear as a reddish-blue swelling

LEARNING OUTCOMES

1. What is the general structure and function of the integumentary system?

2. What terms are used to describe skin lesions?

3. What points are important to preventing skin breakdown and preventing the spread of infection?

Preventing Skin Breakdown	Preventing Spread of Infection

4. What are the symptoms, treatment, and nursing care for clients with infectious skin disorders?

Symptoms	Treatment	Nursing Care

5. What are the manifestations, treatment, and nursing care of clients with fungal skin disorders?

Manifestations	Treatment	Nursing Care

6. What are the different types of parasitic skin disorders, how are they treated, and what are the nursing considerations?

Types	Treatment	Considerations

7. How would the nurse care for the client with a chronic skin condition?

8. What information about skin cancer recognition and prevention would the nurse provide to a client?

9. What are the types of plastic or reconstructive surgery?

APPLY WHAT YOU LEARNED

You are giving a report to the nursing assistant who will be providing care for an elderly immobile client. You must provide her with instructions on care for this client. Before you begin, the nursing assistant says, "I know what to do. I'll turn her when I get to it, do a two-person transfer to the chair, try to feed her breakfast and lunch, order a doughnut for her to sit on when she is up, and massage those areas that look red." After listening to the nursing assistant, you realize that you must provide specific instructions and a rationale for each action, as well as an explanation for those statements on tasks that would be inappropriate or contraindicated for this client.

1. Maintaining skin integrity is critical. Identify specific tasks targeting prevention of the formation of pressure ulcers to be completed for this client.

2. Provide a rationale for each of the delegated tasks.

3. Review the nursing assistant's comments and provide an explanation for those statements on tasks that would be inappropriate for the client.

MULTIPLE CHOICE QUESTIONS

Circle the answer that best completes each of the following statements.

1. The skin, the largest organ of the body, protects the body and helps to maintain health. It is often called the:
   A. First line of defense against infection.
   B. Primary site of autonomic regulation.
   C. Area where most infection takes place.
   D. Site for manufacture of vitamin.

2. The epidermis replaces itself approximately every:
   A. Year
   B. Four weeks
   C. Six months
   D. Day

3. Which of the following substances helps to give skin its color?
   A. Bilirubin
   B. Melatonin
   C. Melanin
   D. Creatinine

4. The nurse is caring for a client who has experienced an allergic reaction with hives on the trunk and upper extremities that appear as round slightly reddened irregular edematous areas accompanied by intense itching. The nurse documents these hives as:
   A. Cysts
   B. Erosions
   C. Pustules
   D. Wheals

5. Which of the following factors contributes to skin breakdown?
   A. Excessive amounts of exercise
   B. Malnutrition
   C. Standing in one place for extended periods of time
   D. A diet in which the largest percentage is carbohydrates

6. You are caring for an elderly immobile client who is at risk for impaired skin integrity. The priority nursing care for this client is:
   A. Encourage the client to consume extra fluids.
   B. Encourage or assist with frequent position changes.
   C. Helping to place the client in a chair for the day.
   D. Encouraging a high protein diet.

7. The nurse, working in a pediatrician's office, admits a toddler with a ruptured vesicle covered with a honey colored crust that the mother says is easily removed but keeps reappearing. The nurse suspects the child has:
   A. Psoriasis
   B. Impetigo
   C. Furuncles
   D. Herpes zoste

8. Tinea unguium or onychomycosis would be commonly observed in or on the:
   A. Feet
   B. Head
   C. Groin
   D. Nails

9. Psoriasis can be best described as a(n):
   A. Chronic genetic inflammatory, noninfectious, noncontagious dermatosis.
   B. Disorder of the sebaceous glands often treated with Accutane.
   C. Infestation of the itch mite transferred by sexual or person-to-person contact.
   D. Lesion caused by the human papillomavirus transmitted by skin contact.

10. During the skin assessment, the nurse lightly pinches the skin and then releases it. The skin tents and does not rebound. The nurse suspects that the client is:
   A. Malnourished
   B. Hypertensive
   C. Edematous
   D. Dehydrated

Chapter 31

Clients with Musculoskeletal System Disorders

KEY TERMS

Match each of the following key terms to its proper definition.

_____ 1. Gangrene

_____ 2. Contractibility

_____ 3. Scoliosis

_____ 4. Elasticity

_____ 5. Strain

_____ 6. Fracture

_____ 7. Extensibility

_____ 8. Gout

_____ 9. Osteoporosis

_____ 10. Osteoarthritis

A. Caused by overuse and/or injury to the joint

B. Any disruption in the bone itself

C. Enables the muscle to lengthen or "extend" in response to a stimulus

D. Allows the muscle to receive a stimulus and act on that stimulus

E. An inflammatory disorder that causes uric acid crystals to form in a joint

F. Causes the shortening of the muscle in response to a stimulus

G. A nonflexible encasement of a fractured extremity

H. Method of providing a steady and continuous pull that maintains the fractured bone in good alignment

I. Occurs when a ligament is twisted in an unusual fashion

J. Causes the muscle to return to its normal shape and form after contracting or extending

_____	11.	Sprain	K.	Necrosis or tissue death
_____	12.	Excitability	L.	Occurs when the end of the bone is no longer articulated in the joint capsule
_____	13.	Cast	M.	Muscle that has been extended through more than the normal range of motion
_____	14.	Traction	N.	A lateral curve of the spine
_____	15.	Dislocation	O.	Occurs in older adults and is characterized by loss of bone mass

LEARNING OUTCOMES

1. List the primary functions of the musculoskeletal system.

2. List diagnostic tests for disorders of the musculoskeletal system.

3. List types of skeletal trauma, treatment, potential complications, and nursing care.

Skeletal Trauma	Treatment	Potential Complications	Nursing Care

4. Define osteoporosis and describe prevention, treatment, and nursing care for a client with osteoporosis.

Definition
Prevention
Treatment
Nursing Care

5. Identify disorders of bone tissue and describe proper nursing care for each.

6. Explain nursing care required by a client in a cast or traction.

Cast	Traction

7. List four inflammatory disorders of the musculoskeletal system and nursing care for each.

8. List the common nursing interventions for a client post joint replacement surgery.

9. Describe the care of clients with spinal disorders.

10. List the most common joint and muscle disorders and nursing interventions for each.

11. List advantages and disadvantages of heat and cold therapy for clients with musculoskeletal disorders.

Type of Therapy	Advantages	Disadvantages
Heat applications		
Cold applications		

12. Describe nursing care for clients with systemic lupus erythematosus or fibromyalgia.

APPLY WHAT YOU LEARNED

Joan Markum is a 72-year-old woman living in a custodial care facility. She visits the doctor's office for a follow-up visit. She has recently been diagnosed with osteoporosis, is stoop shouldered, and is participating in outpatient rehabilitation following a fractured right femur. On discharge following repair of the fracture she was prescribed alendronate (Fosamax), calcium, and vitamin D supplements. She reports feeling frightened of falling because she worries about breaking another bone.

1. What foods would you recommend Ms. Markum add to her diet in order to improve her calcium intake?

2. What foods could Ms. Markum add to her diet to increase her vitamin D intake?

3. What strategies would you suggest to Ms. Markum to help her reduce the risk of falling?

MULTIPLE CHOICE QUESTIONS

Circle the answer that best completes each of the following statements.

1. Which of the following is not a basic property of skeletal muscles?
   A. Elasticity
   B. Connectivity
   C. Excitability
   D. Extensibility

2. This test is performed to obtain fluid for diagnostic purposes and to remove excess fluid.
   A. Arthroscopy
   B. CT scan
   C. Arthrogram
   D. Arthrocentesis

3. A greenstick fracture can best be defined as:
   A. Incomplete break along the length of the bone.
   B. Usually occurring when the extremity is twisted as in a sports injury.
   C. A fracture that has not caused skin to be disrupted.
   D. Occurring when the ends of the fracture are forced into each other.

4. Which classification of medication is *not used* to treat clients diagnosed with osteoporosis?
   A. Bisphosphonates
   B. Polypeptide hormone
   C. Immune system modifiers
   D. Vitamin supplement

5. When providing proper care for a client in traction, the nurse should never:
   A. Provide diversionary activities for immobile clients.
   B. Clean pins placed in bone with hydrogen peroxide and Betadine.
   C. Make sure that the weights are hanging freely.
   D. Pick the weight up onto the bed in order to reposition the client in bed.

6. Which disease is caused by overuse and/or injury to the joint?
   A. Osteoarthritis
   B. Rheumatoid arthritis
   C. Osteomyelitis
   D. Osteomalacia

7. While providing care for clients with total hip replacement, teach client not to flex hip more than _____ degrees, as to not dislocate the hip prosthesis.
   A. 60
   B. 100
   C. 90
   D. 45

8. A client with a herniated disk has had a lumbar laminectomy. When providing care, the LPN/LVN notices the presence of drainage on the dressing with a halo sign. Which of the following tests should be performed on the drainage to determine if CSF is present?
   A. Erythrocyte sedimentation rate (ESR)
   B. Glucose
   C. Phosphorus
   D. Alkaline phosphatase (ALP)

9. A client presents with numbness and tingling of the index finger, thumb, and middle finger. The pain may disrupt the client's sleep. Which joint or muscle disorder would you suspect the client of having?
   A. Temporomandibular joint disorder
   B. Strains
   C. Lyme disease
   D. Carpal tunnel syndrome

10. Which of the following statements is an advantage of cold application therapy?
    A. Increases suppuration
    B. Limits postinjury swelling and bleeding
    C. Causes vasoconstriction
    D. Promotes soft tissue healing

Chapter 32

Clients with Respiratory System Disorders

KEY TERMS

Create a word search puzzle with the key terms and provide definitions as clues:

1.	A pulmonary condition characterized by overinflation and destruction of the alveolar walls	A.	Hemothorax
2.	A surgical incision in the trachea just below the larynx through which a tracheostomy tube is inserted	B.	COPD
3.	An accumulation of air or gas in the pleural space that causes partial or complete collapse of the lung on the affected side	C.	Emphysema
4.	The collapse of a lobe or of an entire lung	D.	Hypoxia
5.	An accumulation of blood in the pleural space that causes partial or complete collapse of the lung on the affected side	E.	Atelectasis
6.	A lung disorder characterized by airway obstruction caused by chronic bronchitis or emphysema	F.	Tracheostomy
7.	Condition of insufficient oxygen anywhere in the body	G.	Pneumothorax

8.	Inward movement of the tissues over the chest	A.	Asthmaticus
9.	Breathing	B.	Hypercapnia
10.	The inflammation of one or more bronchi.	C.	Mesothelioma

11. A rare tumor of the pleura or peritoneum membranes that may develop as a result of asbestos exposure

    D. Ventilation

12. A severe, prolonged asthma attack that is unresponsive to treatment is known as status _____

    E. Retractions

13. Condition caused by long-term lack of oxygen

    F. Bronchitis

14. Excess of carbon dioxide in the blood

    G. Clubbing

LEARNING OUTCOMES

1. What is the structure and function of the respiratory system?

2. What are the processes of breathing and gas exchange?

3. What factors influence respiratory function and oxygenation?

4. What are the three major alterations in respiratory function and their manifestations?

5. What are the common tests performed to diagnose respiratory disorders?

6. What therapeutic measures are used to promote respiratory function?

7. What are the measures used by the nurse to promote oxygenation?

8. What are the common disorders, manifestations, diagnostic measures, treatment, and nursing care for infections and inflammation of the upper respiratory system?

Disorders	Manifestations	Diagnostic Measures	Treatment	Nursing Care

9. What are the common disorders, manifestations, diagnostic measures, treatment, and nursing care for trauma, obstruction, and tumors of the upper respiratory system?

Disorders	Manifestations	Diagnostic Measures	Treatment	Nursing Care

10. What are the common disorders, manifestations, diagnostic measures, treatment, and nursing care for pulmonary embolism, pulmonary hypertension, chest trauma, inhalation injury, and near drowning of the lower respiratory system?

Disorders	Manifestations	Diagnostic Measures	Treatment	Nursing Care

11. What are the common disorders, manifestations, diagnostic measures, treatment, and nursing care for infections and inflammation of the lower respiratory system?

Disorders	Manifestations	Diagnostic Measures	Treatment	Nursing Care

12. What are the obstructive disorders of the lower respiratory system, including manifestations, diagnostic measures, treatment, and nursing care?

Disorders	Manifestations	Diagnostic Measures	Treatment	Nursing Care

13. What are the manifestations, diagnostic measures, treatment, and nursing care for clients with lung cancer and interstitial disorders?

Disorders	Manifestations	Diagnostic Measures	Treatment	Nursing Care

A client has been diagnosed with tuberculosis (TB). He has been living in homeless shelters for the past year and also has diabetes mellitus and hypertension. He tells you he has lost about 35 pounds in the last three to four months, becomes easily fatigued, coughs up bloody sputum, and is having night sweats. You are the LPN/LVN working with the RN to provide care for this client. You begin your planning by answering the following questions.

1. Discuss the nature of TB, its prevalence, and risk factors.

2. Identify the clinical manifestations of secondary TB.

3. Explain the diagnostic tests used to determine the presence of TB.

4. Discuss the nurse's responsibilities when caring for a client with TB.

5. Identify four common nursing diagnoses for clients with lower respiratory disorders such as TB.

6. Identify one outcome for your client.

7. Identify pertinent nursing actions/interventions for this client.

MULTIPLE CHOICE QUESTIONS

Circle the answer that best completes each of the following statements.

1. The primary function of the respiratory system is to:
   A. Eliminate waste products.
   B. Protect the airway from infection.
   C. Maintain acid-base balance.
   D. Exchange gases.

2. The upper respiratory system includes the:
   A. Larynx
   B. Trachea
   C. Bronchi
   D. Alveoli

3. The pharynx is commonly known as the:
   A. Voice box
   B. Throat
   C. Esophagus
   D. Adam's apple

4. The respiratory centers that control breathing are found in the:
   A. Brainstem
   B. Cerebrum
   C. Lungs
   D. Limbic system

5. The movement of gases or other particles from an area of greater pressure or concentration to an area of lower pressure or concentration is known as:
   A. Inhalation
   B. Expiration
   C. Diffusion
   D. Perfusion

6. The amount of blood pumped by the heart, also known as *cardiac output*, is approximately _____ liters per minute.
   A. 2
   B. 3
   C. 4
   D. 5

7. When the carbon dioxide or hydrogen ion concentration increases, the brain:
   A. Decreases the rate and depth of respirations.
   B. Increases the rate and depth of respirations.
   C. Increases the cardiac output to 7 liters per minute.
   D. Decreases the pulse rate to approximately 60 beats per minute.

8. The stimulus for respiration in clients with emphysema or chronic obstructive pulmonary disease is:
   A. Decreased oxygen concentration
   B. Increased oxygen concentration
   C. Hypercapnia
   D. Hypercarbia

9. Which of the following classes of medications would cause a decreased rate and depth of respirations?
   A. Anticonvulsants
   B. Narcotics/barbiturates
   C. Antihypertensives
   D. Bronchodilators

10. A client with a high fever, metabolic acidosis, pain, or hypoxemia would experience:
   A. Tachypnea
   B. Bradypnea
   C. Eupnea
   D. Apnea

11. A pulse oximeter is a noninvasive device that measures:
   A. Oxygen saturation
   B. Hypercapnia
   C. Carbon monoxide levels
   D. Expiratory tidal volume

12. Which of the following statements about oxygen is true?
   A. Oxygen is extremely flammable and will burn easily.
   B. Oxygen by itself will not burn or explode, but it facilitates combustion and burning.
   C. Low concentrations of oxygen will rapidly start fires, making them difficult to extinguish.
   D. Oxygen is stored in cylinders as a liquid under pressure and is released as a gas.

13. Which of the following items is kept at the bedside of a client with a tracheostomy in case the tube becomes dislodged and needs to be reinserted?
   A. A hemostat
   B. An obturator
   C. A suction kit
   D. An outer cannula

14. Which of the following breathing exercises will help the client develop control over breathing by creating resistance to the air flowing out of the lungs, prolonging exhalation and preventing airway collapse by maintaining positive airway pressure?
   A. Abdominal breathing
   B. Diaphragmatic breathing
   C. Pursed-lip breathing
   D. Saying "eeeeeeee" between breaths

15. When suctioning a client using the nasopharyngeal route, it is recommended that you apply suction:
   A. For 5 to 10 seconds while slowly withdrawing the catheter.
   B. For 5 to 10 seconds while inserting the catheter.
   C. For 1 minute while slowly withdrawing the catheter.
   D. For 30 seconds while inserting the catheter.

Chapter 33

Clients with Cardiovascular System Disorders

KEY TERMS

Match each of the following key terms to its proper definition.

_____ 1. Pericarditis

A. Chest pain caused by reduced oxygen supply to the heart

_____ 2. Dysrhythmias

B. Open sores that appear on the lower legs due to poor circulation to the legs

_____ 3. Valvular insufficiency

C. A symptom of ischemia that causes cramping pains and weakness in the calves of the legs while walking

_____ 4. Venous stasis ulcers

D. Pulse with an irregular rhythm

_____ 5. Angina pectoris

E. Failure of the valves to close completely, forcing blood back into the previous chamber when the heart contracts

_____ 6. Intermittent claudication

F. An inflammation, acute or chronic, of the sac that encloses and protects the heart

---

_____ 7. Ischemia

A. A buildup of fatty plaque on the inside of the arteries that causes narrowing of the lumen to the point of blockage

_____ 8. Arteriosclerosis

B. Condition in which the blood pressure elevates rapidly and progressively until the diastolic pressure is greater than 120 mm Hg

_____ 9. Congestive heart failure

C. A deficiency in the blood supply to the tissue

_____ 10. Pericardiocentesis

D. Condition in which the elastic and muscular tissues of the arteries are replaced with fibrous tissue

_____ 11. Malignant hypertension

E. Inability of the heart to function effectively as a pump

_____ 12. Atherosclerosis

F. Surgical drainage of the pericardium

_____ 13. Stroke volume

A. Percentage of blood in the ventricle

_____ 14. Cardiac cycle

B. A regular heartbeat that originates in the sinoatrial node, or pacemaker, of the heart

_____ 15. Ejection fraction

C. Contraction and relaxation of the heart

_____ 16. Sinus rhythm

D. A device used to restore an effective heart rate when the heart's natural pacemakers fail

_____ 17. Cardiac output

E. Amount of blood ejected from the heart in one contraction

_____ 18. Pacemaker

F. The amount of blood pumped by the ventricles in 1 minute

_____ 19. Inotropics

A. Swollen, knotted, and tortuous veins with poorly functioning valves

_____ 20. Telemetry

B. A noninvasive therapy that attempts to restore the heart's natural pacemaker, the sinoatrial node

_____ 21. Aneurysm

C. A life-threatening complication of left-sided congestive heart failure

_____ 22. Cardioversion

D. Remote monitoring

_____ 23. Varicose veins

E. Drugs that increase the force of contraction of the heart

_____ 24. Pulmonary edema

F. A weakening and dilation in the wall of a blood vessel

_____ 25. Myocarditis

A. A condition of abnormally high blood pressure in the arterial system

_____ 26. Cardiomyopathy

B. Conditions of the arteries, veins, and lymph vessels outside the heart

_____ 27. Primary hypertension

C. The inflammation of the valves and lining of the heart

_____ 28. Myocardial infarction   D.   Elevated blood pressure due to another medical diagnosis

_____ 29. Peripheral vascular disease   E.   A group of diseases that affect the heart muscle

_____ 30. Secondary hypertension   F.   Condition that occurs when blood flow through one of the coronary arteries is completely blocked

_____ 31. Endocarditis   G.   The inflammation of the heart muscle

LEARNING OUTCOMES

1. What are the structures and function of the cardiovascular system?

2. What are the factors that affect cardiovascular system function?

3. What are the tests for cardiovascular disorders?

4. What are the major heart disorders, and what is the nursing care for them?

5. What are the normal and the abnormal heart sounds?

6. What are the disorders that affect the heart and lungs, and what is the nursing care for them?

7. What are the valvular and inflammatory heart disorders, and what is the nursing care of them?

8. What are the conduction disorders, and what is the nursing care of them?

9. What are the disorders affecting the central circulation, and what are the nursing interventions for them?

10. What are the disorders affecting peripheral circulation, and what is the nursing care of them?

APPLY WHAT YOU LEARNED

You are working in a long-term care facility, and one of the clients is in congestive heart failure (CHF). You know there are many nursing considerations when providing care for this client. Begin planning by answering the following questions to increase your understanding of CHF.

1. Define CHF.

2. Discuss factors that impact the client's recovery.

3. Describe the target of treatment.

4. Identify three aspects of treatment.

5. Identify three common diuretics used to treat CHF.

6. Identify two common drugs that slow and strengthen the heart rate.

7. Identify three common nursing diagnoses for clients with CHF.

8. Identify nursing interventions for a client with CHF and provide a rationale for each.

MULTIPLE CHOICE QUESTIONS

Circle the answer that best completes each of the following statements.

1. The upper chambers of the heart are known as the:
   A. Right and left ventricles
   B. Right and left atria
   C. Tricuspid valves
   D. Semilunar valves

2. Which of the following best describes what happens when the ventricle contracts?
   A. Deoxygenated blood passes through the pulmonary valve into the large pulmonary artery, taking the blood to the lungs for oxygenation.
   B. The blood travels through the heart and enters the right atrium from the vena cava.
   C. The electrical stimulus passes through internodal pathways in the atria to the atrioventricular node located near the junction of the atria and ventricles.
   D. The initial electrical stimulation starts the heartbeat, passes through the septum, and stimulates the bundle of His.

3. Cardiac output is determined by four major factors: heart rate, preload, afterload, and contractility. Which of the following best defines *afterload*?
   A. When the heart rate increases, it causes increased cardiac output.
   B. The amount of blood in the ventricles before contraction.
   C. The force required for the ventricles to push blood out of the heart and into the circulation.
   D. The natural ability of the cardiac muscle fibers to shorten during contraction.

4. The aorta is the major artery of the body and carries oxygen:
   A. Toward the heart
   B. Away from the heart
   C. To the lungs
   D. Toward the atria

5. Which of the following procedures would be done to visualize the coronary arteries, atria, ventricles, and valves?
   A. An echocardiogram
   B. A thallium scan
   C. An electrocardiogram
   D. A cardiac catheterization

6. A myocardial infarction occurs when blood flow through one of the coronary arteries is completely blocked, causing:
   A. Ischemia and necrosis
   B. Cor pulmonale
   C. Pulmonary edema
   D. Valvular insufficiency

7. When there is an acute or chronic inflammation of the sac that encloses and protects the heart, the client is said to have:
   A. Pericarditis
   B. Myocarditis
   C. Endocarditis
   D. Cardiomyopathy

8. A surgical separation of valve leaflets of the heart is known as:
   A. Cardioversion
   B. Intracoronary streptokinase therapy
   C. Coronary artery bypass grafting
   D. Commissurotomy

9. Sinus bradycardia is the name for a regular heart rhythm rate:
   A. Above 100 beats per minute
   B. Below 60 beats per minute
   C. Between 60 and 100 beats per minute
   D. At 80 beats per minute

10. Which of the following terms is used to describe a blood pressure that elevates rapidly and progressively until the diastolic pressure is greater than 120 mm Hg?
    A. Orthostatic hypertension
    B. Secondary hypertension
    C. Primary hypertension
    D. Malignant hypertension

11. Aneurysms are classified by their location and shape. The most common locations are the thoracic or the abdominal aorta. One of the three common shapes is *fusiform*, which can be best described as an aneurysm where:
    A. The walls of the artery dilate about equally, causing a tubular pouching.
    B. One side of the wall of the artery pouches out.
    C. The lining of the artery pulls away from the pouch itself, allowing blood to flow between the artery layers.
    D. The pressure within the wall is too great, causing retraction of the wall.

12. Signs and symptoms of emboli include:
    A. Sudden pain in an affected area.
    B. Tingling of the extremity.
    C. Absent pulses distal to the blockage.
    D. All of the above.

13. Which of the following nursing actions would be most appropriate when working with a client with a thrombus or embolus?
    A. Teach the client how and when to monitor blood pressure.
    B. Instruct the client to avoid crossing the legs.
    C. Assess the skin for intactness, ulcerations, or breakdown.
    D. Provide gentle massage and range-of-motion exercises.

14. The circulatory system includes the
    A. Heart
    B. Lungs
    C. Blood vessels
    D. All of the above

15. The three biggest risk factors for cardiovascular disease are:
    A. Smoking, high blood pressure, high blood cholesterol.
    B. Gender, high blood pressure, heredity.
    C. High-fat diet, sedentary lifestyle, alcohol consumption.
    D. Smoking, gender, heredity.

Chapter 34

Clients with Hematologic and Lymphatic System Disorders

KEY TERMS

Match each of the following key terms to its proper definition.

_____ 1. Sickle cell trait

_____ 2. Sickle cell crisis

_____ 3. Graft versus host disease

_____ 4. Sickle cell anemia

_____ 5. Agranulocytosis

_____ 6. Sickle cell disease

A. An inherited defect in the formation of hemoglobin

B. The absence of any white blood cells

C. An inherited disorder that distorts red blood cells, causing chronic anemia

D. Acutely painful condition that occurs when sickled red blood cells become lodged in capillaries, occluding blood flow to the affected area

E. Sickle hemoglobin, a factor that, if inherited from both parents, results in sickle cell anemia

F. A very serious complication of a bone marrow transplant where the client's own body attacks itself

_____ 7. Lymphedema

A. Occurs when the donor's red cells rupture or hemolyze and release their hemoglobin, with dangerous or even lethal results

_____ 8. Anemia

B. Inflammation of a lymphatic vessel

_____ 9. Transfusion reaction

C. Enlargement of lymph nodes

_____ 10. Lymphangitis

D. The inability of the lymph system to remove all the lymph fluid from the interstitial tissues

_____ 11. Thrombocytopenia

E. A deficiency of red blood cells or hemoglobin caused by decreased production or increased destruction of red blood cells, or by blood loss

_____ 12. Lymphadenopathy

F. A decrease in the platelet count to lower than 100,000/mL of blood

LEARNING OUTCOMES

1. What is the structure and function of blood and of lymph?

	Structure	Function
Blood		
Lymph		

2. What are the common diagnostic tests for hematologic or lymphocytic disorders?

3. What are the compatible cross-matches for different types of blood donors and recipients?

4. What are the different types of anemia, and what are the treatment and nursing care for each?

Types of Anemia	Treatment	Nursing Care

5. What are the platelet and coagulation disorders, and what are the nursing interventions for them?

6. What are the white blood cell disorders, and what is the treatment for them?

7. What are the four types of lymphatic disorders, and what is the description of each?

8. What are the nursing considerations for clients with lymphatic disorders?

APPLY WHAT YOU LEARNED

A 17-year-old African American client is admitted to the hospital with a diagnosis of sickle cell crisis. The client is experiencing severe pain and shortness of breath. You are working with the RN to assess and plan for this client. The RN suggests that you begin by answering the following questions.

1. Discuss the cause of sickle cell anemia.

2. Provide a rationale for the client's pain and shortness of breath.

3. Identify the two highest-priority nursing diagnoses for the client.

4. Identify one expected outcome based on the above nursing diagnoses.

5. Discuss cultural considerations for this client's care.

MULTIPLE CHOICE QUESTIONS

Circle the answer that best completes each of the following statements.

1. Which of the following elements is required for the formation of hemoglobin?
   A. Potassium
   B. Sodium
   C. Iron
   D. Magnesium

2. The function of monocytes in the body is to:
   A. Transport hemoglobin
   B. Respond to inflammation
   C. Respond to the presence of foreign material.
   D. Promote a healthy immune system

3. Platelets in the blood are necessary for:
   A. Proper blood coagulation
   B. Response to allergic reactions
   C. Transportation of oxygen
   D. Destruction of red blood cells

4. Abnormal levels of any of the types of white blood cells may indicate which of the following?
   A. Anemia.
   B. Leukemia
   C. Sickle cell anemia
   D. Polycythemia

5. Disseminated intravascular coagulation is an acute condition that causes:
   A. Increased peripheral resistance
   B. Disruptions in clotting
   C. Impaired stem cell production
   D. High risk of infection

6. Polycythemia is a disorder in which:
   A. The number of red blood cells is significantly less than normal.
   B. The white blood cell level is elevated, causing fever.
   C. The number of red blood cells is much greater than normal.
   D. The red blood cells assume a sickle shape when put under stress.

7. A client is being treated for leukemia. She is currently undergoing intensive and aggressive chemotherapy to destroy all of the leukemic cells and, as a result, is experiencing bone marrow suppression. This client is in which stage of treatment?
   A. Stage I—Induction
   B. Stage II—Consolidation
   C. Stage III—Maintenance
   D. Stage IV—Ongoing

8. Lymph nodes become enlarged due to:
   A. Inflammation
   B. Infection
   C. Malignancy
   D. All of the above

9. A client shows the nurse a painful red streak running up his arm. He says he has had a fever for the past several days. From the subjective and objective data given by the client, the nurse can conclude that the client is experiencing:
   A. Lymphedema
   B. Lymphoma
   C. Lymphangitis
   D. Lymphadenopathy

10. As multiple myeloma progresses and the tumor grows, the bones become very brittle. The client is at risk for which electrolyte imbalance?
    A. Hypocalcemia
    B. Hypercalcemia
    C. Hypernatremia
    D. Hyperkalemia

11. Which of the following nursing diagnoses would be most appropriate for a client with a disorder of the hematopoietic or lymphatic systems?
    A. Risk for infection
    B. Risk for injury
    C. Fatigue
    D. All of the above

12. Nursing interventions for clients with hematopoietic and lymphatic disorders center on the client's level of:
    A. Fatigue
    B. Pain
    C. Consciousness
    D. Alertness

13. A client with agranulocytosis would be placed in:
    A. Protective isolation
    B. Strict isolation
    C. A negative pressure room
    D. Droplet isolation

14. The *most* important nursing action when caring for a client with a low white blood cell count is to:
    A. Be meticulous with hand washing
    B. Gown, glove, and wear a mask
    C. Turn the client often
    D. Check the skin frequently

15. Indicators of a hemolytic reaction to a blood transfusion would include:
    A. Itching, hives, fatigue
    B. Hypertension, vomiting, abdominal pain
    C. Diplopia, dysuria, polydipsia
    D. Headache, nausea, flushing, chest pain

Chapter 35

Caring for Clients with Immune System Disorders

KEY TERMS

Match each of the following key terms to its proper definition.

_____ 1. Raynaud's phenomenon

    A. A toxin that has been treated so that its toxic property is destroyed but its ability to stimulate production of antibodies remains

_____ 2. HIV

    B. Living and replicating within the host

_____ 3. Seroconversion

    C. The final stage of disease caused by the human immunodeficiency virus

_____ 4. Vaccines

    D. Results in the hands or feet turning white and cold, and then turning blue

_____ 5. AIDS

    E. Medications that cause a person to develop active immunity against a specific organism

_____ 6. Toxoid

    F. A virus that damages and destroys cells of the body's immune system

_____ 7. Retrovirus

    G. Detectable levels of antibodies against the virus in the blood

_____ 8. Autograft

    A. The abnormal growth of connective tissue that supports the skin and internal organs

_____ 9. Seropositive

    B. A lack of protection

_____ 10. Anaphylaxis

    C. The transplant of the client's own tissue

_____ 11.	Isograft	D.	A process that determines the ability of the cells to be compatible and lessens the risk of rejection
_____ 12.	Scleroderma	E.	Tissue and organ transplants that are from the same species
_____ 13.	Tissue typing	F.	Identical twin
_____ 14.	Allograft	G.	A person's blood contains antibodies for HIV

LEARNING OUTCOMES

1. What are the components of the immune system, and what are functions?

2. What is the relationship between antigens and antibodies?

3. What differentiates between active immunity and passive immunity?

4. What are the factors that affect immunity, and what tests are used to determine the status of the immune system?

5. What are the different types of immunizations, and what are the nursing considerations when providing them?

Types	Nursing Considerations

6. What is anaphylaxis, how is it treated, and what is the nursing care for a client with anaphylaxis?

Definition	Treatment	Nursing Care

7. Describe what the care of clients with HIV/AIDS would be?

8. What are the important aspects of care for clients with organ transplants?

9. Describe what the care of clients with autoimmune disorders would be?

10. What are the manifestations of the four levels of hypersensitivity reaction and what would be the treatment and nursing considerations for clients with allergies?

Level	Treatment	Nursing Considerations

APPLY WHAT YOU LEARNED

You are working with another staff nurse on the P.M. shift and during the report period, this nurse, who is assigned to care for a client with HIV, says, "That patient with AIDS did that to himself. Those people need to just stop having anal sex with one another. They deserve what they get when they engage in such immoral behavior." At first you cringe at what you hear, but then realize you must respond to her statement.

1. Discuss the prevalence of HIV/AIDS in the world and the United States.

2. Describe the modes of transmission for HIV.

3. Identify one psychosocial nursing diagnosis appropriate for a client with HIV/AIDS.

4. Discuss the nurse's role in prevention of and education about HIV/AIDS.

5. Construct an appropriate statement to your coworker that would help her understand the epidemic of HIV/AIDS.

MULTIPLE CHOICE QUESTIONS

Circle the answer that best completes each of the following statements.

1. A vaccination stimulates antibodies and memory cells and conveys:
   A. Natural active immunity
   B. Artificial active immunity
   C. Natural acquired immunity
   D. Acquired passive immunity

2. After receiving a purified protein derivative (PPD), the client returns to the clinic 48 hours later and the nurse tells him that she needs to assess the injection site for redness and induration. The client asks, "What does induration mean?" The nurse's best response would be:
   A. "The site would be hardened and raised."
   B. "If you are positive, you'd have a fluid-filled pustule."
   C. "Induration looks like pinkish-blue macules."
   D. "Induration indicates that a cell-mediated response has taken place."

3. For a client undergoing an acute transplant rejection, which of the following lab test results would be elevated?
   A. BUN
   B. Creatinine
   C. Liver and cardiac enzymes
   D. All of the above

4. The nurse taking care of a client who has had transplant surgery must:
   A. Assess the incision site for signs of inflammation.
   B. Maintain hand washing and aseptic technique during delivery of care.
   C. Continue to observe for side effects of medications.
   D. All of the above.

5. Client teaching needed to ensure the effectiveness of latex condoms must include which of the following?
   A. Condoms can safely be stored in a wallet or glove compartment of a car.
   B. Excessive heat and cold can destroy the effectiveness of the condom.
   C. If needed, an oil-based lubricant should be used.
   D. Condoms can be used beyond the expiration date on the package.

6. As the immune system is disrupted by HIV, a client would be prone to develop which of the following opportunistic diseases?
   A. Myasthenia gravis
   B. Systemic lupus erythematosus
   C. *Pneumocystis carinii* pneumonia
   D. Seroconversion

7. A client with HIV says, "The doctor told me that HIV is caused by a retrovirus. I don't know what that means." The nurse's best response would be:
   A. "A retrovirus lives and replicates within the host."
   B. "Replication of the virus takes place outside of the host."
   C. "The virus causes a high level of CD4 or an elevated T-cell count."
   D. "The virus's cell pattern copies DNA into RNA."

8. When caring for a client with AIDS, the nurse must follow standard precautions and use good hand washing techniques before and after care. Which of the following statements provides the *best* rationale for these nursing actions?
   A. A primary risk is infection with an opportunistic disease, and hand washing protects against nosocomial infections.
   B. Early detection of signs of infection helps the physician institute treatment as soon as possible.
   C. The client's body recognizes normal cells, perceives them as foreign, and initiates an immune response, targeting normal cells to be destroyed.
   D. Treatment is focused on controlling the disease, in which familial, environmental, and hormonal factors may play a role.

9. When caring for a client with systemic lupus erythematosus, the nurse would expect which of the following signs and symptoms on assessment?
   A. Pinkish-blue macules that develop into reddish-purple or dark reddish-brown, painful lesions on the body
   B. Watery diarrhea, abdominal cramping, and fever
   C. Ptosis, slurred speech, and shortness of breath
   D. A butterfly-shaped facial rash across the bridge of the nose and cheeks

10. During the initial assessment and data collection, the client tells you that she has been experiencing arthritic pain, fatigue, and pitting edema. She goes on to explain, "When I go out in the cold or get really anxious, my hands and feet turn white and cold and then get blue. When the blueness disappears, my fingertips get quite red." These signs and symptoms would be consistent with which of the following immune system disorders?
    A. Myasthenia gravis
    B. Progressive systemic sclerosis
    C. Systemic lupus erythematosus
    D. Kaposi's sarcoma

11. The highest priority nursing diagnosis for a client who has had organ transplant surgery would be:
    A. Risk for infection
    B. Disturbed body image
    C. Ineffective coping
    D. Impaired gas exchange

12. Following transplant surgery, the client begins to develop antibodies resulting in narrowing of the vessel lumen and diminished blood flow to the transplant; the organ loses functional ability and fails. This client is experiencing which type of rejection?
    A. Hyperactive
    B. Acute
    C. Chronic
    D. Graft-versus-host

13. Which of the following immunosuppressive medications would the nurse expect to administer to a transplant client?
    A. Solu-Medrol
    B. Cyclosporin
    C. Imuran
    D. Celebrex

14. An autoimmune disorder can best be described as one in which:
    A. The body is unable to recognize normal cells and perceives them as foreign.
    B. Autoantibodies attack the body, causing inflammation and damage to the cells, tissues, and organs.
    C. The disorder is more prevalent in females and prevalence increases with age.
    D. All of the above.

15. When assisting the RN in providing teaching and support for the client with an autoimmune disorder, it is important to:
    A. Instruct the client to take over-the-counter medication as needed.
    B. Discourage verbalization of anxiety and past coping strategies used.
    C. Focus on instruction concerning stress reduction, nutrition, and medication.
    D. Encourage the client to keep busy as a way to refocus pain and discomfort.

Chapter 36

Clients with Neurosensory System Disorders

PEARSON
EXPLORE **mynursingkit**™

MyNursingKit is your one stop for online chapter review materials and resources. Prepare for success with additional NCLEX®-style practice questions, interactive assignments and activities, web links, animations and videos, and more!

Register your access code from the front of your book at
www.mynursingkit.com

KEY TERMS

Match each of the following key terms to its proper definition.

_____ 1. Spinal shock

A. Most often seen in mid- or later stages of dementia

_____ 2. Transient ischemic attack

B. Numbness, burning, prickling, tingling, pain

_____ 3. Neuropathy

C. Acute dizziness and lack of balance

_____ 4. Sundowning

D. Temporary loss of reflex activity below the level of spinal cord injury

_____ 5. Vertigo

E. Any disease of the nerves

_____ 6. Paresthesia

F. A temporary loss of blood supply to an area of the brain

_____ 7. Intracranial pressure

A. Sudden, explosive, disorderly discharge of cerebral neurons characterized by an abrupt, transient alteration in brain function

_____ 8. Photophobia

B. Involuntary movement of the eyes

_____ 9. Meningitis

C. The abnormal accumulation of fluid or water in the intracellular space, extracellular space, or both

_____ 10. Seizure

D. The pressure normally exerted by the cerebrospinal fluid that circulates around the brain and spinal cord and within the cerebral ventricles

_____ 11.	Cerebral edema	E.	Sensitivity to light
_____ 12.	Nystagmus	F.	An inflammation of the meninges of the brain and spinal cord

_____ 13.	Chorea	A.	Ringing in the ears
_____ 14.	Tic douloureux	B.	Involuntary, spasmodic movements of the limbs and face
_____ 15.	Aura	C.	Extreme pain in the area of the maxillary and/or mandibular division of the trigeminal sensory root
_____ 16.	Trigeminal neuralgia	D.	A single seizure that lasts more than 30 minutes
_____ 17.	Status epilepticus	E.	A transient neurologic event lasting 5 to 30 minutes and consisting of a visual disturbance
_____ 18.	Tinnitus	F.	Trigeminal neuralgia

_____ 19.	Encephalitis	A.	An exaggerated sympathetic response in spinal cord injuries at or above the T6 level
_____ 20.	Partial seizure	B.	Jerky, alternately contracting and relaxing
_____ 21.	Hemiplegia	C.	A general term for the primary condition that causes seizures
_____ 22.	Autonomic dysreflexia	D.	Event that begins with focal or local discharges in one part of the brain, unilaterally
_____ 23.	Tonic-clonic	E.	An inflammation of the gray and white matter of the brain and the spinal cord
_____ 24.	Epilepsy	F.	Involve neurons bilaterally
_____ 25.	Generalized seizures	G.	Paralysis of one-half of the body when it is divided along the median sagittal plane

_____ 26.	Deceleration	A.	The progressive loss of cognitive and intellectual functions without impairment of perception or consciousness
_____ 27.	Cerebrovascular accident	B.	An infection that has extended into the cerebral tissue
_____ 28.	Contrecoup	C.	Injury that occurs when the head hits an immovable object
_____ 29.	Coma	D.	A focal cerebral injury directly under the area of impact
_____ 30.	Dementia	E.	A sudden, nonconvulsive focal neurologic deficit
_____ 31.	Brain abscess	F.	A cerebral injury that occurs opposite the point of impact
_____ 32.	Coup	G.	A prolonged or irreversible period of unconsciousness

202 Chapter 36

© 2010 Pearson Education, Inc.

LEARNING OUTCOMES

1. What are the structures and functions of the central and peripheral nervous systems?

Nervous System	Structure	Function
Central		
Peripheral		

2. What are the common tests and procedures for diagnosis and treatment of client with neurosensory disorders?

	Tests	Procedures
Diagnosis		
Treatment		

3. What considerations are important in the collection of data about neurosensory disorders?

4. What considerations are important in nursing care of the client with neurosensory disorders?

5. What are the signs and symptoms of increased intracranial pressure?

6. What are the nursing interventions for clients with increased intracranial pressure?

7. What are the common types of cerebrovascular disorders, and what is the nursing care for them?

8. What are the different types of seizures, and what is the nursing care for a client with seizures?

9. What are the infections of the nervous system, and what is the nursing care for them?

10. What injuries are common to the nervous system, and what are their treatments and nursing care?

Injury	Treatment	Nursing Care

11. What are the different types of tumors, and what are the treatments and the nursing care for them?

Types	Treatment	Nursing Care

12. What are four degenerative neurological diseases, and what is the nursing care for them?

13. What are the manifestations and nursing care for peripheral and cranial nerve disorders?

Nerve Disorder	Manifestations	Nursing Care
Peripheral		
Cranial		

14. What are the common visual and hearing disorders, and what are their treatments?

Disorders	Treatments
Visual	
Hearing	

APPLY WHAT YOU LEARNED

You are caring for a 20-year-old college student admitted to the medical unit with probable bacterial meningitis. To plan effectively for this client, you must understand the nature of bacterial meningitis, its etiology, signs and symptoms, treatment options, and nursing considerations. You begin by answering the following questions.

1. Define bacterial meningitis.

2. Identify the major organisms that are known to cause bacterial meningitis.

3. Identify the primary signs and symptoms of bacterial meningitis.

4. Discuss treatment options.

5. Identify primary nursing considerations for a client with bacterial meningitis or other infections of the neurologic system.

MULTIPLE CHOICE QUESTIONS

Circle the answer that best completes each of the following statements.

1. A rapidly progressing, degenerative disease of the upper and lower motor neurons resulting in progressive muscle weakness that leads to respiratory failure and death 2 to 5 years after onset of symptoms is known as:
   A. Parkinson's disease
   B. Multiple sclerosis
   C. Amyotrophic lateral sclerosis
   D. Myasthenia gravis

2. A client with a chronic autoimmune disease that affects the transmission of nerve impulses to muscles, resulting in alterations in mobility and facial expression, would most likely have a medical diagnosis of:
   A. Parkinson's disease
   B. Guillain-Barré syndrome
   C. Huntington's chorea
   D. Myasthenia gravis

3. When caring for a client with trigeminal neuralgia, the nurse's *primary* focus is:
   A. Pain management
   B. Fluid and electrolyte balance
   C. Safety
   D. Nutrition

4. During a recurrent attack of rotational or whirling vertigo caused by Meniere's disease, which activity level would be most therapeutic?
   A. Up ad lib
   B. Up as tolerated
   C. Bed rest
   D. Up with assistance

5. Which of the following disease processes is the most common cause of metabolic neuropathy?
   A. Diabetes mellitus
   B. Coronary artery disease
   C. Parkinson's disease
   D. Hypertension

6. Migraine headaches, though not life-threatening, can severely affect a person's:
   A. Self-esteem
   B. Quality of life
   C. Sexual performance
   D. Mobility

7. A client experiencing *photophobia* is sensitive to:
   A. Light
   B. Odors
   C. Sound
   D. Cold

8. The brainstem contains the midbrain, pons, and medulla oblongata, providing a pathway for ascending and descending tracts. The brainstem is the center for:
   A. Fight-or-flight response
   B. Visual and auditory reflexes
   C. Pleasure and pain responses
   D. Nutrient exchange and waste

9. Which protective membrane covers the outer layer of the brain?
   A. Dura mater
   B. Pia mater
   C. Arachnoid mater
   D. Myelin

10. When there is damage to the cerebellum, the client would experience which of the following signs and symptoms?
    A. Lack of muscle control and balance.
    B. Inability to chew and difficulty swallowing.
    C. Cognitive distortions and thought disturbances.
    D. Difficulty forming words and slurred speech.

11. You are caring for a client who underwent a myelogram. Which of the following nursing actions would be *most* important when the client returns to his room?
    A. Have the client sit up in the chair for 2-hour periods.
    B. Elevate the head of the bed to 16–30 degrees for 12 hours.
    C. Obtain a lunch tray as soon as possible.
    D. Turn the client every 2 hours for the next 24 hours.

12. You are assisting the RN to obtain a history and conduct a neurologic examination on a newly admitted client. Which of the following assessment data would be *most* important?
    A. Cranial nerve function
    B. Ability to understand and use language
    C. Level of consciousness
    D. Reaction to sensory stimulation

13. Which of the following would be the *highest-priority* nursing diagnosis for a client with a neurologic deficit, regardless of the underlying cause of the deficit?
    A. Risk for injury
    B. Balanced nutrition
    C. Fluid balance
    D. Ineffective coping

14. When caring for a client who has just had a seizure, the nurse *must* assess the client's:
    A. Level of consciousness
    B. Pupillary response for equality and reactivity to light
    C. Ability to move all extremities and response to commands
    D. All of the above

15. When a seizure occurs, the nurse must:
    A. Time any seizure activity.
    B. Protect the client from injury.
    C. Keep the environment calm and quiet.
    D. All of the above.

Chapter 37

Clients with Gastrointestinal System Disorders

KEY TERMS

Match each of the following key terms to its proper definition.

_____ 1. The expelling of gas from the stomach through the mouth

A. Steatorrhea

_____ 2. Drugs that induce defecation

B. Emesis

_____ 3. Infection of the peritoneal cavity

C. Achalasia

_____ 4. A _____ hernia is a condition that occurs when part of the stomach moves through an opening in the diaphragm into the chest cavity

D. Encephalopathy

_____ 5. An upper gastrointestinal regurgitation of gastric contents

E. Cathartics

_____ 6. Washing out the stomach through a tube

F. Valsalva

_____ 7. Vomit

G. Dyspepsia

_____ 8. Condition that occurs when the cardiac sphincter of the stomach does not relax to allow food to pass into the stomach

H. Lavage

_____ 9. Straining to have a bowel movement accompanied by holding the breath is known as a _____ maneuver

I. Hiatal

_____ 10. A chronic disease that leads to the development of scar tissue in the liver

J. Eructation

_____ 11. "Fatty stools" that occur when there is inadequate breakdown of fats

_____ 12. The condition that occurs when ammonia and nitrogen levels in the blood affect the central nervous system is known as hepatic _____

_____ 13. Surgical enlargement of the pylorus or gastric outlet

_____ 14. Protuberance of an organ through a defect in the wall of the abdomen

_____ 15. Fluid accumulations in the abdomen

_____ 16. This type of tenderness is caused by pain on release of pressure over McBurney's point in a person with appendicitis

_____ 17. An opening into the colon

_____ 18. The inflammation of the oral cavity; caused by a bacteria, virus, or systemic disease

_____ 19. Procedure involves the insertion of a needle through the abdominal wall to drain the fluid

_____ 20. Abnormally loud, intense, frequent bowel sounds usually caused by hunger

_____ 21. The _____ sign is when the client is unable to take a deep breath while the physician applies pressure under the ribs on the right side

_____ 22. Intense hunger and appetite

_____ 23. A telescoping of the bowel into itself

_____ 24. An inflammation of the gallbladder

_____ 25. A condition characterized by an outpouching of bowel mucosa

_____ 26. Inflammation of the stomach caused by chemotherapy, radiation therapy, food contaminated with toxins, significant alcohol intake, or food allergies

K.   Peritonitis

L.   Cirrhosis

M.   Murphy's

N.   Paracentesis

O.   Polyphagia

P.   Gastritis

Q.   Cholecystitis

R.   Hernia

S.   Diverticulosis

T.   Pyloroplasty

U.   Rebound

V.   Ascites

W.   Colostomy

X.   Stomatitis

Y.   Borborygmi

Z.   Intussusception

LEARNING OUTCOMES

1.   What is the structure and function of the GI system?

2. What are the oral cavity and esophageal disorders, and what is the nursing care for them?

Upper GI	Disorders	Nursing Care
Oral Cavity		
Esophageal		

3. What are the common gastric disorders, and what are the prevention, treatment, and nursing care for each?

Gastric Disorder	Prevention	Treatment	Nursing Care

4. What tests are used to diagnose gastrointestinal disorders, and what is the nursing care before and after those tests?

Tests	Nursing Care Before	Nursing Care After

5. What are the factors that affect defecation, and what is the nursing care for common elimination disorders?

6. What are the common infectious or inflammatory disorders, and what are the nursing considerations when caring for clients with these disorders?

7. What are the structural disorders of the GI system and what are their treatments?

8. What are the nursing interventions that are used to assist clients with colorectal cancer and other disorders of the lower GI tract?

9. What are the common accessory organ disorders, and what are treatment and nursing care for them?

10. What are the important procedures for clients who have undergone surgery for disorders of the gastrointestinal tract?

APPLY WHAT YOU LEARNED

A 65-year-old client is admitted for a diagnostic workup and possible surgery after experiencing weight loss, malaise, abdominal distention, vomiting, and a positive occult blood screen. The physician suspects a large bowel obstruction, possibly related to a cancerous lesion, and has ordered the following:

- NPO
- Nasogastric tube for intermittent suction
- Occult blood screen of any stool
- IV fluids
- Pain medications as directed
- Cleansing enemas
- Barium studies of the colon

1. Define both a mechanical and a functional bowel obstruction.

2. Discuss the physiology of a large bowel obstruction.

3. Identify the focus of treatment of a large bowel obstruction.

4. Discuss the use of a nasogastric tube to treat a large bowel obstruction.

5. Identify the nurse's primary care focus for this client.

6. Identify two psychosocial nursing diagnoses for this client.

7. Identify four specific nursing interventions when caring for clients with lower gastrointestinal disorders.

8. Identify the purpose, client preparation, and postdiagnostic test care for a client receiving a barium enema.

9. Discuss nursing interventions for administration of a cleansing enema.

MULTIPLE CHOICE QUESTIONS

Circle the answer that best completes each of the following statements.

1. The walls of the small intestine absorb nutrients and secrete hormones, mucus, and enzymes. The tiny projections that increase the absorptive surface area within the small intestine are called:
   A. Rugae
   B. Villi
   C. Diverticula
   D. Lumen

2. The Valsalva maneuver can best be described as:
   A. A test used to diagnose peptic ulcer disease.
   B. Treatment aimed at decreasing proton pump inhibitors.
   C. Straining to have a bowel movement accompanied by holding the breath.
   D. A type of cleansing enema used to prepare the intestine for visualization.

3. Cathartics are drugs used to induce:
   A. Vomiting
   B. Labor
   C. Volvulus
   D. Defecation

4. You are auscultating the abdomen of a client admitted for severe wavelike gastrointestinal pain, nausea, and vomiting. The client says, "I haven't been able to pass any stool, just mucus and some blood." You suspect that the client has a mechanical obstruction of the small bowel. Which of the following assessment data would substantiate your suspicions?
   A. Bowel sounds are high-pitched proximal to the obstruction and absent below it.
   B. Bowel sounds are absent, causing increased peristaltic waves.
   C. It's too early to determine any cause of the pain, nausea, and vomiting.
   D. Bowel sounds are low-pitched and audible in all four quadrants of the abdomen.

5. An early sign of colon cancer is:
   A. Daily defecation
   B. Brown, formed stools
   C. Occult blood in the stool
   D. Anal itching

6. When caring for a client experiencing cholecystitis, the nurse's primary focus must be:
   A. Pain relief
   B. Dietary modifications
   C. Skin care
   D. Oral hygiene

7. Which vitamin, when deficient, may cause epistaxis, bruising, and petechiae and is often lacking in a person with cirrhosis of the liver?
   A. Vitamin C
   B. Vitamin D
   C. Vitamin B
   D. Vitamin K

8. Esophageal varices are enlarged veins that occur in the esophagus when there is:
   A. Constant exposure to alcohol
   B. Decreasing blood flow through the liver
   C. Primary hypertension
   D. Hepatic encephalopathy

9. Postprocedure nursing care for a client undergoing a liver biopsy would include:
   A. Auscultation of bowel sounds.
   B. Confirmation of return of the gag reflex.
   C. Palpation of the epigastric region and abdomen.
   D. Application of pressure at the puncture site and monitoring for bleeding.

10. The physician has requested that you measure a client's abdominal girth daily. This measurement helps to determine the presence of:
    A. Ascites
    B. Cholelithiasis
    C. Flatulence
    D. Dyspepsia

11. When the nurse provides care for clients with inflammatory and infectious intestinal disorders, the nursing priorities will involve:
    A. Managing pain and diarrhea.
    B. Helping to identify triggers.
    C. Monitoring electrolyte levels.
    D. All of the above.

12. Gastroesophageal reflux disease (GERD) is more prevalent among:
    A. African Americans
    B. Asians
    C. Hispanics
    D. Caucasians

13. Following gastric surgery, a client may experience dumping syndrome after eating. To prevent dumping syndrome, the nurse should include which of the following statements in the teaching plan?
    A. Drink at least 50 mL of liquid with each bite of food.
    B. Eat foods high in carbohydrates.
    C. Eat smaller, more frequent meals.
    D. Assume a supine position immediately after eating.

14. Numerous factors affect defecation. Which of the following statements should the nurse include when teaching a client how to improve bowel regularity?
    A. A daily fluid intake of 2000 to 3000 mL is necessary to promote a normal soft, formed stool.
    B. Low-residue foods such as rice, eggs, and lean meats stimulate peristalsis.
    C. Bowel patterns are established at an early age and change as a person ages.
    D. Diets high in cabbage, onions, and cauliflower are laxative producing.

15. When assessing a stoma, the nurse should report which of the following?
    A. Complaints of a burning sensation under the faceplate of the ostomy device.
    B. Any redness and irritation of the peristomal skin.
    C. Stomal swelling that remains after 6 weeks postop.
    D. All of the above.

Chapter 38

Clients with Endocrine System Disorders

KEY TERMS

Match each of the following key terms to its proper definition.

_____ 1. Exophthalmos

    A. Build-up of ketones in the blood, signaling high blood sugar level and breakdown of fats for energy

_____ 2. Pheochromocytoma

    B. The thyroid gland does not make enough thyroid hormone

_____ 3. Diabetic ketoacidosis

    C. A benign tumor located in the adrenal medulla that causes excessive amounts of epinephrine and norepinephrine to be produced

_____ 4. Hormones

    D. Bulging eyes resulting from enlarging tissue behind the eyes

_____ 5. Myxedema

    E. Chemical messengers that function individually

_____ 6. Polyphagia

    A. Condition in which the pituitary secretes too much growth hormone prior to closure of the epiphyses in the bones

_____ 7. Cretinism

    B. Intense hunger and appetite

_____ 8. Gigantism

    C. Loss of consciousness that occurs when the client with Type 2 diabetes has extreme hyperglycemia

_____ 9.	Ketones	D.	The thyroid gland does not make enough thyroid hormone in infancy
_____ 10.	Hyperosmolar hyperglycemic nonketotic coma	E.	Products of the breakdown of fatty acids

_____ 11.	Endocrine glands	A.	Body's cells are affected by increased weight and are unable to use the insulin
_____ 12.	Hyperglycemia	B.	Secrete hormones directly into the blood
_____ 13.	Insulin resistance	C.	Glands that secrete substances through ducts that reach the epithelial surface inside the body or on the skin
_____ 14.	Hypoglycemic	D.	The secretion of too much growth hormone that occurs after the client is an adult
_____ 15.	Exocrine glands	E.	Low glucose levels
_____ 16.	Acromegaly	F.	High blood sugar caused by lack of an adequate amount of insulin or insufficient insulin action

_____ 17.	Goiter	A.	Clients drink large amounts of fluid
_____ 18.	Polyuria	B.	A method by which hormone production is decreased
_____ 19.	Polydipsia	C.	A severe form of hyperthyroidism that can occur when clients' hyperthyroidism is left untreated or after thyroid surgery
_____ 20.	Thyrotoxicosis	D.	Painless enlargement of the thyroid gland
_____ 21.	Addisonian crisis	E.	A severe form of Addison's disease that causes a life-threatening medical situation
_____ 22.	Negative feedback	F.	Diuresis; excessive urination

LEARNING OUTCOMES

1. What are homeostasis and negative feedback mechanisms?

2. What is the structure and function of the endocrine system?

3. What are the disorders of the pituitary gland and what are the nursing interventions for clients with pituitary disorders?

4. What are the thyroid and the parathyroid disorders?

5. What is the nursing care needed for clients with thyroid and parathyroid disorders?

6. What are the different types of diabetes mellitus, and what is the treatment for each type?

7. What are the topics that need to be included when teaching clients with diabetes mellitus about self-care?

8. What are the complications of diabetes, and how can the risk be decreased?

9. What are the disorders of the adrenal glands, and what nursing care is needed for them?

APPLY WHAT YOU LEARNED

You are caring for a 62-year-old African American male who was recently diagnosed with Type 2 diabetes mellitus. He is overweight and hypertensive. The client says, "Boy, I don't know how I will manage the new diet. Everything I like I'm not supposed to eat. The doctor also said I had to exercise, which I really don't have time to do. Will I really have to take this medication the rest of my life?"

1. Describe Type 2 diabetes, including its etiology and onset.

2. Identify the three most common signs and symptoms of Type 2 diabetes that you would teach to the client.

3. Discuss cultural considerations for this client.

4. Discuss the importance of diet, exercise, and medications in the control of Type 2 diabetes.

5. Discuss the role of the LPN/LVN when working with this client.

MULTIPLE CHOICE QUESTIONS

Circle the answer that best completes each of the following statements.

1. Which of the following is considered a tropic hormone secreted by the anterior pituitary?
   A. Luteinizing hormone
   B. Insulin
   C. Thymosin
   D. Cortisol

2. Seasonal affective disorder, caused by a lack of sunlight in winter, is thought to be related to increased melatonin secretion from which gland?
   A. Pituitary
   B. Hypothalamus
   C. Pineal
   D. Pancreas

3. Insulin is secreted by the
   A. Alpha cells of the pancreas.
   B. Beta cells of the pancreas.
   C. T lymphocytes of the thymus.
   D. Glucocorticoids of the adrenal glands.

4. A client has been diagnosed with diabetes insipidus. He says, "I just don't know where I got this disease from. I don't eat a lot of sweets or sugar. I really shouldn't have sugar in my blood." What is the nurse's best response to this client?
   A. "Well, you'll have to watch your diet even more closely now that you have diabetes. You'll have to eliminate all sweets and sugars from your diet and count calories carefully."
   B. "Do you know of any family members who had diabetes and needed to take insulin? Diabetes does run in families, and if you can identify a family history, it will help your doctor determine your treatment."
   C. "It doesn't matter where you got it from, just that you know you have it and can do something about it. We can't help a lot of what happens to us and shouldn't really worry about those things over which we have no control."
   D. "Actually, diabetes insipidus is not the same as diabetes mellitus. The diabetes that relates to blood sugar is caused by a lack of insulin production by the pancreas, whereas diabetes insipidus is caused by lack of the hormone ADH produced by the pituitary gland."

5. Primary hyperthyroidism is caused by an oversecretion of:
   A. Insulin
   B. T_3 and/or T_4
   C. Calcitonin
   D. Parathormone

6. Along with a positive Chvostek's sign, which of the following signs and symptoms would be consistent with hypocalcemia?
   A. Continuous muscle spasms and tremors
   B. Diaphoresis and headache
   C. Polyuria and polyphagia
   D. Weight loss and heat intolerance

7. Hyperglycemia results from a lack of
   A. Insulin
   B. Thyroxine
   C. Cortisol
   D. Calcium

8. The LPN/LVN must know about different insulins and understand the onset, peak, and duration of the prescribed insulin. Which of the following statements best describes *peak* time? It:
   A. Refers to the time the insulin begins to take effect.
   B. Occurs when the medication is most effective.
   C. Is the length of time that the insulin effect lasts.
   D. Is the time that the insulin must be administered.

9. Most oral hypoglycemic agents should be administered:
   A. Thirty minutes prior to a meal
   B. One hour after the meal
   C. Along with the meal
   D. One hour before beginning to eat

10. A client reports feeling shaky, weak, and dizzy. When you talk with him, he becomes easily irritated and says, "I haven't eaten all day. I'm so hungry I could eat a horse. Get me something to eat!" From these assessment data, which of the following interventions would be *most* appropriate?
   A. Check the client's blood sugar and provide a snack.
   B. Have the client lie down and administer oxygen.
   C. Monitor the client for orthostatic hypotension.
   D. Call the physician for an order for an IV.

11. You are caring for a client with myxedema. Which of the following symptoms is consistent with the client's diagnosis?
   A. Weight loss
   B. Hair loss
   C. Tachycardia
   D. Hypertension

12. Clients with hyperparathyroidism experience low back pain, pathologic fractures, and renal calculi. These symptoms are related to:
   A. Decalcification of the bone and increased blood calcium.
   B. Deficient production of parathormone by the parathyroid glands.
   C. Lack of an adequate amount of insulin or insufficient insulin action.
   D. Inhibition of gonadotropins secreted by the pineal gland.

13. When caring for a client with pheochromocytoma, the nurse *must:*
   A. Monitor blood glucose
   B. Administer oxygen
   C. Monitor blood pressure
   D. Assess for signs of infection

14. Which of the following disorders occurs when the adrenal glands do not secrete enough corticosteroids?
   A. Addison's disease
   B. Cushing's disease
   C. Pheochromocytoma
   D. Thyroid toxicosis

15. Which of the following symptoms would be consistent with a diagnosis of Cushing's disease?
   A. Bronze color of the skin; hypotension
   B. Pounding headache; diaphoresis
   C. Increased glucose levels; fatty tissue deposits
   D. Intolerance to cold; lethargy

Chapter 39

Clients with Urinary System Disorders

KEY TERMS

Match each of the following key terms to its proper definition.

_____ 1. Micturition   A. Incomplete emptying of the bladder

_____ 2. Peritoneal dialysis B. The process of emptying the urinary bladder

_____ 3. Anuria   C. Urine remaining in the bladder following the voiding

_____ 4. Retention   D. Dysfunction of nerves supplying the bladder

_____ 5. Neurogenic bladder   E. A process to remove extra fluid and waste products wherein the dialyzing solution is instilled directly into the abdomen

_____ 6. Residual urine   F. Low amounts of urine or no urine

---

_____ 7. Frequency   A. Low amounts of urine or no urine

_____ 8. Azotemia   B. Excessive nighttime urination

_____ 9. Pyuria   C. Pain on urination

_____ 10. Nocturia   D. Need to void more than usual

_____ 11. Oliguria   E. Increased nitrogenous wastes in the blood including urea and creatinine

_____ 12. Dysuria   F. Pus in the urine

_____ 13.	Polyuria	A.	A slow, progressive deterioration in kidney function
_____ 14.	Chronic renal failure	B.	An inflammation of the urethra and causes redness, irritation, edema of the mucosa, and urethral discharge
_____ 15.	Pyelonephritis	C.	A sudden decrease in or total lack of kidney function
_____ 16.	End-stage renal disease	D.	A condition in which the kidneys are unable to carry out the normal functions necessary to eliminate waste products and maintain fluid and electrolyte balance
_____ 17.	Acute renal failure	E.	An inflammation that affects the kidney pelvis and parenchyma
_____ 18.	Renal failure	F.	Diuresis; excessive urination
_____ 19.	Urethritis	G.	Stage of failure in which the kidneys ultimately lose the ability to excrete waste products and regulate fluid and electrolytes

_____ 20.	Urgency	A.	Urinary incontinence after voluntary control has normally been reached
_____ 21.	Enuresis	B.	A familial disease characterized by an enlarged kidney with multiple fluid-filled cysts
_____ 22.	Hemodialysis	C.	Feeling that voiding must occur immediately
_____ 23.	Uremia	D.	An inflammatory disease of the glomerulus affecting kidney function; can be acute or chronic
_____ 24.	Glomerulonephritis	E.	Distention of the renal pelvis caused by increased pressure due to urine backup
_____ 25.	Polycystic kidney disease	F.	A process of removing waste products, excess fluids, and electrolytes from the blood
_____ 26.	Hydronephrosis	G.	A toxic state marked by an accumulation of urea and other nitrogenous wastes in the blood

LEARNING OUTCOMES

1. What is the structure and function of the urinary system, and what factors affect urinary function?

2. What are the characteristics of normal and abnormal urine?

3. What are the factors associated with altered urinary elimination?

4. What tests are used to check renal function, and what are the basic nursing skills needed for urinary care?

5. How is the collection of data related to urinary function?

6. What are the manifestations, diagnosis, treatment, and nursing care for disorders of the kidneys?

Manifestations	Diagnosis	Treatment	Nursing Care

7. What is the treatment and nursing care for clients with renal failure and end-stage renal disease?

	Treatment	Nursing Care
Renal Failure		
End-stage Renal Disease		

8. What are the common disorders of the ureters, bladder, and urethra, and what is the treatment and nursing care for each?

	Disorders	Treatment	Nursing Care
Ureters			
Bladder			
Urethra			

APPLY WHAT YOU LEARNED

You are caring for an 85-year-old female client in a long-term care facility who is incontinent of urine and also experiences involuntary defecation. Her urine is dark amber and foul-smelling. Her appetite is diminished, and her fluid intake is less than the daily recommended amount of at least 1500 mL. Vital signs: T 99.6F oral, BP 90/56, P 68, and R 20. Upon review of her record, you determine that, in collaboration with the RN, you must institute additional nursing actions. You begin by answering the following questions.

1. Identify changes in urinary elimination for an older adult.

2. Identify possible factors that may contribute to incontinence.

3. Describe characteristics of normal and abnormal urine.

4. Discuss client-related factors for prevention of urinary tract infections.

5. Discuss the relationship between incontinence and skin integrity.

6. Identify three appropriate nursing diagnoses.

7. Identify nursing interventions/actions necessary for this client.

MULTIPLE CHOICE QUESTIONS

Circle the answer that best completes each of the following statements.

1. Special sensory nerve endings in the bladder called *stretch receptors* respond when the adult bladder contains between:
   A. 150 and 200 mL of urine
   B. 250 and 450 mL of urine
   C. 300 and 500 mL of urine
   D. 350 and 600 mL of urine

2. Normal urine consists of 96% water and 4% solutes. Inorganic solutes include:
   A. Sodium
   B. Creatinine
   C. Ammonia
   D. Uric acid

3. Clients who are at risk for urinary tract infections or urinary calculi should consume a significant amount of fluid daily. When planning care, the nurse must ensure that the client will consume how many milliliters of fluid in a 24-hour period?
   A. 1500 mL per day
   B. 1500 mL per shift
   C. 2000 to 3000 mL daily
   D. 4000 to 5000 mL daily

4. Urine is normally slightly acidic. Which of the following would reflect an average (normal) pH for urine?
   A. 5.5
   B. 6.0
   C. 7.3
   D. 8.0

5. You are caring for a client whose urinalysis indicates the presence of ketone bodies. Which of the following statements would *best* explain this finding?
   A. The client is pregnant.
   B. The client has been dieting.
   C. The client has a normal urinalysis.
   D. The client has kidney damage.

6. A client with polycystic kidney disease would exhibit which of the following signs and symptoms?
   A. Pain in the flank area.
   B. Pain upon urination.
   C. Little or no urine output.
   D. Retention of sodium and fluid.

7. Clients in chronic renal failure with an underlying autoimmune disease such as lupus erythematosus may experience which complication?
   A. Nephrosclerosis
   B. Azotemia
   C. Neuropathy
   D. Glomerulonephritis

8. A client undergoing hemodialysis will have an arteriovenous (AV) fistula that is created by surgically joining an artery and a vein, usually in the forearm, with graft tubing. When providing care for this client, it is *most* important that the nurse:
   A. Take the blood pressure on the extremity opposite the shunt.
   B. Monitor vital signs, fluid I&O, and level of alertness.
   C. Collect urine specimens using sterile technique.
   D. Observe the skin for color, texture, and tissue turgor, and for the presence of edema.

9. Which of the following nursing actions would be a *priority* action for a client with a urinary diversion device?
   A. Ensure adequate fluid intake and monitor I&O.
   B. Assess the level of pain and administer analgesics as needed.
   C. Assess the condition of the stoma and surrounding skin.
   D. Assist the client to the most comfortable position.

10. Which causative agent is responsible for most urinary tract infections?
    A. Escherichia coli
    B. Staphylococcus aureus
    C. Pseudomonas
    D. Candida

11. Cholinergic drugs such as bethanechol chloride (Urecholine) may be ordered for a client with urinary retention. The action of this medication is thought to:
    A. Reduce pain
    B. Stimulate bladder contraction
    C. Decrease acidity
    D. Relax smooth muscles

12. When teaching women about prevention of urinary tract infections, which of the following statements should the nurse include?
    A. Avoid bubble baths and feminine hygiene products.
    B. Void immediately after sexual intercourse.
    C. Wear cotton or cotton-lined underwear.
    D. All of the above.

13. Twenty-four hours following a prostatectomy, the client's urine is pink colored and clot free. As the nurse assessing the color and clarity of the output, you know that this finding is:
    A. Abnormal and must be reported to the physician immediately.
    B. Abnormal; the catheter must be removed to prevent further bleeding.
    C. Normal; the catheter may be removed at this time.
    D. Normal for the first 24–48 hours after surgery.

14. When providing care for a client with a disorder of the penis or testicles, the nurse must:
    A. Be sensitive.
    B. Be professional.
    C. Avoid making comments that could embarrass the client.
    D. All of the above.

15. You are caring for a 75-year-old female client who is experiencing frequent urinary incontinence. The client says, "I am so embarrassed when I have urine leaking. I'm so afraid I will have an odor or my clothing will become wet. Is there anything you can do?" You decide to develop a plan targeting ways to reduce the number of episodes of incontinence. Which of the following interventions would be most effective?

    A. Have the client wear adult-sized diapers such as Depends.
    B. Instruct the client to reduce her fluid intake, especially when she plans to appear in public.
    C. Ask the physician to write an order for an indwelling catheter which can be connected to a leg drainage collection device.
    D. Develop and adhere to a bladder training schedule.

Chapter 40

Clients with Reproductive System Disorders

KEY TERMS

Match each of the following key terms to its proper definition.

_____ 1. Pelvic inflammatory disease

_____ 2. Dilatation and curettage

_____ 3. Menopause

_____ 4. Uterine prolapse

_____ 5. Polycystic ovary syndrome

_____ 6. Fibroadenoma

A. Permanent cessation of menstruation

B. The condition that occurs when the uterus descends into or out of the vaginal canal

C. A freely movable, rounded mass with well-defined borders and a solid rubbery texture

D. Opening of the cervix and scraping of the lining of the uterine walls

E. An infection usually involving the fallopian tubes, ovaries, cervix, uterus, and peritoneum

F. Endocrine disorder resulting from numerous follicular cysts, and characterized by higher than normal LH, estrogen, and androgen levels, and low FSH levels

_____ 7. Menarche

_____ 8. Metrorrhagia

_____ 9. Endometriosis

_____ 10. Conization

A. Bleeding between periods

B. Condition that occurs when endometrial tissue grows outside the uterine cavity

C. Repetitive, excessive, or prolonged menstruation flow

D. The beginning of menstrual cycles during puberty

_____ 11. Menorrhagia

E. A plastic device shaped like a ring, arch, or ball that is placed in the vagina to support the uterus

_____ 12. Pessary

F. Removal of a cone-shaped wedge of cervical tissue

_____ 13. Dysmenorrhea

A. Removal of the fallopian tubes

_____ 14. Oophorectomy

B. Painful menses

_____ 15. Intrauterine device

C. Removal of tumor and surrounding myometrium

_____ 16. Myomectomy

D. Surgical removal of the ovaries

_____ 17. Salpingectomy

E. Termination of the reproductive period in the female

_____ 18. Climacteric

F. A small T-shaped piece of metal covered with copper or levonorgestrel placed in the uterus, used for contraception

---

_____ 19. Ectopic

A. Hernial protrusion of part of the rectum into the vagina

_____ 20. Tenesmus

B. Condition of excessive hair growth

_____ 21. Amenorrhea

C. Dilated blood vessel in the testis

_____ 22. Varicocele

D. Absence of menstruation

_____ 23. Hirsutism

E. Painful straining to defecate

_____ 24. Rectocele

F. Occurring outside of the uterus

LEARNING OUTCOMES

1. What is the structure and function of the male and female reproductive systems?

Reproductive System	Structure	Function
Male		
Female		

2. What are the important points to cover in obtaining a comprehensive sexual history?

3. What is the normal sexual response cycle, and what are the possible causes of reproductive issues?

4. What are the common breast disorders, and what are their treatments and the nursing interventions for them?

Disorders	Treatment	Interventions

5. What are the common uterine disorders and changes with menopause? What are the treatments and appropriate nursing care for them?

Disorders	Changes with Menopause	Treatment	Nursing Care

6. What tumors are associated with the female reproductive system, and what are the treatments and appropriate nursing care of them?

Tumors	Treatments	Nursing Care

7. What are the other disorders of the female reproductive system not already defined, and what is the appropriate nursing care for them?

8. What are the common disorders of the male reproductive system, and what are the treatments and nursing interventions for them?

Disorders	Treatment	Nursing Interventions

9. What are the three infectious disorders that have an impact on family planning issues?

10. What are the common contraceptive methods, and what is the effectiveness of each?

11. What are the issues involved in infertility and what are the possible methods of treatment?

APPLY WHAT YOU LEARNED

Read the following situation. Unscramble the words and define each term. Answer the following questions.

A 58-year-old client has been diagnosed with *vaseniiv caromanic* of the left breast. Inspection reveals a *puae d'rangeo* skin texture, *pilenp tractioner,* and a nipple discharge in the left breast. The physician tells the client that the most effective way to manage this cancer is to perform *beastr-vinecronsg* surgery. The client is unsure about the surgery and asks for more options.

1. Which nursing diagnosis best reflects the client's concern?

2. List four nursing interventions that would assist the client in deciding on an option.

3. The client finally agrees to the partial mastectomy. What information should be provided to the client and her family?

4. What information should you document in your nurse's notes relating to your teaching session?

MULTIPLE CHOICE QUESTIONS

Circle the answer that best completes each of the following statements.

1. Which of the following is considered an internal structure of the female reproductive system?
   A. The clitoris
   B. The vaginal introitus
   C. The endometrium
   D. The labia majora

2. When obtaining a comprehensive sexual history, the nurse should do which of the following? (Select all that apply.)
   A. Elicit data while being nonjudgmental and non-threatening.
   B. The client should feel somewhat uncomfortable.
   C. Privacy should be honored.
   D. Be sensitive to and aware of sexual concerns of people from non-Western backgrounds.
   E. Closed-ended questions are less threatening to clients.

3. Which cause of reproductive disorders can be prevented through client teaching by the nurse?
   A. Infections
   B. Tumors
   C. Structural changes
   D. Blockage

4. The nurse teaches the client with what breast disorder to reduce intake of chocolate in order to reduce impact of the disorder?
   A. Intraductal papillomas
   B. Fibroadenoma
   C. Breast cancer
   D. Fibrosis

5. The nurse suspects which of the following in the female athlete who has been training for the Olympics?
   A. Metrorrhagia
   B. Amenorrhea
   C. Menorrhagia
   D. Dysmenorrhea

6. The nurse would consider the client with which of the following at greater risk for cervical cancers?
   A. Unprotected sex
   B. Poor diet
   C. HPV
   D. HIV infection

7. Which of the following items would the nurse find in a rape kit? (Select all that apply.)
   A. Microscopic slides
   B. Hairbrush
   C. Mirror
   D. Large paper bags
   E. Bible

8. What male reproductive disorder would the nurse administer Alprostadil injections for?
   A. Testicular cancer
   B. Epispadias
   C. Erectile dysfunction
   D. Hydrocele

9. After abstinence, which of the following is the most reliable method of contraception?
   A. Diaphragm
   B. Female condom
   C. Vaginal sponge
   D. Intrauterine device

10. What percentage of cases involving infertility issues are shared problems with the male and the female?
    A. 10 percent
    B. 15 percent
    C. 20 percent
    D. 25 percent

Chapter 41

Clients with Sexually Transmitted Infections

EXPLORE **PEARSON** **mynursingkit**™

MyNursingKit is your one stop for online chapter review materials and resources. Prepare for success with additional NCLEX®-style practice questions, interactive assignments and activities, web links, animations and videos, and more!

Register your access code from the front of your book at
www.mynursingkit.com

KEY TERMS

Match each of the following key terms to its proper definition.

_____ 1. Gumma

_____ 2. Salpingitis

_____ 3. Chancre

_____ 4. Neurosyphilis

_____ 5. Adenopathy

A. Tertiary syphilis that can appear from 1 to 40 years following the onset of the infection

B. Generalized lymph node swelling

C. Infectious granuloma

D. Hard ulcer

E. Inflammation of the uterine tube

_____ 6. Papillomata

_____ 7. Jarisch-Herxheimer reaction

_____ 8. Condylomata lata

_____ 9. Vesicles

A. A small, circumscribed elevation of the skin containing fluid

B. Flat papules in the anal area or skin folds

C. Warts

D. A transient immunologic reaction to antibiotic therapy of syphilis and certain other diseases, characterized by fever, headache, myalgia, and significant chancre changes

1. What are the prevalence of and risks for STIs?

2. What are the methods of transmission and prevention of STIs?

3. What tests are used to diagnose STIs?

4. What are the common STIs and what are their clinical manifestations, potential complications, diagnoses, and treatment of them?

STI	Manifestations	Complications	Diagnoses	Treatment

5. What is the appropriate nursing care for clients with STIs using the nursing process?

6. What are the key concepts in client teaching for STIs?

APPLY WHAT YOU LEARNED

A young woman undergoing an elective surgery is tested for HIV as a part of the preoperative screening. The results of the blood test are positive for HIV. She is currently asymptomatic for HIV or AIDS. As you discuss this test result with her, she begins to cry, saying, "I thought only homosexual men got HIV. How in the world did I get it? What am I going to do?"

1. Provide this client with an explanation focusing on the transmission and treatment of HIV.

2. Explain the pathophysiology of HIV and AIDS.

3. Identify four discharge considerations important for this client.

MULTIPLE CHOICE QUESTIONS

Circle the answer that best completes each of the following statements.

1. The Centers for Disease Control and Prevention (CDC) requires that healthcare personnel report identified cases of:
   A. Herpes genitalis
   B. Gonorrhea neisseria
   C. Condylomata acuminata
   D. Trichomonas vaginalis

2. Symptoms of secondary syphilis are typically present:
   A. Within 3 weeks of initial sexual contact.
   B. 1 to 40 years following the onset of infection.
   C. 6 weeks after appearance of the initial chancre with flu-like symptoms.
   D. 6 to 8 days after the incubation period.

3. Due to the rapid destruction of spirochetes during treatment with penicillin, clients may develop:
   A. Anaphylactic shock
   B. Wernicke's encephalopathy
   C. Jarisch-Herxheimer reaction
   D. Hypertensive crisis

4. After sexual contact and exposure to Chlamydia trachomatis, a female would most likely experience which of the following?
   A. Interruption of the menstrual cycle
   B. Single or multiple painless chancres
   C. Dysuria, urinary frequency, and pelvic pain
   D. Fever, headache, malaise, and myalgias

5. A fungal or yeast infection may be caused by:
   A. Candida albicans
   B. Trichomonas vaginalis
   C. Human papillomavirus
   D. Herpesvirus type 2

6. Herpes genitalis can be cured with:
   A. Antibiotic therapy
   B. Antiviral agents
   C. Rest, fluids, and nonsteroidal anti-inflammatory drugs (NSAIDs)
   D. It cannot be cured

7. After infection with the human immunodeficiency virus (HIV), acquired immunodeficiency syndrome (AIDS) may not occur for up to:
   A. 1 year
   B. 2 years
   C. 5 years
   D. 10 years

8. A male exposed to gonorrhea during sexual contact would most likely experience:
   A. No symptoms
   B. Urethritis
   C. Epididymitis
   D. Chancres

9. A 25-year-old female client reports having a frothy, foul-smelling vaginal discharge, pruritis, and lower abdominal pain. From her signs and symptoms, you conclude that she probably has been exposed to:
   A. Candidiasis
   B. Chlamydia
   C. Gonorrhea
   D. Trichomoniasis

10. Which of the following diagnostic measures would be used to identify gonorrhea?
    A. Cytology
    B. Gram stain
    C. Tissue culture
    D. Serology

11. The physician has prescribed Acyclovir 400 mg po, t. i. d. Acyclovir is an effective drug for which sexually transmitted disease?
    A. Herpes
    B. Gonorrhea
    C. Syphilis
    D. Chlamydia

12. Metronidazole (Flagyl) is effective against which sexually transmitted disease?
    A. Candidiasis
    B. Chlamydia
    C. Human papillomavirus
    D. Trichomoniasis

13. One of your peers tells you that her physician has recommended that she undergo cryotherapy for treatment of a sexually transmitted disease. As a nursing student studying this chapter, you conclude that she probably has been exposed to:
    A. Gonorrhea
    B. Trichomoniasis
    C. Human papillomavirus
    D. Syphilis

14. A client states, "I had no idea I could catch all these nasty diseases from having sex." Which of the following nursing diagnoses would be most appropriate for this client?
    A. Risk for injury
    B. Sexual dysfunction
    C. Impaired social interaction
    D. Deficient knowledge

15. Discharge teaching must be a priority nursing intervention for clients experiencing a sexually transmitted disease. Which of the following is important to include in the teaching plan?
    A. Discuss the transmission methods of sexually transmitted diseases.
    B. Explain that the entire course of treatment prescribed must be completed.
    C. Explain the importance of refraining from sexual contact until treatment is completed.
    D. All of the above.

Chapter 42

Health Promotion of Older Adults

KEY TERMS

Match each of the following key terms to its proper definition.

_____ 1. Nocturnal myoclonus   A. A disease that destroys sharp, central vision

_____ 2. Benign prostatic hyperplasia   B. Sudden, repetitive kicking or jerking movements of the lower extremities

_____ 3. Gerontology   C. Change in the alignment of a bone to relieve stress on the bone or joint

_____ 4. Macular degeneration   D. Enlarged prostate gland in the older male

_____ 5. Osteotomy   E. Health specialty that focuses on care of the older adult

_____ 6. Geriatrics   A. Difficulty focusing on close objects

_____ 7. Cataracts   B. An uncontrollable movement of the lower extremities

_____ 8. Presbyopia   C. A health specialty that focuses on care of the older adult

_____ 9. Presbycusis   D. A clouding of the lens in the eye that limits vision

_____ 10. Restless leg syndrome   E. Low bone mass

_____ 11. Osteopenia   F. Atrophic changes to the muscles that support the tympanic membrane related to the aging process

LEARNING OUTCOMES

1. What is the definition of gerontology, and why is it important as a specialty?

2. What are the factors that affect the aging process?

3. What are the normal physiologic changes of older adults by body system, including sensory changes and adaptations?

Physiologic Changes	Sensory Changes	Adaptations

4. What are the ways of maintaining or restoring urinary continence?

5. What are the psychosocial challenges confronting older adults?

6. What are the special health concerns of older adults?

7. What the important safety issues of older clients?

8. What is caregiver stress, and what are the factors that contribute to elder abuse? What client teaching would be helpful to prevent elder abuse?

Caregiver Stress	Factors	Client Teaching

APPLY WHAT YOU LEARNED

A 90-year-old friend knows you are a nursing student studying the care of elderly clients and asks you to speak at a meal site for older adults. She tells you that many of the attendees talk regularly about growing older. They apparently argue about what is considered a normal consequence of aging and what is not. Your friend thinks you could help them recognize and understand the changes. You agree to speak to the group on Friday.

1. Identify cultural considerations when speaking to this group.

2. Identify two age-related sensory changes that need to be considered when planning for this group.

3. Identify three key points applicable to a diverse group of aging adults.

MULTIPLE CHOICE QUESTIONS

Circle the answer that best completes each of the following statements.

1. According to Erikson, the developmental stage for a person over age 60 is:
   A. Trust vs. mistrust
   B. Generativity vs. stagnation
   C. Role identity vs. role confusion
   D. Ego integrity vs. despair

2. Which of the following alterations is considered a normal change of aging?
   A. Slower immune response
   B. Folic acid deficiency
   C. Thrombus formation
   D. Angina pectoris

3. Intermittent claudication is caused by which of the following?
   A. Arterial occlusive disease
   B. Coronary artery disease
   C. Varicose veins
   D. Venous stasis

4. The most common age-related abnormality of the endocrine system in the older adult is:
   A. Hyperthyroidism
   B. Diabetes mellitus
   C. Addison's disease
   D. Hypocalcemia

5. Older women often experience an increased incidence of yeast infections. Which physiologic change contributes to this increase?
   A. Cessation of menstruation
   B. Change in vaginal pH
   C. Decreased thyroid hormone
   D. Increased sexual activity

6. Older adults are at increased risk for heat stroke or heat exhaustion. Which of the following statements provides the best rationale for this increase?
   A. Older adults frequently do not have air conditioning.
   B. Older adults dress warmer than is appropriate or necessary.
   C. Older adults have increased sebaceous gland activity.
   D. Older adults have fewer and less active sweat glands.

7. The older adult experiences significant hair changes. Which of the following is considered a normal change?
   A. Loss of most body hair
   B. Loss of pigment cells from hair bulbs
   C. Increased thickness and texture
   D. Increased axilla and pubic hair

8. Which of the following is considered a normal change of the musculoskeletal system of the older adult?
   A. Inflammation of the lining of the joints.
   B. Decreased muscle tone and flexibility.
   C. Excessive loss of calcium from the bone.
   D. Spontaneous fractures of the bones.

9. The nursing assistant has been assigned to give an elderly client a bath. Which of the following statements should be included in your instructions to the nursing assistant?
   A. "Be sure to test the temperature of the bath water carefully since touch sensation and sensitivity decrease with age and the client may not realize it is too hot."
   B. "Because the client knows what temperature he can tolerate, tell the client to step into the bathtub to check the temperature of the bath water."
   C. "Run a nice hot bath and let the client soak in it for 20 minutes."
   D. "You've been at this nursing assistant thing for a long time, so just go ahead and do what you normally do."

10. The client says, "I'm so cold all the time. Years ago, I was usually too hot, but now I always need an extra blanket or a sweater. I just don't understand it." Which of the following would be the best explanation for this change?
   A. The immune system is less efficient, contributing to increased frequency of illness.
   B. With aging, the efficiency of the body's temperature-regulating mechanism decreases.
   C. The older adult's ability to adapt to changes in environmental temperature decreases.
   D. B and C

11. Kegel exercises will help to:
   A. Maintain movement in the joints.
   B. Reduce the risk of presbyopia.
   C. Strengthen the pelvic floor muscles.
   D. Lose and/or maintain weight.

Chapter 43

Nursing Care of Ill Older Adults

KEY TERMS

Match each of the following key terms to its proper definition.

_____ 1. Diabetic retinopathy   A. Hardening of the stapes to the oval window in the ear

_____ 2. Mitral valve prolapse   B. Backflow of blood from the left ventricle into the left atrium

_____ 3. Cardiomegaly   C. Condition in diabetics wherein circulatory changes in the blood vessels of the eye cause small blood vessels to hemorrhage into the vitreous humor of the eye

_____ 4. Polypharmacy   D. Displacement of the mitral valve, usually due to benign proliferative changes of the valve leaflets

_____ 5. Otosclerosis   E. Enlargement of the heart

_____ 6. Mitral regurgitation   F. A condition that occurs when a client takes many different medications that interact with each other and create side effects

---

_____ 7. Glaucoma   A. Double vision

_____ 8. Retinal detachment   B. The onset of delirium during the evening or night with impairment or disappearance during the day, most often seen in mid- or later stages of dementia

	9.	Gout	C.	A disease progression in the eye character-ized by increased intraocular pressure
_____	10.	Diplopia	D.	A separation of the retina from the choroids
_____	11.	Sundowning	E.	An inflammatory disorder that causes uric acid crystals to form in a joint

LEARNING OUTCOMES

1. What is the role of the LPN/LVN in providing care for ill older adults?

2. What are the common disorders of older adults by body system?

3. What are the specific needs and the appropriate nursing interventions for the ill older client with an acute illness?

4. What are the specific issues related to medication administration for older clients?

APPLY WHAT YOU LEARNED

Read the following situation. Unscramble the words and define each term. Answer the following questions.

Gagin brings about *yscpialh* changes as well as the strong probability of *spycohcislao* changes. Nursing care promotes health in older adults and includes teaching healthy *vibrehosa* and encouraging healthy *fesyletlsi*.

1. Name five illnesses noted in older adulthood.

2. What nursing diagnoses go along with those illnesses?

3. Discuss healthy lifestyle and behavioral issues of the older adult.

MULTIPLE CHOICE QUESTIONS

Circle the answer that best completes each of the following statements.

1. Which of the following are considered roles of the LPN/LVN in providing nursing care for the ill older adult? (Select all that apply.)
   A. Balancing the need to complete tasks quickly with the client's need to feel a measure of control over their life
   B. Basic nursing care will change based on client's age.
   C. Caregiving conditions are simplified and special attention is not required.
   D. Additional time may be required for ADLs.
   E. The nurse will need to have patience due to the extra time that may be required due to cognitive deficits.

2. What abnormal change in the integumentary system of an older adult can progress to swelling and enlargement of the nose and may also cause conjunctivitis if left untreated?
   A. Basal cell carcinoma
   B. Dermatitis
   C. Rosacea
   D. Pressure ulcers

3. Which musculoskeletal system abnormality most commonly affects the great toe?
   A. Gout
   B. Bunions
   C. Bursitis
   D. Hammertoe

4. Which of the following would be a specific nursing concern related to care of the older adult who is being hospitalized?
   A. Metabolism is faster and their bodies will be quicker to clear drugs than a younger person.
   B. Pressure ulcers are a constant danger for immobilized older adults.
   C. Older clients require more assistance with ADLs.
   D. Assistive devices are not recommended due to risk of falls.

5. What might the client be diagnosed with when presenting with the symptoms of nausea, jaundice, confusion, and changes in elimination patterns?
   A. Urinary tract infections
   B. Gastroesophageal reflux disease
   C. Peripheral vascular disease
   D. Polypharmacy

6. Which nervous system abnormality would show diminished levels of norepinephrine and dopamine?
   A. Alzheimer's disease
   B. Sundowner's syndrome
   C. Parkinson's disease
   D. Transient ischemic attacks

7. Which cardiovascular system abnormality is caused by hypertrophy of the left ventricle in an attempt to improve oxygenation?
   A. Congestive heart failure
   B. Mitral valve prolapse
   C. Thrombophlebitis
   D. Cardiomegaly

8. Diplopia is associated with which body system?
   A. Ears
   B. Nervous
   C. Eyes
   D. Gastrointestinal

9. What nervous system abnormality can affect younger persons as well as older adults, and may be caused not only by organic means but also by drug overdoses?
   A. Dementia
   B. Sundowning
   C. Depression
   D. Cerebrovascular accidents

10. Obese, inactive older adults, as well as older adults who spend a lot of time on their feet, are at increased risk for which cardiovascular system abnormality?
    A. Hypertensive disease
    B. Peripheral vascular disease
    C. Varicose veins
    D. Arterial occlusive disease

Chapter 44

Caring for Chronically or Terminally Ill Clients

EXPLORE PEARSON **mynursingkit**™

MyNursingKit is your one stop for online chapter review materials and resources. Prepare for success with additional NCLEX®-style practice questions, interactive assignments and activities, web links, animations and videos, and more!

Register your access code from the front of your book at www.mynursingkit.com

KEY TERMS

Match each of the following key terms to its proper definition.

_____ 1. Livor mortis

_____ 2. Living will

_____ 3. Do not resuscitate

_____ 4. Algor mortis

_____ 5. Durable power of attorney for health care

_____ 6. Rigor mortis

A. An order to prevent interventions the client does not wish to have performed when death approaches

B. Discoloration of surrounding tissues caused after blood circulation has ceased

C. The stiffening of the body that begins about 2 to 4 hours after death

D. A written statement appointing someone else to manage healthcare treatment decisions when the client is unable to do so

E. The gradual decrease of the body's temperature after death

F. A document that provides specific instructions about what medical treatment the client chooses to omit or refuse in the event that he or she is unable to make those decisions

_____ 7. Hospice

_____ 8. Palliative care

A. Irreversible damage to the cerebral cortex

B. An unconscious response of professionals in which they hold back emotionally

—— 9.	Cerebral death	C.	Care that incorporates the holistic concepts of palliative care and is provided for terminally ill clients with a prognosis of 6 months or less survival time
—— 10.	Vegetative state	D.	A shift in treatment goals from curing a disease to providing relief from suffering
—— 11.	Distancing	E.	The set of skills and activities applied to client care to assist the individual to return to his or her maximum level of functioning
—— 12.	Rehabilitation	F.	Irreversible state of unconsciousness

LEARNING OUTCOMES

1. What are the characteristics of chronic illness?

2. What are the factors associated with chronic illness, and what can be done to prevent chronic illness?

3. What is the role of the LPN/LVN in caring for chronically ill clients?

4. What are the definitions of terminal illness, palliative care, and hospice?

5. What is the LPN/LVN's role in caring for dying clients and their families?

6. What are the common nursing diagnoses used in end-of-life care?

7. What are the interventions the LPN/LVN can perform in caring for the dying person and their family?

8. What are the clinical signs of impending death?

9. What are the legal issues involved in terminal illness, and what are the essential aspects of the Patient Self-Determination Act?

10. What are the definitions and clinical indications of death?

11. What are the special pediatric and cultural concerns related to dying?

12. What are the nursing measures for the care of the body after death?

APPLY WHAT YOU LEARNED

Lambert Montgomery, 52, was admitted to the hospital last week for removal of a tumor that was blocking the esophagus. The client has terminal lung cancer and the surgery was performed as palliative treatment so he could eat and drink. Mr. Montgomery is married with three adult children. His wife arrives every morning and stays until late in the evening, sitting at his bedside talking and knitting. When his children visit, one of his daughters will encourage Mrs. Montgomery to join her for dinner in the cafeteria while the others stay with the client; otherwise, she takes her meals with her husband. Mr. Montgomery is not expected to survive to go home, and Mrs. Montgomery says she wants to spend as much time with him as possible while he is still here.

1. What signs would make you aware the client is within hours of death?

2. If Mrs. Montgomery told you she was going to go to dinner in the cafeteria with her daughter after you noted these signs of impending death in the client, what would you do and say?

3. Mrs. Montgomery informs you she plans to stay all night with her husband because she doesn't want him to die alone. How would you respond to this?

MULTIPLE CHOICE QUESTIONS

Circle the answer that best completes each of the following statements.

1. Which of the following factors are associated with the development of chronic illness? (Select all that apply.)
    A. Age
    B. Culture
    C. Pain tolerance
    D. Genetics
    E. Education

2. What factors can the client adjust to prevent chronic illnesses?
    A. Race
    B. Culture
    C. Lifestyle
    D. Increase income

3. What is the role of the LPN/LVN in caring for the chronically ill?
    A. Early treatment of decubitus before they become debilitating
    B. Encouraging independence
    C. Repositioning client every four hours to prevent decubitus
    D. Providing complete physical hygiene

4. Which of the following is a principle of palliative care?
   A. All diagnostic tests and other invasive procedures are exhausted.
   B. Heroic treatment measures are encouraged.
   C. The physician is the expert on whether pain and symptoms are adequately relieved.
   D. Death is regarded as a natural process, to be neither hastened nor prolonged.

5. What is the role of the nurse when caring for clients with a terminal illness and their families?
   A. Allow the family to express their fears.
   B. Provide clients with multiple opportunities to socialize.
   C. Enforce all facility policies regarding visitation.
   D. Inform the family that updates on client condition must come from the provider.

6. Which of the following are common signs and symptoms in the terminal client? (Select all that apply.)
   A. Increased thirst
   B. Agitation, confusion, and restlessness
   C. Frequent urination
   D. Fever and chills.

7. What priority nursing interventions can the nurse perform when caring for the dying person and their families?
   A. Help families to understand changes in the client's condition.
   B. Tell the family how they should respond to given situations.
   C. Position the client to improve perfusion.
   D. Support urinary elimination by supplying plentiful fluids.

8. Which of the following would be considered a clinical sign of impending death?
   A. Increasing blood pressure
   B. Extremities are warm and flushed
   C. Increased appetite
   D. Weak pulse

9. Which of the following indicates that only palliative care is to be administered?
   A. Durable power of attorney for health care
   B. Do not resuscitate order
   C. Comfort measures only order
   D. Living will

10. Which of the following is a clinical indication of death if the client is dependent on a mechanical ventilator?
    A. Irreversible destruction of the spinal cord
    B. Total lack of response to external stimuli
    C. Lack of involuntary reflexes
    D. Absence of electric current from the brain

Chapter 45

Caring for Clients with Cancer

KEY TERMS

Match each of the following key terms to its proper definition.

_____ 1. Carcinogenesis

_____ 2. Oncology

_____ 3. Adjuvant

_____ 4. Biotherapy

_____ 5. Nadir

A. The manipulation of the immune system to restore, augment, or modulate its function

B. The lowest point that the blood cell counts reach before they begin to rebound following chemotherapy

C. The study of cancer

D. A type of therapeutic treatment used to enhance the result of another therapy

E. The production of cancer

_____ 1. Neoplasm

_____ 2. Metastasis

_____ 3. Oncogenes

_____ 4. Cachexia

_____ 5. Anaplastic

A. Physical wasting and weight loss

B. Any abnormal growth of new tissue that may be harmless or cancerous

C. Lacking structural differentiation

D. Genes found in the chromosomes of tumor cells

E. Cancerous cells that have traveled from the primary site to a distant site

LEARNING OUTCOMES

1. What are the basic terms that describe cancer and what it does?

2. What are the differences between normal and malignant cells?

3. What are the important concepts in cancer prevention?

4. What are the factors that affect a client's choice of evaluation for cancer?

5. What are the nursing concerns when caring for clients receiving a cancer diagnosis?

6. What are the ways of classifying and staging cancer, and what are the tests used to determine whether a client has cancer?

7. What are the treatment options for cancer, and what are their common effects on the client?

8. What nursing interventions are appropriate for clients receiving cancer treatments?

9. What are the important considerations when caring for the very young or very old client with cancer?

APPLY WHAT YOU LEARNED

Matthew's mother says he is a very happy, curious baby. He started walking at 10 months and is now 18 months old and, as his mother says, "is into everything he can reach." However, he has been falling down a lot in the last two weeks, and today he had a clonic-tonic seizure that lasted for more than five minutes. His parents called 911 and he was brought to the emergency department. They stopped the seizure activity with medications and then performed diagnostic tests, including an MRI. The emergency room physician explained to the parents that Matthew has a large growth in an area that is not operable. Judging by the appearance of the cancer and the suspected rapidity with which it is growing, they believe the condition will be terminal; however, they arrange for a pediatric neurologic oncologist to speak with them and care for Matthew, who is admitted to the pediatric unit. You and the supervising RN receive report on the client and the RN asks you to begin collecting data on Matthew. His parents are tearful and look very frightened. Matthew is just watching his parents, but is lethargic from the medications he was given in the emergency room.

1. What are your priorities of care for this client?

2. What type of treatment might be appropriate for this client?

MULTIPLE CHOICE QUESTIONS

Circle the answer that best completes each of the following statements.

1. Which of the following occurs in the growth of cancer tumors?
   A. Cancer cells divide only 50 to 60 times before they die.
   B. Cancer cells require an anchoring point in order to grow.
   C. Cancer cells form a single layer of growth on the bottom of a petri dish.
   D. Cancer cells never enter the resting phase in the cell cycle.

2. What are the genes called that are found in the chromosomes of tumor cells?
   A. Neoplasm
   B. Carcinogenesis
   C. Oncogenes
   D. Neutropenia

3. Which of the following are concepts for preventing cancer?
   A. Having unprotected sex with only one partner at a time
   B. Wearing SPF 10 sunscreen for protection from sunlight
   C. Limiting drinks to two alcoholic drinks per day
   D. Getting at least 30 minutes of physical activity every day

4. Which factors affect the client's choice of evaluation for cancer? (Select all that apply.)
   A. Client's history of comorbid conditions
   B. Tolerance to invasive tests
   C. Goal of palliative treatment
   D. Biological characteristics of the tumor
   E. Insurance restrictions

5. What concerns might the nurse consider priorities when caring for the client who has received a cancer diagnosis? (Select all that apply.)
   A. Distancing themselves from the client
   B. Exploring the needs of the family
   C. Getting too close to the client
   D. Providing proper referrals or assisting with appointments
   E. Being a source of comfort for the client

6. What staging system is used to classify colorectal cancer?
   A. Duke's staging system
   B. Clark level
   C. Tumor-node-metastasis (TNM) staging
   D. Tumor markers

7. What factors influence the decision regarding the appropriateness of a surgical approach to cancer? (Select all that apply.)
   A. Metastatic potential
   B. Quality of life
   C. Mental status
   D. Tumor cell kinetics
   E. Growth rate

8. When caring for a client receiving chemotherapy for colon cancer that has metastasized to the liver, the nurse would consider which of the following goals appropriate?
   A. The client will remain asymptomatic of infection until normal immune response returns.
   B. The client will reduce activity level to lowest level possible throughout chemotherapy treatment.
   C. The client will increase caloric intake by increasing the amount of fat eaten daily.
   D. The client will avoid public places in order to prevent infections until chemotherapy treatment is completed.

9. When planning care for a client diagnosed with cancer, the nurse recognizes that an important factor in the client's recovery is: (Select all that apply.)
   A. Family support
   B. Chemotherapy
   C. Nutrition
   D. Radiation therapy
   E. Surgery

10. Which of the following are side effects of radiation? (Select all that apply.)
    A. Rapid hair growth
    B. Temporary or permanent alterations of taste
    C. Increased blood coagulation
    D. Fibrosis of lung tissue
    E. Susceptibility to infection

Chapter 46

Long-Term Care and Rehabilitation Nursing

KEY TERMS

Match each of the following key terms to its proper definition.

_____ 1. Custodial

A. A disturbance in structure or function resulting from physiologic or psychological abnormalities

_____ 2. Aphasia

B. The degree of observable and measurable impairment

_____ 3. Rehabilitation

C. Facilities in which clients require specialized care are known as _____-care facilities.

_____ 4. Handicap

D. Reduced ability or inability to speak or understand verbal or written language

_____ 5. Impairment

E. The _____ Budget Reconciliation Act is the law passed to improve nursing homes and extended-care facilities.

_____ 6. Disability

F. The total adjustment to disability that limits functioning at a normal level

_____ 7. Skilled

G. Term for ongoing, maintenance care

_____ 8. Omnibus

H. The set of skills and activities applied to client care to assist the individual to return to his or her maximum level of functioning

LEARNING OUTCOMES

1. What are the differences between skilled and custodial care in a long-term care facility, and why are these differences important?

Long-Term Care	Differences	Importance
Skilled		
Custodial		

2. What are the roles and responsibilities of the LPN/LVN in long-term care?

3. What is the LPN's/LVN's role in supervising and delegating to nursing assistants and aides?

4. What is the multidisciplinary approach to long-term client care, and how is it important to the family?

5. What are the specialized needs of young adult clients receiving care in a skilled nursing or rehabilitation facility?

6. What are the roles of the LPN/LVN in rehabilitation?

7. What are the legal and ethical concerns related to long-term care and rehabilitation?

8. What rules apply to Medicare, Medicaid, and insurance reimbursement for long-term care and rehabilitation?

Medicare	Medicaid	Insurance Reimbursement

APPLY WHAT YOU LEARNED

Martha King, 74, lost her husband six months ago to lung cancer. She lives alone in a home she lived in with her husband since their children were small. Her bedroom is on the top floor and the laundry is in the basement. She is no longer able to climb the stairs comfortably secondary to arthritis and congestive heart failure, so her son has been trying to convince her to sell her home and move into an assisted living facility. Mrs. King says she loves her home and has too many happy memories to leave, and can get along just fine with a little bit of help and organization. Unfortunately, while climbing the stairs carrying a laundry basket full of clean clothes, she lost her balance and fell down the stairs. She was brought to the emergency room with hypothermia from lying on the cold cement for 2 hours before she was found and x-rays revealed a fractured left humerus and left femur. She is admitted for repair of the left hip and the left arm is casted. You are the nurse taking care of this client.

1. What can you do to help her prepare for admission to the rehabilitation center following discharge?

2. How can you help her to explore her feelings regarding assisted living after rehabilitation?

3. What suggestions would you make if she insists on returning to her home that would reduce the risk of injury and create a safer environment for her to live in?

MULTIPLE CHOICE QUESTIONS

Circle the answer that best completes each of the following statements.

1. Which of the following would be considered custodial care?
   A. Occupational therapy
   B. Administering eye drops to a client
   C. Assisting clients to bathe
   D. Performing dressing changes

2. Which of the following are appropriate roles for the LPN/LVN working in a long-term care facility? (Select all that apply.)
   A. Administering IV push medications
   B. Supervising and delegating tasks to UAPs
   C. Developing care plans for clients
   D. Setting up appointments for clients
   E. Driving clients to doctor's visits

3. Which of the following tasks could be delegated to unlicensed personnel? (Select all that apply.)
   A. Notification to the funeral home of a deceased client
   B. Range of motion procedures
   C. Tube feeding a client
   D. Changing client's positions
   E. Glucose readings

268   Chapter 46   © 2010 Pearson Education, Inc.

4. What member of the healthcare team would normally be the one to order the use of an adaptive device?
   A. Physical therapist
   B. Occupational therapist
   C. Pharmacist
   D. Registered Nurse supervisor

5. Which of the following is unique when providing care to a child requiring rehabilitation or long-term care?
   A. Socialization with peers
   B. Incorporating school into the environment
   C. Including the family in providing a positive environment
   D. Occupational therapy

6. The role of the LPN/LVN includes which of the following when working in rehabilitation nursing?
   A. Developing an appropriate rehabilitation program.
   B. Providing age-appropriate schoolwork to the pediatric client.
   C. Providing complete care to clients to allow them to rest in preparation for PT.
   D. Preventing complications through early recognition of symptoms.

7. The nurse working at the elder care facility observes a coworker's care of a client to be abrupt and rough. The nurse's responsibility is to:
   A. Notify the supervisor.
   B. Counsel the coworker.
   C. Notify the board of nursing.
   D. Investigate the event.

8. Where does the bulk of the reimbursement for skilled care in the first 100 days come from for people over 65 years old?
   A. Out of pocket
   B. Private insurance
   C. Medicaid
   D. Medicare

9. What law was passed to improve nursing homes and extended-care facilities?
   A. Nurse Practice Acts
   B. Omnibus Budget Reconciliation Act
   C. Prospective payment system
   D. Supplemental Security Income

10. Which of the following procedures may be performed by the LPN/LVN?
    A. Treatments for pressure ulcers
    B. Tele-checks for pacemaker function
    C. Drawing blood for lab testing
    D. Pushing IV medications
    E. Digital fecal disimpaction

Chapter 47

Emergency Room and Urgent Care Nursing

KEY TERMS

Match each of the following key terms to its proper definition.

_____ 1. Third spacing

_____ 2. Full-thickness burns

_____ 3. Superficial burns

_____ 4. Titration

_____ 5. Partial-thickness burns

A. Chemical or thermal damage that does not involve all the skin layers

B. Burns that injure only the epidermis and may be caused by everyday events

C. Determination of the correct volume for administration

D. Involvement of all layers of skin in a burn

E. Shunting of fluids into the extracellular space

_____ 6. PALS

_____ 7. Urgent care

_____ 8. Triage

A. A center where staffing is maintained around the clock to provide care for high-acuity cases, such as trauma

B. Life-threatening condition of inadequate tissue perfusion

C. A specialized training course that prepares the healthcare professional to perform advanced lifesaving skills or techniques on the pediatric client

_____ 9. Emergency care

    D.   Care for minor injuries and acute illnesses when clients cannot see their primary care provider or if they do not have a designated healthcare provider

_____ 10. Shock

    E.   System of prioritizing victims' care needs, from most severe to least injured or ill

LEARNING OUTCOMES

1. What are the roles and safety issues for the LPN/LVN in emergency care/urgent care nursing?

2. Why is triage used in the EC/UC setting?

3. What are the important components involved in the initial contact with clients and admission to the EC/UC setting?

4. What is the description of airway management and CPR in emergency nursing care?

5. List the different types of shock, including a description of each and how they are managed.

Types	Description	Management

6. What factors are important when caring for clients with trauma?

7. What are the other conditions that would require urgent or emergency care, and what nursing considerations apply to each?

8. What are the important concepts to remember when dealing with the effects of bioterrorist or terrorist attacks in the EC setting?

9. What is the nursing care for different types of burns in the EC/UC setting?

10. What are the appropriate nursing actions after the death of a client in the EC/UC setting?

11. What are the steps in nursing procedures that may be performed in an EC/UC setting for clients with a sprain or fracture?

APPLY WHAT YOU LEARNED

Lisa Rice, 36, is admitted to the emergency department. When asked what brought her to the ED, the client says, "I really don't feel very well. I feel dizzy when I stand up, I have a fever, and I am really sweaty. I've had an earache for the last few days, so maybe that's the problem?" The nurse examines the client and finds vital signs 98.8 oral – 56-22 84/46, the client's extremities are cold and clammy and the skin is very pale.

1. What diagnosis do you suspect for this client?

2. What immediate nursing interventions will you initiate while waiting for the provider to examine this client?

3. What orders will you anticipate from the provider?

MULTIPLE CHOICE QUESTIONS

Circle the answer that best completes each of the following statements.

1. Which of the following would the trained LPN/LVN be responsible for in an EC/UC setting? (Select all that apply.)
   A. Performing nursing interventions.
   B. Creating client discharge plans.
   C. Administering IV piggyback medication.
   D. Compiling information so the RN can input information in the ED information system.
   E. Reinforcing client teaching.

2. What situation would the nurse be in if they were working in an incident command center?
   A. Triaging clients in EC.
   B. Confining hazardous waste spill to an operating room.
   C. Practicing disaster training.
   D. Attending a Board of Nurses hearing regarding confidentiality infringement.

3. Which of the following clients may the nurse triaging in the EC administer Tylenol to before they meet the primary care provider?
   A. An adolescent who has an earache.
   B. An adult who has an inflamed laceration on the leg.
   C. An adolescent who has fallen down a stairway.
   D. An adult with head wounds from an automobile accident.

4. Which of the following would be an example of a low-flow device used in oxygen therapy?
   A. Non-rebreather
   B. Bag-valve-mask units
   C. Endotracheal tubes
   D. Venturi masks

5. A client presents with severe diaphoresis and oliguria following a diagnosis of pneumonia a few days ago. What type of shock should the nurse be concerned the client might have?
   A. Hypovolemic shock
   B. Anaphylactic shock
   C. Septic shock
   D. Neurogenic shock

6. In which type of trauma would the acronym RICE be useful for regarding treatment?
   A. Chest trauma
   B. Soft tissue injuries
   C. Abdominal trauma
   D. Head trauma

7. The nurse admits a client whose lab results are positive for *Bacillus anthracis*. The nurse recognizes this as indicative of:
   A. Inhaled poison
   B. Ingested poison
   C. Bioterrorism
   D. Snake bite

8. The nurse admits a client who was burned and assesses third-degree burns on the front of the client's right leg, anterior trunk, and anterior aspects of both arms. What percentage of the client's body is burned?
   A. 18%
   B. 27%
   C. 36%
   D. 45%

9. What are the responsibilities of the nurse in the EC when a client dies?
   A. Notify the family by phone and tell them of the death.
   B. Prepare the body for donation of organs if indicated.
   C. Counsel the family.
   D. Call the morgue to arrange care for the deceased client.

10. Which of the following are the nurse's responsibilities in regard to a sprain or fracture?
    A. Apply a splint.
    B. Apply a cast.
    C. Position client against a wall to measure for crutches.
    D. Instruct client to place weight on axilla when crutch walking.

Chapter 48

Community Nursing

KEY TERMS

Match each of the following key terms to its proper definition.

_____ 1. Ambulatory care nursing

_____ 2. School-based health clinic

_____ 3. Mental health clinic

_____ 4. Urgent care office

_____ 5. Same-day surgery clinic

A. Walk-in medical facility where clients can obtain treatment for minor injuries and acute illnesses

B. Health facility in which the client arrives early in the day, has a surgical procedure, and returns home after he or she is fully recovered from anesthesia

C. Facility that meets the needs of the ambulatory older adult; various degrees of personal care assistance may be provided

D. Ambulatory care centers, located in a number of inner city school districts, whose professionals perform a higher level of care than the typical school nurse's office

E. Medical facilities whose focus is on psychosocial issues and the mental health status of its clients

_____ 6. Assisted living facility

A. A licensed nurse who works for a company that contracts with healthcare agencies to provide them with staff

    _____ 7. Traveling nurse
                                      B. Facilities that give residents independence to be in their own apartments or condominiums but that offer nursing or medical care on the grounds

    _____ 8. Adult day care facility
                                        C. Nurse who provides for the health care of inmates

    _____ 9. Correctional nurse
                                        D. Center that provides health and social services to the older adult who is still living at home

LEARNING OUTCOMES

1. What are the common community nursing care settings?

2. What is the LPN's/LVN's scope of practice in a physician's office or outpatient surgery center?

3. What are the important aspects of nursing care in the school health office or clinic?

4. What are the nursing responsibilities in home care and hospice?

5. What does the admission process and preparation of a client for examination include in a physician's office or clinic?

6. How can the LPN/LVN assist with office surgical procedures?

7. How can the LPN/LVN perform or assist with office screening and testing procedures?

APPLY WHAT YOU LEARNED

The nurse accepts a full-time position working in a physician's office and is hired by the office manager, Malik McNamara, MA. The nurse is one of three nurses and five medical assistants working in the five-physician practice, including a pediatrician, a family practice doctor, an obstetrician, and two internal medicine doctors.

1. The nurse admits a client who reports chest pain and shortness of breath. Who would the nurse report these symptoms to and why would they choose that person?

2. The office manager tells the nurse to increase the flow of oxygen from 2 liters by nasal cannula to 5 liters. What should the nurse do?

3. The nurse has questions about benefits, requesting time off, and scheduling. Who would the nurse discuss these concerns with? Why would they make that choice?

MULTIPLE CHOICE QUESTIONS

Circle the answer that best completes each of the following statements.

1. What type of facility meets the needs of the ambulatory older adult and also may provide various degrees of personal care?
   A. Ambulatory care nursing
   B. Adult day care facility
   C. Urgent care office
   D. Assisted living facility

2. Which of the following are considered within the LPN's/LVN's scope of practice in the physician's office? (Select all that apply.)
   A. Reporting to the office manager.
   B. Admitting new clients.
   C. Performing lab tests.
   D. Conducting electrocardiograms.
   E. Performing diagnostic and simple surgical procedures.

3. Which of the following are important aspects of nursing care in a school health office or clinic? (Select all that apply.)
   A. Provides aspirin to students with headaches
   B. Administers basic first aid
   C. Reports to the principal of the school
   D. Provides client teaching to parents about drug use
   E. Contacts the principal when an issue outside of protocol presents itself

4. Which of the following statement is accurate regarding the LPN's/LVN's responsibilities in home care and hospice care settings?
   A. The LPN/LVN cannot work in these healthcare settings.
   B. The LPN/LVN makes the initial visit to do the admission.
   C. The LPN/LVN requires well-developed observational and critical thinking skills.
   D. The nurse assesses the client and the situation collaboratively.

5. Which of the following are components of the process of admitting a new client in a physician's office? (Select all that apply.)
   A. Have black and red pens for charting.
   B. Ask appropriate questions using medical terminology.
   C. Thank the client for cooperating.
   D. Use open-ended questions to obtain all data.
   E. Stand in front of the client while obtaining medical information.

6. What are the ways the LPN/LVN may assist with office surgical procedures? (Select all that apply.)
   A. Suture the wound closed when the physician indicates the procedure is completed.
   B. Document events that occurred during the procedure.
   C. Wear sterile gloves and hand instruments to the surgeon during the procedure.
   D. Dispose of any biohazards into their proper containers.
   E. Have container ready to receive specimen if required.

7. Which of the following can the LPN/LVN perform independently? (Select all that apply.)
   A. Sigmoidoscopy
   B. Scoliosis screening
   C. Capillary blood sample
   D. 12-lead electrocardiograms
   E. Audiometric testing

8. Which immunization is given first to a newborn usually before 2 months?
   A. DTaP
   B. Polio
   C. Pneumococcal conjugate
   D. Hepatitis B

9. Which of the following are parts of the emergency procedures for clients in acute distress?
   A. Keep the client in a high Fowler's position.
   B. Give the client cold water to drink.
   C. Administer slow-acting inhalers.
   D. Do not leave the client alone.

10. What equipment is needed to measure visual acuity for near vision? (Select all that apply.)
   A. Plus lens glasses
   B. Ishihara test plates
   C. Snellen chart
   D. Hardy Rand-Rittler pseudoisochromatic plates

Chapter 49

Mental Health Disorders

PEARSON

EXPLORE **mynursingkit™**

MyNursingKit is your one stop for online chapter review materials and resources. Prepare for success with additional NCLEX®-style practice questions, interactive assignments and activities, web links, animations and videos, and more!

Register your access code from the front of your book at
www.mynursingkit.com

KEY TERMS

Match each of the following key terms to its proper definition.

_____ 1. Psychomotor retardation

_____ 2. Personality

_____ 3. Flat affect

_____ 4. Prodromal phase

_____ 5. Anhedonia

A. Lack of ability to feel pleasure

B. Warning phase of a condition or disease

C. Lack of activity

D. Absence of facial expressions or other body language indicating feelings

E. The relatively stable way that a person thinks, feels, and behaves

_____ 6. Pressured speech

_____ 7. Stigma

_____ 8. Alogia

_____ 9. Psychosis

_____ 10. Hallucinations

A. Restriction in the fluency and productivity of speech

B. Sensory perceptions that seem very real but occur without external stimulus

C. Fast and determined speech that is hard to interrupt

D. Negative cultural attitude that marks people with disgrace

E. A major feature of schizophrenia

_____ 11. Disorganized behavior   A.   Fixed false beliefs

_____ 12. Avolition   B.   An enduring pattern of inner experience and behavior characterized by a lack of self-identity and maladaptive, rigid thinking that lead to self-defeating behaviors

_____ 13. Delusions   C.   A marked decrease in response to the environment

_____ 14. Personality disorder   D.   Inability to sort and interpret incoming sensory information or respond appropriately

_____ 15. Catatonic behavior   E.   Lack of goal orientation

_____ 16. Disorganized thinking   F.   A lack of motivation

LEARNING OUTCOMES

1. What are the characteristics of a mentally healthy person?

2. What are the key concepts about mental disorders that make them difficult to diagnose and treat?

3. What are the mental health disorders seen in children?

4. What are the three major types of treatment used for clients with major mental health disorders?

5. What is the nurse's role in promoting mental health?

6. What are the diagnostic criteria, treatment, and nursing care for clients with schizophrenia?

Diagnostic Criteria	Treatment	Nursing Care

7. What are the different types of mood disorders, their treatments and nursing care for each?

Types	Treatments	Nursing Care

8. What are the key aspects of personality disorders, and what is the nursing care for clients with each type of disorder?

APPLY WHAT YOU LEARNED

The nurse, working in a same-day surgery center, admits a client scheduled for an inguinal hernia repair. When gathering data for the nursing history, the client is quiet and withdrawn, often looking off into the distance and sighing. The client's wife reports he has not been sleeping, has no appetite, and always seems sad lately. She says he no longer has any interest in social activities, declines sex, and never plays with his children. She expresses concern about his condition.

1. What diagnosis do you suspect may be appropriate for this client? Why?

2. What is the most important question you would want to ask this client?

3. What action will you take based on your suspicions regarding this client's condition?

MULTIPLE CHOICE QUESTIONS

Circle the answer that best completes each of the following statements.

1. Which of the following are characteristic of a mentally healthy person?
   A. Ability to control others
   B. False evaluation of reality
   C. Rigidity toward change and conflict
   D. A sense of the meaning of life

2. What percentage of people in the United States will have a psychiatric or substance abuse problem at some point in their lives?
   A. 15%
   B. 40%
   C. 50%
   D. 25%

3. Half of all cases of mental illnesses begin at what age?
   A. 12 years
   B. 14 years
   C. 8 years
   D. 10 years

4. What type of inpatient mental health treatment is associated with creating a safe, structured environment in which to do mental health work?
   A. Psychosocial rehabilitation
   B. Psychopharmacology
   C. Cognitive rehabilitation
   D. Milieu therapy

5. Which of the following would be an example of the nurse's role in providing tertiary mental health care?
   A. Calling schizophrenic clients to remind them to attend group therapy.
   B. Teaching drug abuse prevention to grammar school children.
   C. Screening for depression at sporting events.
   D. Screening the postpartum woman for postpartum psychosis or depression.

6. Which manifestation of schizophrenia would be categorized as a negative symptom?
   A. Somatic hallucination
   B. Delusion of reference
   C. Catatonic behavior
   D. Anhedonia

7. Which of the following antidepressants can cause a hypertensive crisis when combined with foods containing the amino acid tyramine?
   A. Tricyclic antidepressants (TCAs) and related cyclic agents
   B. Selective serotonin reuptake inhibitors (SSRIs)
   C. Novel antidepressants
   D. Monoamine oxidase inhibitors (MAOIs)

8. The client diagnosed with a personality disorder characterized by difficulty forming satisfying relationships, excessive emotionality, and attention-seeking behavior would be diagnosed with:
   A. Schizoid Personality Disorder
   B. Borderline Personality Disorder
   C. Histrionic Personality Disorder
   D. Avoidant Personality Disorder

9. Which of the following would be a desired outcome for clients with mood disorders? (Select all that apply.)
   A. Be independent with activities of daily living
   B. Sleep uninterrupted for 5 to 6 hours
   C. Enter into a no-self-harm agreement
   D. Suppress feelings of anger
   E. Be able to fall asleep within 30 minutes of going to bed

10. Which of the following findings are related to the likelihood of diagnosis of schizophrenia? (Select all that apply.)
    A. No genetic predisposition
    B. Urban living increases risk of diagnosis
    C. Increased immune function and a decrease in cytokines
    D. Inflammatory abnormalities
    E. People born in January

Chapter 50

Substance Abuse and Eating Disorders

EXPLORE PEARSON mynursingkit™

MyNursingKit is your one stop for online chapter review materials and resources. Prepare for success with additional NCLEX®-style practice questions, interactive assignments and activities, web links, animations and videos, and more!

Register your access code from the front of your book at
www.mynursingkit.com

KEY TERMS

Match each of the following key terms to its proper definition.

_____ 1. Denial

_____ 2. Binge

_____ 3. Relapse

_____ 4. Abstinence

_____ 5. Dichotomous thinking

_____ 6. Withdrawal

_____ 7. Purging

A. Complete lack of drug use

B. Condition that occurs due to discontinuing or reducing use of a substance that has been heavy and prolonged and that results in significant distress or impairment in social or occupational functioning

C. Thought process in which something is either all one way or all its opposite

D. Return to drug use after abstinence

E. Self-induced vomiting or abuse of laxatives or diuretics

F. An attempt to ignore unacceptable realities by refusing to acknowledge them

G. Eating in a limited period of time an amount of food that is definitely larger than most individuals would eat under similar circumstances

_____	8.	Diabulimia	A. A maladaptive pattern of substance use despite adverse outcomes
_____	9.	Substance dependency	B. Filling in gaps in memory with imagined or made-up events
_____	10.	Intoxication	C. A need for increased amounts of the substance to achieve the same effect, or diminished effect with continued use of the same amount of the substance
_____	11.	Tolerance	D. A reversible set of physical, psychologic, and behavioral symptoms caused by use of a substance
_____	12.	Confabulation	E. Involves tolerance, withdrawal, and compulsive use of substances
_____	13.	Substance abuse	F. An eating disorder in which clients with Type 1 diabetes deliberately give themselves less insulin for the purpose of weight loss

LEARNING OUTCOMES

1. What are the issues and terms related to substance abuse and dependency?

Issues	Terms

2. What are the effects of alcohol and other CNS depressants?

3. What are the effects of commonly abused substances?

4. What are the treatments and nursing interventions for clients with problems related to substance abuse and dependency?

5. What is the philosophy of the 12-step program for treatment of substance abuse?

6. What is the appropriate response when substance abuse issues impair a colleague at work?

7. What are the three major types of eating disorders?

8. What treatment and nursing care is appropriate for clients with eating disorders?

APPLY WHAT YOU LEARNED

Andy Johnson is a 26-year-old man who is addicted to alcohol. He drinks every day and drinks to get drunk at least 3 times a week. He is divorced and his wife has obtained an order of protection to keep him away from her and their children because he often becomes angry and abusive when he is drunk. Andy calls his family physician's office and says, "I admit I'm a drunk and I want help. I'm ruining my life and I know it can't get better until I stop drinking."

1. If you were the nurse who received this phone call, what would you say to this client when he finished speaking?

2. What actions would you take to help this client break his dependence and addiction to alcohol?

MULTIPLE CHOICE QUESTIONS

Circle the answer that best completes each of the following statements.

1. The client who attempts to quit smoking finds it impossible to concentrate because all they can think about is smoking a cigarette. This is the result of:
   A. Dependence
   B. Addiction
   C. Tolerance
   D. Lack of willpower

2. What ethnic group has the lowest levels of alcoholism due to a specific variant of a gene that causes the body to break down the alcohol in such a way that the person experiences symptoms known as the flushing response?
   A. African American
   B. Islamic
   C. Latino
   D. Asians

3. The person using these drugs commonly presents with high energy, may be very talkative, and often has extreme weight loss or anorexia.
   A. Barbiturates
   B. Methadone
   C. Amphetamines
   D. Benzodiazepines

4. The nurse caring for a client with substance abuse would provide a low-stimulation environment if the nursing diagnosis is:
   A. Ineffective coping
   B. Ineffective protection
   C. Deficient knowledge
   D. Ineffective denial

5. Which of the following would be associated with Alcoholics Anonymous?
   A. Self-help program for alcoholics based on 10 steps
   B. Groups offer a sense of community
   C. People with unique problems share experiences, strengths, and hope
   D. Unconditional support is offered, if individual follows steps

6. The nurse suspects a coworker has a substance abuse problem. What should the nurse do?
   A. Communicate concerns to the nurse asked to be in charge today.
   B. Confront the coworker with your concerns.
   C. Notify the state board of nursing.
   D. Notify a hospital supervisor.

7. What type of eating problem is characterized by episodes of compensatory behaviors?
   A. Nonpurging type—Bulimia nervosa
   B. Diabulimia
   C. Binge eating disorder
   D. Restricting type—Anorexia nervosa

8. What can improve the chance of success in long-term maintenance of weight loss?
   A. Changes in eating patterns to include less nutrient-dense, low-energy foods
   B. High physical activity on most, if not all, days
   C. Realistic weight loss goals (25 to 30% of initial body weight)
   D. Social support

9. What would be the BMI of the client who is 215 pounds and 5 feet, 11 inches tall?
   A. 35.83
   B. 29.98
   C. 21.71
   D. 33.02

10. What prescription drug has a street name of pancakes and syrup?
    A. Flunitrazepam
    B. Propoxyphene
    C. Codeine
    D. Barbiturates

Chapter 51

Care of Women During Normal Pregnancy

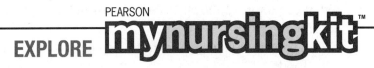

EXPLORE PEARSON mynursingkit™

MyNursingKit is your one stop for online chapter review materials and resources. Prepare for success with additional NCLEX®-style practice questions, interactive assignments and activities, web links, animations and videos, and more!

Register your access code from the front of your book at
www.mynursingkit.com

KEY TERMS

Match each of the following key terms to its proper definition.

_____ 1.	Let-down reflex	A.	Absence of neural tissue in the cranium
_____ 2.	Amniocentesis	B.	The ability to live outside the uterus
_____ 3.	Colostrum	C.	White, cheesy covering of the fetal or newborn skin
_____ 4.	Viability	D.	The withdrawal of amniotic fluid through a needle inserted into the abdomen and the uterus
_____ 5.	Vernix caseosa	E.	A yellowish fluid rich in antibodies, secreted in the last trimester and the first few days following delivery
_____ 6.	Anencephaly	F.	Release of milk after delivery

_____ 7.	Nullipara	A.	A woman who has produced viable young, whether or not the child was living at birth
_____ 8.	Ballottement	B.	A woman who has had two or more pregnancies that resulted in viable fetuses, whether or not the offspring were alive at birth
_____ 9.	Primipara	C.	A dark line on the abdomen from the umbilicus to the pubis

_____ 10. Multipara   D. A woman who has had one pregnancy that resulted in a viable child, regardless of whether the child was living at birth, and regardless of whether it was a single or multiple birth

_____ 11. Para   E. Rebounding against the fingers by the fetus if the examiner puts two fingers into the vagina and pushes upward on the uterus

_____ 12. Linea nigra   F. A woman who has never borne a viable child

---

_____ 13. Multigravida   A. Soft downy hair present on the fetus's or newborn's face, arms, and back

_____ 14. Primigravida   B. A woman who has never conceived

_____ 15. Lanugo   C. A woman who has been pregnant several times

_____ 16. Meconium   D. A pregnant woman

_____ 17. Gravida   E. A woman pregnant for the first time

_____ 18. Nulligravida   F. Newborn's first stool

_____ 19. Chadwick's sign   A. First fetal movements felt by the mother

_____ 20. Wharton's jelly   B. Painless contractions

_____ 21. Goodell's sign   C. An incomplete closure of the vertebra and neural tube

_____ 22. Spina bifida   D. Softening of the lower uterine segment

_____ 23. Braxton-Hicks contractions   E. A bluish-purple discoloration of the cervix and vagina

_____ 24. Quickening   F. A softening of the cervix

_____ 25. Hegar's sign   G. White gelatinous tissue

LEARNING OUTCOMES

1. What healthcare concerns are important related to preconception care?

2. Describe the processes of fertilization and fetal development.

3. What are the signs of pregnancy, and what tests are used to determine pregnancy?

4. What are the maternal changes anticipated to occur throughout pregnancy?

5. What is the nursing care required by a pregnant woman?

6. What are the common maternal discomforts during pregnancy, and how will you treat each one?

7. What client teaching should the nurse provide during delivery of prenatal care?

8. What are the normal signs and warning signs seen during pregnancy?

9. What are the steps performed when obtaining a fetal heart rate using a Doppler ultrasound?

10. What are the ways the LPN/LVN can assist with fetal testing procedures?

APPLY WHAT YOU LEARNED

Anne Collins, 31 years old, is seen in the obstetrician's office and determined to be 6 weeks pregnant with her first child. She is very excited about being pregnant and is anxious to call her boyfriend and share the good news.

1. What topics will you cover when providing her with prenatal teaching?

2. Would you provide teaching before or after she calls her boyfriend? Why did you make that choice?

MULTIPLE CHOICE QUESTIONS

Circle the answer that best completes each of the following statements.

1. Good eating patterns are paramount in promoting early fetal health. The nutrients required by the pregnant woman are found in high numbers in certain foods. Which of the following foods are high in folic acid? (Select all that apply.)
    A. Liver
    B. Brown rice
    C. Milk
    D. Kidney beans
    E. Fruit juices

2. What area of the trophoblast secures the blastocyst to the uterus?
    A. Chorion
    B. Morula
    C. Villus
    D. Amnion

3. Amenorrhea would be characterized as what type of sign related to a diagnosis of pregnancy?
    A. Objective sign
    B. Probable sign
    C. Positive sign
    D. Presumptive sign

4. What can an increase in platelets, fibrin, fibrinogen, and other coagulation factors coupled with venous stasis cause?
    A. Anemia
    B. Thrombus formation
    C. Hyperemesis gravidarum
    D. Ductus arteriosus

5. What client teaching may the nurse provide to the pregnant woman complaining of heartburn?
   A. Eat small amounts of food.
   B. Take antacids after eating fried or spicy foods.
   C. Increase fiber from fruits and vegetables.
   D. Lie down for 30 minutes after eating.

6. How much weight would be appropriate for the pregnant client to gain?
   A. 40 to 50 pounds
   B. 30 pounds
   C. 35 to 45 pounds
   D. 25 to 35 pounds

7. Which of the following should the nurse teach the pregnant client?
   A. Drinking 1500 to 2000 mL of water, milk, or coffee every 24 hours is recommended.
   B. Douching on days when not showering or bathing is encouraged due to an increase in vaginal secretions.
   C. Fluid leakage from the nipples should be rubbed into it to lubricate the skin and promote breast health.
   D. Physical fitness is encouraged and clients should perform strenuous exercises during the first trimester.

8. When the pregnant client calls the obstetrician's office to report double vision, the nurse suspects the possibility of:
   A. Pregnancy-induced hypertension.
   B. Ectopic pregnancy.
   C. Spontaneous abortion.
   D. Abruptio placenta.

9. Which of the following is accurate information regarding assessing the fetal heart rate with a Doppler?
   A. Apply gel to the abdomen of the client to aid with sound transmission and help maintain contact between the Doppler and the abdomen.
   B. Position the diaphragm to the left of midline halfway between the umbilicus and the symphysis pubis.
   C. When pulse is heard, check it against the mother's pulse. If they are the same, reposition the mother to a side-lying position.
   D. FHR should be assessed any time the mother accesses health care for any reason during pregnancy.

10. Which of the following is NOT a way the nurse may assist with fetal testing procedures?
   A. Instruct the woman on symptoms to report after testing.
   B. Attach proper labels on samples collected.
   C. Perform fetal ultrasounds as ordered by the physician.
   D. Assist with applying a dressing over puncture site.

Chapter 52

Care of Women During High-Risk Pregnancy

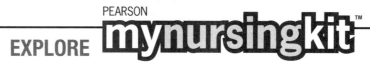

KEY TERMS

Match each of the following key terms to its proper definition.

_____ 1. Eclampsia

_____ 2. Incompetent cervix

_____ 3. Hydatidiform mole

_____ 4. Preeclampsia

_____ 5. Cerclage

A. Surgical placement of sutures in the cervix to hold the cervix closed

B. A disease in which the trophoblast develops into hydropic vesicles instead of normal embryonic tissue

C. Condition in which the cervix is weak, dilates in the second trimester, and expels the fetus

D. Severe hypertensive disorder with pregnancy, evidenced by grand mal seizures

E. Most common hypertensive disorder that occurs with pregnancy

_____ 6. Hydramnios

_____ 7. Abruptio placentae

_____ 8. Placenta previa

A. Pregnancy in which a blastocyst implants low in the uterus, allowing the placenta to grow partially or totally across the cervical opening

B. Pregnancy in which a blastocyst implants outside the uterine cavity

C. Acronym for characteristics of severe preeclampsia with liver damage

_____ 9. Ectopic pregnancy   D. Premature separation of the placenta

_____ 10. HELLP syndrome   E. Excessive amniotic fluid

LEARNING OUTCOMES

1. What are the risk factors that create a high-risk pregnancy?

2. What are the physical, psychological, and sociologic risks faced by the adolescent who is pregnant?

Physical	Psychological	Sociologic

3. What are the tests performed to assess maternal and fetal well being?

4. What are the complications of pregnancy, and what are the treatments and nursing care for each of them?

Complications	Treatments	Nursing Care

5. What are the medical conditions that are complicated by pregnancy, and what are the appropriate measures to support the pregnant woman with these medical conditions?

6. What nursing care is needed for the woman with a high-risk pregnancy?

APPLY WHAT YOU LEARNED

Jennifer McNamara, 24, has always dreamed of having a baby. When she became involved in a serious committed relationship, she and her partner started talking about having children almost immediately. Her life partner, Susan, has a career that wouldn't easily adapt to pregnancy, so it was decided Jennifer would undergo artificial insemination to become pregnant. When that was unsuccessful, she saw a doctor specializing in infertility and was placed on hormone therapy to help her conceive. When she became pregnant, an ultrasound was performed that confirmed the presence of triplets. Jennifer is now 28 weeks pregnant and has been placed on complete bed rest and terbutaline to stop preterm contractions. Her obstetrician is trying to maintain the pregnancy as long as possible, with a goal of reaching at least 32 weeks gestation to improve the likelihood of a good outcome for the babies. Susan spends evenings and weekends with Jennifer, and they play board games or do crossword puzzles. Jennifer keeps her laptop computer handy and says she's been keeping in touch with all of her friends via e-mail. They are both willing to do whatever is necessary to improve the chances of delivering healthy babies, and Susan is busy preparing the nursery at home for when they arrive.

1. What assessments would you perform when caring for Jennifer to determine the health of both her and the babies?

2. When listening to fetal heart tones, how would you ensure you were hearing all three heartbeats and not just listening to one heartbeat three times?

3. What interventions would you anticipate for this client?

MULTIPLE CHOICE QUESTIONS

Circle the answer that best completes each of the following statements.

1. The nurse caring for a pregnant client who is unmarried identifies what risk factor grouping for this client in regard to risk categories?
   A. Biophysical factors
   B. Psychosocial factors
   C. Sociodemographic factors
   D. Environmental factors

2. Which of the following adolescent mothers would be at the most risk during pregnancy?
   A. A 15-year-old who receives early prenatal care.
   B. A sexually active 15-year-old practicing safe sex.
   C. A 15-year-old who stops smoking and drinking after missing a menstrual period.
   D. A 15-year-old who has experimented with narcotics.

3. What test would be preformed on the Rh-negative woman at 28 weeks?
   A. Maternal hemoglobin test
   B. One-hour glucose screen
   C. Triple screen test
   D. Indirect Coombs' test

4. The pregnant woman presents at 10 weeks of pregnancy with decreased urinary output, electrolyte imbalance, increase in blood urea nitrogen, and complaints of frequent vomiting. What diagnosis does the nurse suspect?
   A. Hyperemesis gravidarum
   B. Ectopic pregnancy
   C. Placenta previa
   D. Gestational trophoblastic disease

5. Which medication administered to pregnant women may produce side effects including GI upset and the possibility of seizure?
   A. Sulfadiazine
   B. Azidothymidine
   C. Acyclovir
   D. Pyrimethamine

6. When assessing the high-risk mother and fetus, the nurse cannot collect which of the following data without a physicians order?
   A. Protein in the urine
   B. Cervical exam
   C. Fetal heart rate
   D. Fetal ultrasound

7. The pregnant client in her 28th week presents with edema of the hands and face, hyperreflexia, scotoma, and a blood pressure of 35mmHg systolic above her normal blood pressure reading. What diagnosis does the nurse suspect?
   A. Chronic hypertension
   B. Gestational hypertension
   C. Mild preeclampsia
   D. Polyhydramnios

8. What is the most common complication of pregnancy often seen in primigravidas under 20 or over 35 years of age who have a poor nutritional status?
   A. Preeclampsia
   B. Abruptio placentae
   C. Gestational hypertension
   D. Hydramnios

9. What condition diagnosed at the beginning of labor will mandate performance of a cesarean section?
   A. Cytomegalovirus
   B. Herpes genitalis
   C. Rubella
   D. Toxoplasmosis

10. Which of the following readings of the multiple marker screen test would be considered a precursor for a possible diagnosis of Down syndrome in the fetus?
    A. Low inhibin-A
    B. Low MSAFP
    C. Low hCG
    D. High UE

Chapter 53

Care of Women During Labor and Birth

KEY TERMS

Match each of the following key terms to its proper definition.

_____ 1. Effacement
_____ 2. Cephalopelvic disproportion
_____ 3. Prolapsed umbilical cord
_____ 4. Episiotomy
_____ 5. Breech
_____ 6. Lightening

A. Descent of the fetus into the pelvis that may occur as early as 2 to 4 weeks prior to the onset of labor
B. Umbilical cord positioned between the fetus and the cervix
C. The shortening and thinning of the cervix
D. Buttocks-first position of the fetus
E. Surgical cutting of the perineal tissue
F. Fetal head larger than the maternal pelvis

_____ 7. Fetal attitude
_____ 8. Cephalic presentation
_____ 9. Precipitous birth
_____ 10. Station
_____ 11. Dystocia

A. A birth that occurs rapidly, unexpectedly, and without the attention of a physician or nurse-midwife
B. Body part of the fetus that is closest to the cervix
C. A long, difficult, or abnormal labor pattern
D. Degree of flexion of the fetal head and limbs to the trunk
E. Head-down position of the fetus

| | 12. | Fetal presentation | F. | Relationship between the fetus and the maternal ischial spines |

	13.	Crowning	A.	Medications that inhibit contractions
	14.	Nuchal cord	B.	Entrance of the presenting part into the true pelvis
	15.	Tocolytic agents	C.	Relationship of the presenting part to the four quadrants of the maternal pelvis
	16.	Ferguson's reflex	D.	Umbilical cord
	17.	Engagement	E.	Point when the largest part of the fetal head is past the vulva and remains visible between contractions
	18.	Fetal position	F.	A spontaneous urge to push that occurs when the fetus touches the pelvic floor

LEARNING OUTCOMES

1. What describes the beginning of labor, and what are the variables that affect labor and birth?

Beginning of Labor	Variables

2. What are the stages and mechanisms of labor, and what are the important nursing interventions for each stage?

3. What are the nursing diagnoses, with appropriate nursing interventions, to assist the client in labor?

4. What is the role of the LPN/LVN in preparing the mother for birth and in providing infant care?

5. What are the causes of high-risk labor, and what are the nursing interventions for each?

APPLY WHAT YOU LEARNED

Jenna Cardona is a 22-year-old woman pregnant with her first baby. On her last visit to the obstetrician's office, she told the nurse how nervous she is about labor and delivery, and how glad she will be when it's all over and she's holding the baby. She asked the nurse if it would be possible to schedule a C-section instead of giving birth vaginally, which she thought would be far more convenient and less painful and frightening. The client also asked about delivering using Lamaze or Leboyer methods for delivery.

1. Is it appropriate to allow mothers-to-be to choose how they give birth (vaginal or C-section)? Why or why not?

2. Explain the use of Lamaze in labor and delivery.

3. Use the Internet to learn about the Leboyer method of delivery, and explain why this may be dangerous.

MULTIPLE CHOICE QUESTIONS

Circle the answer that best completes each of the following statements.

1. Which of the following would be a sign of impending labor?
   A. Braxton-Hicks contractions.
   B. The lengthening and thickening of the cervix.
   C. Sudden feelings of fatigue.
   D. The passage of the mucus plug from the cervix.

2. What is the most ideal position for a vaginal delivery?
   A. Occiput ROA
   B. Mentum RMA
   C. Sacrum LSP
   D. Breech

3. Which of the following may occur before the first contraction or during the first stage of labor?
   A. Crowning
   B. Engagement
   C. Extension
   D. Restitution

4. Which of the following nursing interventions would be effective when assisting the client in labor?
   A. Lie in the supine position to relieve pain.
   B. Provide only clear liquids to moisten the mouth late in labor.
   C. Encourage pushing between contractions.
   D. Promote use of breathing techniques.

5. Which of the following are roles of the LPN/LVN in preparing the mother for birth?
   A. Checking the functioning of all equipment in the birthing room.
   B. Providing assistance to the RN, client, and family.
   C. Administering IV push medications for pain control.
   D. Arranging the sterile instruments in the birthing room.
   E. Assessing fetal health.

6. The nurse is attending a high school football game when a pregnant woman, with a history of precipitous delivery, says the baby is coming. What is the nursing priority of care while assisting this woman?
   A. Have someone call EMS, and don't leave the mother if baby is crowning.
   B. Instruct the mother to take slow deep breaths.
   C. Apply firm pressure to the head of the fetus to stop it from being born.
   D. Clamp the umbilical cord but wait for EMS to cut it using sterile techniques.

7. What type of high risk labor and birth would require an immediate Cesarean section? (Select all that apply.)
   A. Precipitous birth
   B. Dystocia
   C. Prolapsed cord
   D. All malpresentation positions
   E. Mother's preference

8. During the recovery stage after labor, which of the following would be considered abnormal?
   A. The mother's fundus is soft, below the umbilicus, and in the midline.
   B. The perineal pad is saturated every 3 hours.
   C. The newborn is being kept in the room with the mother.
   D. The newborn has nasal milia.

9. Which of the following would be considered signs of false labor?
   A. The cervix shows progressive dilatation.
   B. The contractions are felt in the back or abdomen above the umbilicus.
   C. The cervix is in increasing anterior position.
   D. The contractions increase in intensity with walking.

10. Which of the following are achieved through contractions?
   A. The muscle fibers contract and relax in an irregular pattern.
   B. Uterine muscle fibers lengthen; the upper uterine segment relaxes, allowing the fetus to become stationed.
   C. Contractions allow for effacement and dilatation of the sphincter ani muscle.
   D. Begin in response to the posterior pituitary hormone oxytocin.

Chapter 54

Care of Postpartum Women

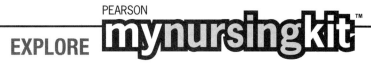

KEY TERMS

Match each of the following key terms to its proper definition.

____ 1.	Kegel	A.	Discomfort from uterine contractions after delivery
____ 2.	Engrossment	B.	Soft and spongy
____ 3.	Boggy	C.	Tissue that lines the uterine wall during pregnancy
____ 4.	Postpartum	D.	A sense of interest and preoccupation
____ 5.	Afterpain	E.	A return to normal size
____ 6.	Decidua	F.	An exercise used for the tightening and lifting of the muscles that cross the pelvic floor
____ 7.	Involution	G.	Discarded blood, mucus, and tissue
____ 8.	Lochia	H.	The period beginning immediately after delivery of the placenta and ending when the body and reproductive organs return to a near prepregnant state

LEARNING OUTCOMES

1. What physical changes occur after a woman delivers the baby and placenta?

2. What psychological changes occur in the postpartum woman?

3. What are the important aspects of support for the postpartum woman?

4. What are the nursing interventions used when providing care for a postpartum woman?

5. What are the methods for providing pain relief for the postpartum woman?

6. What are the crucial areas of client teaching for the postpartum woman?

7. What are the important factors in self-care for women after discharge?

8. What are the postpartum emergencies that the nurse should teach the client?

9. How does postpartum care differ when the client has delivered by Cesarean section?

10. What are the important nursing considerations regarding the new family?

11. What nursing care and teaching should be provided to the client in relation to breastfeeding?

APPLY WHAT YOU LEARNED

Joanne Peoples vaginally delivered an 8-pound, 10-ounce baby boy 3 days ago and is scheduled to go home later today. When the nurse enters her room, she is crying and tells the nurse, "I have decided not to breast feed after all. I don't know whether it's the baby that doesn't know what he's doing or me, but it just isn't working and I end up feeling like a terrible mother. It's a shame because I really looked forward to breast feeding, but I give up."

1. How should the nurse respond to this mother's statement?

2. What can the nurse do to improve this mother's breastfeeding attempts?

MULTIPLE CHOICE QUESTIONS

Circle the answer that best completes each of the following statements.

1. This condition presents itself after childbirth. It is attributed to the increased number of white blood cells being expelled from the uterus, and is white to yellowish in color.
   A. Lochia
   B. Lochia rubra
   C. Lochia alba
   D. Lochia serosa

2. During what stage of the psychological change process would the parents discover they desire social interactions with others?
   A. Taking-in stage
   B. Taking-out stage
   C. Letting-in stage
   D. Letting-go stage

3. How can the nurse help to build a support network for the postpartum woman? (Select all that apply.)
   A. Help the mother realize people want to help her during this time.
   B. Inquire about family and friends who might assist when she returns home.
   C. Explore specific ways that people can help.
   D. Suggest the mother compile a list of people who might help.
   E. Invite the mother to join the nurse for dinner after she feels better.

4. Which mnemonic is used when assessing the postpartum client?
   A. BOBBLE
   B. BUBBLE
   C. BUMBLE
   D. HUMBLE

5. The nurse receives orders from the physician for the postpartum client who delivered by Cesarean section 2 hours ago. Among the orders are several orders for analgesics, including ibuprofen, acetaminophen with codeine, morphine, and Darvocet N-100. While admitting the client to the unit, she reports pain as a 7 on a 1 to 10 scale. What analgesic will the nurse administer?
   A. Ibuprofen
   B. Acetaminophen with codeine
   C. Morphine
   D. Darvocet N-100

6. The nurse is providing discharge teaching for the postpartum client and includes which of the following?
   A. Drink at least 1000 mL of fluid per day.
   B. The breastfeeding mother should consume an additional 700 kcal per day.
   C. The diet should be low in fiber and high in fluids.
   D. The new mother should consume 125 g of protein per day.

7. What client teaching should the nurse provide for the postpartum client regarding self-care?
   A. Rest whenever she feels the need or gets the opportunity.
   B. Eat whenever she is hungry.
   C. Return to normal maintenance routines as soon as possible.
   D. Wait two weeks to begin simple postpartum exercises.

8. Which of the following should be considered a postpartum emergency by the mother?
   A. An axillary temperature of 100.2.
   B. Refusal to feed for 8 hours.
   C. Loose black or green watery stools.
   D. Six wet diapers in a 24-hour period.

9. Which of the following should be considered in the postpartum care of the client after a Cesarean section?
   A. Offer food or fluids immediately to aid in return of bowel sounds.
   B. A few women feel very little pain and require little pain medication.
   C. A complete absence of lochia is normal following a Cesarean section.
   D. The client will usually have an indwelling catheter for 24 to 48 hours.

10. What information should the nurse provide the client about breastfeeding?
    A. Breastfed babies are more likely to experience constipation.
    B. Breast milk can cause allergies in newborns.
    C. Suckling a baby promotes expansion of the uterus after delivery of the placenta.
    D. Breastfeeding provides natural immunity for the newborn because of passed antibodies.

Chapter 55

Care of High-Risk Postpartum Women

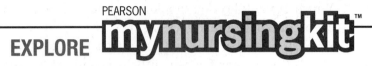

EXPLORE **PEARSON** **mynursingkit**™

MyNursingKit is your one stop for online chapter review materials and resources. Prepare for success with additional NCLEX®-style practice questions, interactive assignments and activities, web links, animations and videos, and more!

Register your access code from the front of your book at
www.mynursingkit.com

KEY TERMS

Match each of the following key terms to its proper definition.

_____ 1. Mastitis

_____ 2. Endometritis

_____ 3. Uterine atony

_____ 4. Clonus

_____ 5. Subinvolution

_____ 6. Postpartum depression

A. Failure of the uterus to contract following birth

B. Failure of the uterus to return to its normal size

C. A major mood disorder that most frequently appears 4 weeks post delivery and upon weaning the child from the breast

D. Infection of the breast

E. Infection usually begins in the vagina and migrates upward into the uterus

F. A series of abnormal reflex movements of the foot in response to sudden dorsiflexion

LEARNING OUTCOMES

1. What are the signs and symptoms of potential complications in the postpartum period?

2. What assessments are indicated for the postpartum client diagnosed with preeclampsia during pregnancy?

3. What are the nursing interventions for clients with postpartum bleeding and other complications?

4. What are the signs and symptoms of postpartum infections?

5. What are the differences among postpartum blues, depression, and psychosis?

Postpartum Blues	Depression	Psychosis

6. What are the family care needs when the mother dies?

APPLY WHAT YOU LEARNED

Natashia O'Donnell is brought to the postpartum unit 4 hours after delivering twins by spontaneous vaginal delivery. These are her first children. She is assisted into bed and says, "Oh, this feels so good. I'm exhausted. I feel like I could sleep for 2 days." After helping her get comfortable, the nurse asks about the babies and learns they are identical twin girls who weighed 6 pounds, 8 ounces, and 8 pounds, 2 ounces.

1. What assessments will the nurse initially perform upon admitting this client to the postpartum unit?

2. If this mother chooses to breast feed, what instructions will the nurse provide specific to nursing twins?

MULTIPLE CHOICE QUESTIONS

Circle the answer that best completes each of the following statements.

1. The nurse checks the urine of the postpartum client diagnosed with preeclampsia for:
   A. Ketones.
   B. Amniotic fluid.
   C. Blood.
   D. Protein.

2. The nurse knows that that the mother's blood pressure may elevate during labor, but should return to prebirth measurement within an hour after birth. If her blood pressure remains elevated after an hour, how often should it be rechecked?
   A. Every 2 hours
   B. Every hour
   C. Every 4 hours
   D. Every 6 hours

3. What can result from prolonged third-stage labor, intrauterine infections, and/or oxytocin administration for labor augmentation?
   A. Postpartum hemorrhage
   B. Subinvolution
   C. Uterine atony
   D. Vaginal hematomas

4. The nurse teaches the mother to report fever of 100.4 or higher, chills, abdominal pain, or foul-smelling lochia because they may indicate:
   A. Laceration infection
   B. Puerperal infection
   C. Episiotomy infection
   D. Thromboembolic disease

5. What score on the Edinburgh Postnatal Depression Scale would be considered the threshold for concern that the client is suffering from postpartum depression?
   A. 12 to 13 out of 30
   B. 6 to 7 out of 30
   C. 15 to 16 out of 30
   D. 10 to 11 out of 30

6. The nurse cared for a woman who died after delivery of a healthy newborn. What actions should the nurse take? (Select all that apply.)
   A. Give detailed explanations of the pathology and treatment provided to the client so the family understands.
   B. Provide referrals to social services to follow up with the family and provide support as needed.
   C. Attend a critical incident debriefing with other team members who provided care to this client.
   D. Offer to help the family by providing child care during the nurse's off hours.
   E. Attend the client's funeral with other members of the healthcare team.

7. The nurse, working in the obstetrician's office, admits a client who is 6 weeks postpartum and reports breast pain. Upon examination, the nurse finds an irregularly shaped area on the outer aspect of the left breast that is red, warm to touch, painful, and edematous. The nurse suspects a diagnosis of:
   A. Mastitis.
   B. Thromboembolic disease.
   C. Milk stasis.
   D. Septicemia.

8. What would be a suggestive sign of subinvolution?
   A. Sanguineous drainage
   B. Lochia rubra that continues longer than 2 weeks
   C. Scarce or black lochia
   D. Headache

9. What type of hemorrhage is considered the most dangerous?
   A. Vulvar hematoma
   B. Vaginal hematoma
   C. Pelvic hematoma
   D. Postpartum hemorrhage

10. What occurs in most women beginning a few days after childbirth and can be related to changes in estrogen, progesterone, and prolactin levels?
   A. Endometritis
   B. Lactation
   C. Uterine atony
   D. Postpartum blues

Chapter 56

Care of Normal Neonates

KEY TERMS

Match each of the following key terms to its proper definition.

_____ 1. Pseudomenstruation

_____ 2. Lanugo

_____ 3. Witch's milk

_____ 4. Retractions

_____ 5. Vernix

_____ 6. Milia

A. Soft downy hair present on the fetus's or newborn's face, arms, and back

B. Inward movement of the tissues over the chest

C. White pinpoint spots resembling whiteheads that appear on the neonate's face a few days after birth

D. White, cheesy covering of the fetal or newborn skin

E. Mucus or slightly bloody vaginal discharge which may be present in female newborns and disappears in a few days; related to the influence of maternal hormones

F. Whitish fluid that may be secreted by newborn's nipples

____ 7.	Moro reflex	A.	Reaction that occurs when the newborn's cheek is stroked; the head will turn to the side that was stroked
____ 8.	Rooting reflex	B.	Reaction that occurs when the sole of the neonate's foot is touched; the toes curl under as if newborns are trying to "grasp" with their feet
____ 9.	Cephalhematoma	C.	Reaction in which newborns step as if walking when their feet touch a hard surface
____ 10.	Tonic neck reflex	D.	Reaction that occurs when newborns have a sense of falling; they will quickly extend the arms with fingers flared and thumb and first finger forming a "C"
____ 11.	Plantar grasp reflex	E.	Reaction that occurs when the head is turned to one side; newborns will extend the arm and leg on that side
____ 12.	Stepping reflex	F.	An accumulation of blood between the periosteum and the skull bone

____ 13.	Epstein's pearls	A.	Periods without breathing
____ 14.	Acrocyanosis	B.	Dark red spots on the eyelids, forehead, or nape of the neck
____ 15.	Mongolian spot	C.	A condition caused by excess bilirubin in the blood
____ 16.	Stork bites	D.	A dark discolored area found over the lower back and sacrum of infants of Black, Hispanic, south Asian, or east Asian descent
____ 17.	Apneic spells	E.	A bluish discoloration of the hands and feet, common for several hours after delivery
____ 18.	Jaundice	F.	Small white cysts that may be present on the newborn's palate but disappear in a few weeks

LEARNING OUTCOMES

1. What are the physiologic adaptations of the neonate?

2. How is the Apgar score used, and by what method is it obtained?

3. What are the aspects of delivery room care and nursing interventions for the neonate?

4. What nursery care will the nurse provide to the neonate?

5. What are the differences that identify the gestational age of the neonate?

6. What are the physical characteristics of the neonate?

7. What are the proper hygiene methods used in caring for a newborn?

8. How do the two methods of providing neonatal nutrition compare, and how do they contrast?

Methods	Pros	Cons
Breast Feeding		
Bottle Feeding		

9. What common procedures are used when caring for the newborn?

10. What client teaching should the nurse provide to the parent of a newborn who is being discharged?

APPLY WHAT YOU LEARNED

The nurse is preparing to discharge several clients from the postpartum unit with their newborns today. One client is Fran Snyder, who has just delivered her fourth child. Her other children are 6 years, 4 years, and 18 months of age. She is married and plans to return to work full-time when the baby is 6 weeks old. Another client to be discharged is Brittany Timberlake, who is 16 years old and delivered her son via Cesarean section. This is her first baby and she will not have the father's involvement.

1. How will client teaching on care of the newborn differ between these two mothers?

2. How will information provided be similar for bother mothers?

MULTIPLE CHOICE QUESTIONS

Circle the answer that best completes each of the following statements.

1. What is the earliest sign that the infant may be having difficulty maintaining gas exchange?
    A. Expiratory grunting
    B. Retraction of the skin over the ribs
    C. Flaring of the nostrils
    D. Retraction of the skin over the sternum

2. What Apgar score would require emergency newborn care?
    A. 4 to 7
    B. 5 to 8
    C. 2 to 3
    D. 8 to 10

3. Which of the following procedures are preformed in the delivery room?
   A. Examine newborn for gestational age and any congenital problems.
   B. Apply identification bands to mother and child verifying identical numbers.
   C. Provide skin care and bathe the infant to remove vernix and secretions.
   D. Obtain length, height, and head circumference of the infant.

4. Which of the following are safety precautions for protecting the neonate in the mother-baby unit? (Select all that apply.)
   A. Limiting access to the nursery and the obstetric unit
   B. Security banding the infant
   C. Holding the infant with both hands when transporting from nursery to mother's room
   D. Teaching parent to not give infant to anyone who doesn't have proper identification
   E. Placing the infant on a radiant warmer to perform all procedures

5. The neonate's gestational age was determined by calculating from the mother's reported last menstrual period. The nurse recognizes this method of calculating gestational age is likely to be how accurate?
   A. 80 to 90%
   B. 65 to 75%
   C. 85 to 95%
   D. 75 to 85%

6. Which of the following are common and normal skin alterations found on the skin of a full-term neonate?
   A. Strabismus
   B. Telangiectatic nevi
   C. Lanugo
   D. Epstein's pearls
   E. Milia

7. When can the newborn be placed in a tub of water?
   A. After the infant's temperature has stabilized
   B. Immediately after birth to remove the vernix from the newborn
   C. After the umbilical cord falls off
   D. Reserve till right before discharge

8. The highest concentration of calories, protein, and immunities are found in:
   A. Witch's milk
   B. Colostrum
   C. Meconium
   D. Chloasma

9. This common procedure is required by law in all 50 states and must be preformed after the neonate has been fed.
   A. Bilirubin test
   B. Serum glucose level
   C. Newborn screening
   D. Newborn urine screening

10. When preparing the parent to take their newborn home, the nurse teaches which of the following? (Select all that apply.)
    A. Placing infant on stomach to sleep.
    B. Umbilical cord care.
    C. Diapering.
    D. Don't leave child unattended on high surfaces unless secured in an infant carrier.
    E. Wake the baby at night to feed every 3 hours.

Chapter 57

Care of the High Risk Neonate

KEY TERMS

Match each of the following key terms to its proper definition.

_____ 1. Meningocele

_____ 2. Circumoral

_____ 3. Logan

_____ 4. Macrosomia

_____ 5. Meningomyelocele

_____ 6. Omphalocele

_____ 7. Talipes

_____ 8. Trisomy

_____ 9. BPD

_____ 10. SGA

A. Also called clubfoot; a twisting of the foot, usually inward

B. Abbreviation for term describing infants who weigh less than anticipated for their gestational age

C. Congenital malformation of abdominal wall, allowing contents to herniate into umbilical cord

D. Chromosomal abnormality involving the 21st chromosome in Down syndrome

E. Herniation of the meninges through a vertebral defect

F. Abbreviation for condition of permanent lung disease resulting from damage to the alveoli

G. Cyanosis around the mouth

H. Conditions of the newborn whose birth weight is over the 90th percentile

I. Herniation of the spinal nerves as well as the meninges through a vertebral defect

J. Type of clamp used in the surgery to close a cleft lip

LEARNING OUTCOMES

1. What factors cause a newborn to be classified as "high risk," and what is the role the LPN/LVN plays in relation to caring for the high-risk neonate?

2. What type of general care is required by the high-risk newborn?

3. Contrast the physiological characteristics of the preterm and postterm newborn.

4. Contrast appearance and nursing considerations for the large-for-gestational-age with the small-for-gestational-age newborn.

5. Describe common respiratory conditions of the high-risk newborn and the nursing care required.

6. Name six congenital heart defects and describe nursing care for each.

7. List common congenital nervous system defects and treatment for each.

8. Identify current treatment for congenital gastrointestinal conditions.

Condition	Treatment
Tracheoesophageal fistula and esophageal atresia	
Omphalocele	
Imperforate anus	

9. Explain special care needed by a newborn with an inborn error of metabolism.

Inborn Error of Metabolism	Special Care Needed
Phenylketonuria	
Galactosemia	
Maple syrup urine disease	

10. Identify congenital genitourinary or musculoskeletal disorders and nursing considerations for each.

11. Explain the special care needed by a drug-exposed newborn.

12. Describe priorities of care for a neonate at risk for infection, and measures to be taken to reduce the risk of infection.

APPLY WHAT YOU LEARNED

Baby Girl Barker was born at 27 weeks' gestation. Within a week of birth, she had surgery to close a persistent ductus arteriosus and flourished after the surgery. She is currently 7 weeks old and has been successfully bottle feeding twice a day, with other feedings given via an indwelling nasogastric feeding tube. She required mechanical ventilation for the first 5 days of life, was given artificial surfactant via the endotracheal tube, and gradually weaned from the ventilator. She is currently receiving oxygen via nasal cannula and experiences periodic apneic episodes, for which she is receiving oral caffeine twice a day.

The neonate is being transferred to the observation nursery where you work to gain weight and prepare for eventual discharge. Answer the following questions about the care you will deliver.

1. What specific strategies will you employ to reduce the risk of infection for this neonate?

2. What teaching will her parents require before they take her home?

3. Shortly after admission you overhear the mother, while holding and rocking the baby, whisper, "I'm so sorry I put you through this. I should have taken more care to prevent delivering early." How will you respond to this mother's statement?

4. Prior to administering a tube feeding, what actions will you take?

MULTIPLE CHOICE QUESTIONS

Circle the answer that best completes each of the following statements.

1. The nurse is caring for a baby who has been vomiting, has diarrhea, doesn't eat well, is hypoglycemic, and has an enlarged liver. What disease does the nurse suspect?
    A. Phenylketonuria
    B. Galactosemia
    C. Maple syrup urine disease
    D. Neonatal abstinence syndrome

2. Which of the following pregnancies would cause the healthcare team to anticipate delivery of a high-risk neonate?
   A. The woman who is expecting the birth of her 5th child.
   B. The woman who is 41 weeks pregnant when she begins labor.
   C. The woman who arrives in labor at 38 weeks pregnant.
   D. The woman who is pregnant with triplets.

3. When caring for an infant who is large for gestational age, a priority nursing action is to:
   A. Place the baby in a heated isolette or on a radiant warmer to maintain temperature.
   B. Avoid bathing the infant to prevent further drying of the skin.
   C. Apply a moisturizing lotion to the skin.
   D. Monitor blood sugar levels.

4. The nurse is providing general care for the high-risk newborn, including which of the following? (Select all that apply.)
   A. Administering tube feedings
   B. Bathing the newborn
   C. Repositioning every 2 hours
   D. Suctioning the airway as needed
   E. Providing wound care

5. The nurse is caring for a premature infant who requires high-percentage oxygen therapy and mechanical ventilation for several weeks. The nurse recognizes this treatment places the infant at increased risk for development of:
   A. Bronchopulmonary dysplasia
   B. Meconium aspiration
   C. Lung cancer
   D. Umbilical hernia

6. The nurse is caring for a newborn who is very irritable, cannot be soothed with usual calming techniques (holding, swaddling, pacifier), temperature instability, diaphoresis, and has a high-pitched cry. The nurse would anticipate which of the following orders?
   A. Increased feeding volume
   B. Drug screen
   C. Metabolic screening
   D. Sedation

7. Which of the following symptoms, if demonstrated by the previously stable newborn, would the nurse interpret as a possible indication of neonatal infection?
   A. Hypothermia, apneic episodes, and lethargy
   B. Increased hunger and extended periods of quiet alert time
   C. Spitting up of small amounts of formula when burped
   D. Jittery movements of the hands and legs

8. The nurse is caring for an infant with a congenital heart defect. When assessing this infant, a priority assessment would include which of the following?
   A. Bowel sounds
   B. Capillary refill time
   C. Gentle palpation of fontanels
   D. Temperature

9. When caring for an infant with a large cleft lip and palate, a priority parent teaching point would be which of the following?
   A. Feeding technique
   B. Diaper care
   C. Use of a car seat
   D. Infection prevention

10. The nurse is examining a neonate recently admitted to the high-risk nursery and finds an absence of creases on the sole of the infant's foot, very flexible cartilage of the earlobe, floppy muscle tone, and extended extremities. These findings lead the nurse to classify this infant as:
    A. Small for gestational age
    B. Postterm
    C. Preterm
    D. Large for gestational age

Chapter 58

Pediatric-Focused Nursing Care

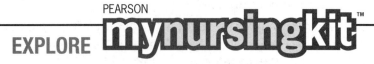

PEARSON
EXPLORE **mynursingkit**™

MyNursingKit is your one stop for online chapter review materials and resources. Prepare for success with additional NCLEX®-style practice questions, interactive assignments and activities, web links, animations and videos, and more!

Register your access code from the front of your book at
www.mynursingkit.com

KEY TERMS

Match each of the following key terms to its proper definition.

_____ 1. Epiphyseal plate   A. Structure that consists of the bones of the arms and legs

_____ 2. Scoliosis   B. Condition in which the sternum protrudes, causing an increase in the anteroposterior diameter

_____ 3. Appendicular skeleton   C. A lateral deviation of the spine

_____ 4. Funnel chest   D. A layer of cartilage in the metaphysis of the bone

_____ 5. Pigeon chest   E. Condition in which the lower portion of the sternum is depressed

---

_____ 6. Autonomy   A. Membranous gaps in the bone structure of the skull

_____ 7. Mainstreaming   B. Information that helps parents prepare for expected physical and behavioral changes during their child's or teen's current and approaching stages of development

_____ 8. Anticipatory guidance   C. Movement to increase community service over institutional service in order to provide the developmentally disabled with the least restrictive environment

_____ 9. Fontanels   D. The right and ability to make one's own decisions

LEARNING OUTCOMES

1. What are the differences between body systems of the pediatric client and the adult client?

2. What are the unique aspects of collecting data for a pediatric assessment by age group?

3. What are effective strategies for collecting data about vital signs, pain, and growth in pediatric clients?

4. What adaptations will you make when providing nursing care to pediatric clients?

5. What are important considerations when providing nursing care to hospitalized pediatric clients and their families?

6. What teaching strategies will you use when caring for children at different developmental ages?

7. What are the physical and psychosocial needs of the terminally ill pediatric client?

8. What are the psychosocial needs of chronically ill pediatric clients and their families?

9. What tools and programs are available for pediatric clients with developmental or cognitive issues?

10. How do the terms *mainstreaming* and *normalization* relate to developmental disabilities?

APPLY WHAT YOU LEARNED

Jay, 8 years old, was diagnosed with leukemia and required a bone marrow transplant when his disease did not respond to traditional treatment. He is now 6 months posttransplant, and is being treated for a life-threatening septicemia that is not responding to antibiotic therapy. The nurse is sitting with Jay's mother when the provider tells her that Jay is not likely to survive the infection. The provider recommends contacting the family and preparing for Jay's imminent death.

1. What is the nurse's role with this family?

MULTIPLE CHOICE QUESTIONS

Circle the answer that best completes each of the following statements.

1. Why are infants and small children more likely to choke than an adult?
   A. Immature swallowing reflex
   B. Excess oral and respiratory secretions
   C. Narrow airways
   D. Immature breathing reflexes

2. Which age group responds particularly well to positive reinforcement used when good behavior is demonstrated?
   A. Toddler
   B. Preschooler
   C. School-age children
   D. Adolescent

3. What type of pulse is difficult to access in an infant?
   A. Apical
   B. Biracial
   C. Carotid
   D. Temporal

4. At what age can children begin to play a role in managing their own long-term drug therapy?
   A. Adolescents
   B. Preschoolers
   C. Teens
   D. School-age children

5. What age group has an increased need for autonomy that must be considered and planned for by the nurse when the child is hospitalized ?
   A. Toddler
   B. Preschooler
   C. School-age child
   D. Adolescent

6. The use of puppets can be an effective teaching strategy when the nurse provides health teaching to what age group?
   A. Toddlers
   B. Preschoolers
   C. School-age
   D. Adolescents

7. When caring for a terminally ill pediatric client, the nurse is best able to meet psychosocial needs by:
   A. Providing detailed explanations of everything that is going to happen.
   B. Asking many questions and probing for more details.
   C. Limiting visitors so the client is more likely to talk to the nurses.
   D. Listening to what the client is saying and what they are not saying.

8. When caring for a child with a chronic illness, the child's psychosocial needs can best be met by which of the following? (Select all that apply.)
   A. Clearly and honestly answer the child's questions.
   B. Provide information they need to know in understandable terminology.
   C. Explore the child's understanding of what is occurring.
   D. Always accompany parents when they talk with the child about healthcare.
   E. Encourage children to participate in their own care.

9. Which developmental screening test focuses on the child's ability to learn rather than what the child already knows?
   A. The DDST II
   B. Vineland Adaptive Behavior Scale
   C. Screening Test for Evaluating Preschoolers
   D. The Early Screening Inventory

10. Which of the following are important in normalization of a child with special needs? (Select all that apply.)
    A. Encourage handicapped behavioral patterns.
    B. Encourage the child to become as self-sufficient as possible.
    C. Expect behavior as normal as possible from the time the child is born.
    D. Use discipline and child management techniques as for any other child.
    E. Console the child by telling them they are special with limited ability when frustrations occur.

Chapter 59

Care and Illnesses of Infants and Toddlers (1 Month to 36 Months)

KEY TERMS

Match each of the following key terms to its proper definition.

_____ 1. Hypospadias
_____ 2. Epispadias

_____ 3. Separation anxiety
_____ 4. Cryptorchidism

_____ 5. Shaken baby syndrome

_____ 6. Hydrocele

A. Undescended testicles
B. Closed head injury that is a result of head trauma, either from an external force such as a fall or an internal force
C. An accumulation of fluid in the scrotal sac
D. Condition in which the urinary meatus opens onto the ventral surface of the penis
E. Condition in which the urethral meatus opens onto the dorsal surface of the penis
F. A state of extreme discomfort an infant or toddler experiences when separated from loved ones

_____ 7. Echolalia

_____ 8. Pica

A. A term representing a group of respiratory illnesses that result from inflammation and swelling of the epiglottis, larynx, trachea, and bronchi
B. Distention of the renal pelvis caused by increased pressure due to urine backup

_____ 9. Colic

_____ 10. Hydronephrosis

_____ 11. Nephroblastoma

_____ 12. Croup

C. A highly metastatic cancerous tumor of the kidney

D. A condition in which words are incessantly repeated

E. Abdominal pain caused by periodic spasm of the intestines

F. A craving to eat substances that are not food

LEARNING OUTCOMES

1. What are the elements of good nutrition for infants and toddlers?

2. What are normal vital sign ranges for infants and toddlers?

3. What are the important intervals for well-child checkups for infants and toddlers?

4. What are the common respiratory, cardiovascular, hematologic, and immune disorders diagnosed in newborns and toddlers, and what nursing care would you provide for each?

	Disorders	Description	Nursing Care
Respiratory			
Cardiovascular			
Hematologic			
Immune Disorders			

5. What are the common neurologic, sensory, and musculoskeletal disorders seen in newborns and toddlers, and what nursing care would you provide for each?

	Disorders	Description	Nursing Care
Neurologic			
Sensory			
Musculoskeletal			

6. What are the common gastrointestinal and endocrine disorders seen in infants and toddlers, and what nursing care would you provide for each?

Gastrointestinal	Endocrine Disorders	Nursing Care

7. What are the common urinary and reproductive disorders seen in newborns and infants, and what nursing care do they require?

	Disorder	Description	Nursing Care
Urinary			
Reproductive			

8. What are common integumentary disorders seen in newborns and toddlers, and what nursing care would you provide?

9. What are common psychosocial disorders seen in newborns and toddlers, and what nursing care would you provide?

APPLY WHAT YOU LEARNED

The nurse, working in a pediatric clinic, admits a 6-month-old with excoriated skin in the diaper area (diaper dermatitis) that is draining a yellow clear fluid. Touching the area, even gently, causes the infant to cry in pain. When questioned about the rash the mother says, "Oh, yeah, I noticed that. I guess it's just one of those things that happen when babies mess their diapers so often." The nurse asks the mother what diapers she has been using and the mother says, "I buy whatever is cheapest or on sale. Diapers are really expensive." The nurse next asks how often the mother is changing the diaper and the mother says, "I change it in the morning and at night before bed, and then maybe once during the day if it stinks."

1. What concerns might the nurse have and what client teaching is required?

MULTIPLE CHOICE QUESTIONS

Circle the answer that best completes each of the following statements.

1. At what age should the infant or toddler begin to use the pincer grasp?
   A. 8 to 10 months
   B. 4 to 6 months
   C. 6 to 8 months
   D. 10 to 12 months

2. Which of the following vital signs in a newborn would be a concern to the nurse?
   A. Temperature – 36.8 degrees Celsius
   B. Pulse – 179
   C. Blood pressure – 70/42
   D. Respirations – 24

3. By the age of 2 months, the infant should have 2 doses of what vaccination?
   A. Measles/mumps/rubella
   B. Polio
   C. Hepatitis B
   D. Diphtheria/tetanus/pertussis

4. What respiratory disorder is diagnosed by a positive sweat test?
   A. Whooping cough
   B. Cystic fibrosis
   C. Respiratory syncytial virus
   D. Bronchopulmonary dysplasia

5. What nervous system disorder can be caused by low birth weight in premature babies, an incompatibility between the blood of the mother and the fetus, or insufficient oxygen reaching the fetus?
   A. Cerebral palsy
   B. Down syndrome
   C. Reye's syndrome
   D. Mental retardation

6. What gastrointestinal disorder is corrected with the aid of a Logan clamp after surgery?
   A. Cleft lip
   B. Gastroesophageal reflux disease
   C. Biliary atresia
   D. Intussusception

7. What reproductive disorder is a diagnosis of balanoposthitis associated with?
   A. Balanoposthitis
   B. Phimosis
   C. Cryptorchidism
   D. Testicular cancer

8. What integumentary disorder would be described if the manifestations were redness, edema, blistering and infection with *Candida albicans* at the site?
   A. Seborrheic dermatitis
   B. Herpes simplex
   C. Diaper dermatitis
   D. Contact dermatitis

9. The nurse is assessing the height and weight of the 10-month-old who is trembling and crying and cannot be consoled by the nurse. The nurse suspects these symptoms indicate (select all that apply):
   A. Shaken baby syndrome
   B. Stranger anxiety
   C. Separation anxiety
   D. Fetal alcohol syndrome
   E. Autism

10. Infants of Native American descent, premature infants with low birth weight, babies exposed to passive smoke, and children born to mothers less than 20 years of age are all at increased risk of:
    A. Sudden infant death syndrome
    B. Myelominingocele
    C. Respiratory syncytial virus
    D. Bronchopulmonary dysplasia

Chapter 60

Care and Illnesses of Preschoolers (3 to 6 Years)

PEARSON

EXPLORE **mynursingkit**™

MyNursingKit is your one stop for online chapter review materials and resources. Prepare for success with additional NCLEX®-style practice questions, interactive assignments and activities, web links, animations and videos, and more!

Register your access code from the front of your book at
www.mynursingkit.com

KEY TERMS

Match each of the following key terms to its proper definition.

_____ 1. Encopresis	A. An increased amount of blood in the conjunctivae
_____ 2. Hyphema	B. Surgical removal of the palatine and pharyngeal tonsils
_____ 3. Tonsillectomy and adenoidectomy	C. Condition associated with constipation and fecal retention in which watery stools bypass the hard fecal mass and may be confused with diarrhea
_____ 4. Conjunctival hyperemia	D. A deficiency in protein in the diet that results in muscle wasting
_____ 5. Kwashiorkor	E. Hemorrhage into the anterior chamber of the eye

_____ 6. Pediculosis	A. Sex-linked recessive disorder carried by mothers and passed to their sons
_____ 7. Ringworm	B. Urinary incontinence after voluntary control has normally been reached
_____ 8. Duchenne's muscular dystrophy	C. Condition that occurs when increased pressure in a limited space compromises circulation and nerve function, leading to possible necrosis

_____ 9. Enuresis

D. Term for some tinea infections

_____ 10. Compartment
syndrome

E. An infestation with lice

LEARNING OUTCOMES

1. What are the growth and development milestones for preschoolers?

2. What are the elements of good nutrition, and what are the normal vital sign ranges for preschoolers?

3. What are the common respiratory and communicable disorders diagnosed in preschoolers, and what nursing care would be appropriate?

Respiratory	Communicable	Appropriate Care

4. What are the common cardiovascular, hematologic, and immune disorders diagnosed in preschoolers, and what is the nursing care appropriate for them?

Cardiovascular	Hematologic	Immune	Nursing Care

5. What are the common neurosensory disorders diagnosed in preschoolers, and what is the appropriate nursing care for them?

6. What are the common musculoskeletal, gastrointestinal, endocrine, and genitourinary disorders diagnosed in preschoolers, and what is the appropriate nursing care for them?

	Disorder	Description	Nursing Care
Musculoskeletal			
Gastrointestinal			
Endocrine			
Genitourinary			

7. What are the integumentary disorders seen in preschoolers, and what is the appropriate nursing care for them?

8. What are the psychosocial conditions commonly diagnosed in preschoolers, and what is the nursing care for them?

Frank is 4 years old and comes home from preschool telling his mother he doesn't feel well. He declines dinner and just seems to want to lie on the couch and watch TV. When getting him ready for bed, his mother notices he feels warm and takes his temperature, obtaining a reading of 101.2 oral. She gives him some ibuprofen before putting him to bed in his summer pajamas and 20 minutes later, hears him vomiting. Frank vomits 6 times in the next 4 hours and also has 12 diarrhea stools. After 4 hours, he seems to feel less sick to his stomach and his episodes of diarrhea reduce to once per hour. The mother calls the clinic and asks what she should do. The doctor tells the nurse to give advice based on suspected gastroenteritis.

1. What information will the nurse provide to this mother?

MULTIPLE CHOICE QUESTIONS

Circle the answer that best completes each of the following statements.

1. Which of the following is a developmental milestone for preschoolers?
   A. Can draw 5-part stick person
   B. Can prepare own food
   C. Gains 7 to 12 kg per year
   D. Uses knife, fork, and spoon

2. What dietary need can lead to interference with the absorption of iron if taken in excess in the preschooler?
   A. Fiber
   B. Calcium
   C. Protein
   D. Sugar

3. The nurse provides special skin care to the child whose skin is sloughing and limits environmental lighting when diagnosed with:
   A. Mumps
   B. Rubella
   C. Measles
   D. Varicella

4. What religion allows organ transplantation as long as all of the blood is drained from the organ prior to transplantation?
   A. Judaism
   B. Seventh-Day Adventists
   C. Jehovah's Witnesses
   D. Christian Scientists

5. What type of brain tumor is categorized by seizures, increased intracranial pressure, and visual disturbances?
   A. Astrocytoma
   B. Brainstem glioma
   C. Ependymoma
   D. Medulloblastoma

6. When caring for a child with this infection of the bone, the nurse recognizes it is very difficult to treat and can lead to amputation.
   A. Legg-Calvé-Perthes disease
   B. Muscular dystrophy
   C. Osteomyelitis
   D. Salter-Harris classification

7. What causes the integumentary disorder of dermatophytes?
   A. Lice
   B. Parasites
   C. Overexposure to low environmental temperatures
   D. Fungal infections

8. What common thought process disorder has the symptoms of repetitive behaviors and sensitivity to tactile stimuli?
   A. Asperger's syndrome
   B. Autism
   C. Rett's syndrome
   D. Down syndrome

9. What nutritional disorder is caused by a lack of vitamin C in the diet?
   A. Kwashiorkor
   B. Scurvy
   C. Rickets
   D. Giardiasis

10. The child in traction with symptoms of deep pain unrelieved by analgesia, lack of sensation, and edema may be suffering from:
    A. Closed reduction
    B. Musculoskeletal trauma
    C. Open reduction
    D. Compartment syndrome

Chapter 61

Care and Illnesses of School-Age Children (6 to 12 Years)

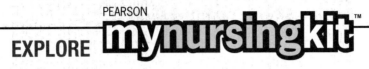

EXPLORE PEARSON mynursingkit™

MyNursingKit is your one stop for online chapter review materials and resources. Prepare for success with additional NCLEX®-style practice questions, interactive assignments and activities, web links, animations and videos, and more!

Register your access code from the front of your book at **www.mynursingkit.com**

KEY TERMS

Match each of the following key terms to its proper definition.

____ 1. Hyperopia	A.	A reduction in vision in which there is no pathology in the eye
____ 2. Rhabdomyosarcoma	B.	Visual disturbances that occur when light rays do not uniformly focus on the eye due to abnormal curvature of cornea or lens
____ 3. Astigmatism	C.	A malignant tumor found most commonly in the femur, pelvis, tibia, fibula, ribs, humerus, scapula, and clavicle
____ 4. Precocious puberty	D.	Visual disturbance that occurs when light is focused behind the retina
____ 5. Amblyopia	E.	Visual disturbance that occurs when light is focused in front of the retina
____ 6. Myopia	F.	The presence of any secondary sex characteristics before the age of 8 in girls and before the age of 9 in boys
____ 7. Ewing's sarcoma	G.	A malignant tumor originating in the muscle around the eye, in the neck, and less commonly in the abdomen, genitourinary tract, and extremities

LEARNING OUTCOMES

1. What are the milestones, nutritional requirements, and normal vital signs for school-age children?

Milestones	Nutritional	Vital Signs

2. What are the common respiratory, cardiovascular, hematologic, and immune disorders, and associated nursing care, that affect school-age children?

	Disorder	Description	Nursing Care
Respiratory			
Cardiovascular			
Hematologic			
Immune			

3. What are the common neurologic and musculoskeletal disorders that affect school-age children, and what is the nursing care for them?

Neurologic	Musculoskeletal	Nursing Care

4. What are the common gastrointestinal and endocrine disorders that affect school-age children, and what is the nursing care for them?

Gastrointestinal	Endocrine	Nursing Care

5. What are the common urinary and reproductive disorders that affect school-age children, and what is the nursing care for them?

Urinary	Reproductive	Nursing Care

6. What are the common integumentary disorders that affect school-age children, and what is the nursing care for them?

7. What are the psychosocial conditions that affect school-age children, and what is the nursing care for them?

APPLY WHAT YOU LEARNED

Michael is an 11-year-old boy who was brought to the doctor's office because he had pain in his upper right thigh. His mother reports that he was playing football with his friends a few weeks ago and assumed the pain was related to that event, but it has not improved and seems to be getting worse. The provider orders an MRI, then performs a biopsy before confirming that Michael has a Ewing's sarcoma in the right femur. The provider explains that the best option to save Michael's life is to amputate the leg, going on to say that traditional cancer therapies have not proven successful with this form of cancer unless amputation is performed to remove the source of the malignant cells. The provider asks if they have any questions and the family just stares at the provider mutely. After the provider leaves the room the family begins to cry and the mother keeps telling Michael she's sorry.

1. Why would Michael's mother feel the need to apologize? How can the nurse explore what she is feeling?

2. Based on Michael's age and development, what special needs will he have after the amputation is completed?

3. How can the nurse best help and support this family right now as they adjust to the news of the need for surgery?

MULTIPLE CHOICE QUESTIONS

Circle the answer that best completes each of the following statements.

1. The nurse is presented with an 8-year-old child whose vital signs are 37 degrees oral, pulse 75, respirations 24, and blood pressure 120/80. Which vital sign would the nurse be most concerned with?
   A. Pulse
   B. Temperature
   C. Blood pressure
   D. Respirations

2. The nurse sees a child with chorea and anticipates a diagnosis of:
   A. Tuberculosis
   B. Acute rheumatic fever
   C. Anemia
   D. Hyperlipidemia

3. Which of the following spinal conditions is associated with the excessive convex curvature of the thoracic spine?
   A. Kyphosis
   B. Lordosis
   C. Scoliosis
   D. Amblyopia

4. The nurse examines a child with symptoms of weight loss, poor wound healing, and polydipsia. The nurse would suspect which of the following diseases?
   A. Hyperlipidemia
   B. Diabetes mellitus
   C. Acute rheumatic fever
   D. MRSA

5. Edema, pale skin, tachycardia, and hypertension are classic symptoms of:
   A. Jaundice
   B. Diabetes mellitus
   C. Precocious puberty
   D. Renal failure

6. What disease is resistant to all penicillins and cephalosporins, and can be easily prevented with hand washing and following standard precautions?
   A. Vaginitis
   B. Appendicitis
   C. MRSA
   D. Myopia

7. The child diagnosed with this disease will often require a sleep study, full blood workup, and a psychological assessment to rule out other diagnoses. The nurse suspects the child has:
   A. Attention deficit-hyperactivity disorder
   B. Anxiety
   C. Dyslexia
   D. Osgood-Schlatter disease

8. What type of musculoskeletal tumor is most likely to affect Caucasians and Hispanics?
   A. Rhabdomyosarcoma
   B. Ewing's sarcoma
   C. Osteosarcoma
   D. Lymphoma

9. What focusing error occurs when the light is focused behind the retina?
   A. Myopia
   B. Astigmatism
   C. Hyperopia
   D. Amblyopia

10. What is the recommended serving size of meat, poultry, fish, dry beans, eggs, or nuts for children aged 6 to 12 years old?
    A. 2 to 3 ounces
    B. 4 to 5 ounces
    C. 6 to 9 ounces
    D. 5 to 6 ounces

Chapter 62

Care and Illnesses of Adolescents

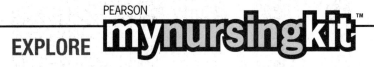

MyNursingKit is your one stop for online chapter review materials and resources. Prepare for success with additional NCLEX®-style practice questions, interactive assignments and activities, web links, animations and videos, and more!

Register your access code from the front of your book at
www.mynursingkit.com

KEY TERMS

Match each of the following key terms to its proper definition.

_____ 1. Migraine

     A.   A group of related metabolic disorders, including obesity, insulin resistance, and complications of Type 2 diabetes

_____ 2. Menarche

     B.   Age when the reproductive organs become functional and secondary sex characteristics develop

_____ 3. Comedo

     C.   The period of growth and development that begins with the appearance of secondary sex characteristics and ends with the cessation of physical growth and emotional maturity

_____ 4. Puberty

     D.   The beginning of menstrual cycles during puberty

_____ 5. Adolescence

     E.   Familial disorder marked by periodic, unilateral pulsating headache that often begins during adolescence and continues into adulthood

_____ 6. Metabolic X syndrome

     F.   Basic acne lesion

LEARNING OUTCOMES

1. What are the growth changes and developmental milestones that occur during the adolescent stage?

2. What is included in healthful nutrition, good hygiene practices, and normal vital signs for adolescents?

Nutrition	Hygiene	Vital Signs

3. What are routine health care needs, and how is confidentiality maintained for adolescents?

4. What are the common health and safety concerns during the adolescent years?

5. What are the respiratory, cardiovascular, hematologic, and immune disorders commonly diagnosed in adolescence?

Respiratory	Cardiovascular	Hematologic	Immune

6. What are the neurologic and musculoskeletal disorders commonly diagnosed in adolescence?

7. What are the gastrointestinal and endocrine disorders commonly diagnosed in adolescence?

8. What are the urinary and reproductive disorders commonly diagnosed in adolescence?

9. What are the integumentary disorders commonly diagnosed in adolescence?

10. What are the psychosocial conditions commonly seen in adolescence, and what nursing care is required?

APPLY WHAT YOU LEARNED

Brittany Fuentez is a 16-year-old Latina who recently passed her driving test and obtained her license. She was so excited to finally have her independence and her parents agreed to let her have the car for the evening. She picked up several of her friends and they drove around town listening to music, laughing and singing along with the tunes. They decided to go to a neighboring town, even though her parents made her promise she would stay off the interstate. Brittany was whipping the steering wheel back and forth to the music and lost control of the car. The car skidded off the highway and rolled several times before finally coming to rest in a ditch upside down. Emergency responders came quickly and pulled three of the girls from the car, including Brittany, but they couldn't find the fourth girl, who was not using her seat belt, and was eventually found under the car, dead. Brittany was diagnosed with several facial lacerations that were deep and jagged, fractured third lumbar vertebrae with cord severance, and a fractured left humerus. The other two girls were admitted with fractures, lacerations, and one of the girls had a fractured skull. Neither are expected to have long-term results from their injuries.

1. What psychological issues will Brittany need to deal with, and how can you, as her nurse, help her to cope with them?

2. What issues will Brittany encounter secondary to her change in physical appearance and ability specific to her age and developmental needs? What can the nurse do to help her?

3. What nursing care will Brittany require to care for her physical needs?

MULTIPLE CHOICE QUESTIONS

Circle the answer that best completes each of the following statements.

1. What happens when the hypothalamus of the brain signals the pituitary gland to increase secretion of estrogens or androgens?
   A. Adolescence
   B. Growth spurts
   C. Puberty
   D. Development of breast buds

2. Which vital sign in teenagers averages lower than that of an adult?
   A. Pulse
   B. Temperature
   C. Blood pressure
   D. Respirations

3. For the nurse to appropriately address issues such as depression, suicide, substance abuse, unintended pregnancy, and sexual orientation, which of the following is required?
   A. Consent from the parent or guardian
   B. Protection of confidentiality
   C. Routine health care
   D. Private environment

4. What is the major cause of death during adolescence?
   A. HIV infection
   B. Substance abuse
   C. Lack of proper nutrition
   D. Accidents and injuries

5. In what disease would staging be part of the diagnostic process?
   A. Hodgkin's lymphoma
   B. Glandular fever
   C. Migraine
   D. Amyotrophic lateral sclerosis

6. What disease would be considered if while flexing the child's head in supine position, there is an involuntary flex of the knees or hips?
   A. Mononucleosis
   B. Fibromyalgia
   C. Brudzinski's sign
   D. Meningitis

7. The nurse admits a child of Jewish descent who presents with recurrent abdominal pain and diarrhea. The nurse suspects the child has:
   A. Hepatitis
   B. Metabolic syndrome
   C. Inflammatory bowel disease
   D. Meningitis

8. What type of disorder is corrected by a radical orchectomy?
   A. Testicular cancer
   B. Hyperthyroidism
   C. Testicular torsion
   D. Amputation of a limb

9. What adolescent disorder would have comedo as part of the manifestation for diagnosis?
   A. Bulimia nervosa
   B. Borderline personality disorder
   C. Acne
   D. Testicular cancer

10. The nurse assesses an adolescent and finds marked weight loss below average levels. The client reports difficulty concentrating and says, "I'm just a waste of space. My mother would be lucky if I just went away." In assessing the teen further, the nurse needs to ask what question?
    A. "Have you been drinking alcohol or taking any illegal drugs?"
    B. "Are you thinking about hurting yourself?"
    C. "What have you been eating?"
    D. "Are you dealing with more stress than usual?"

Chapter 63

Leadership and Professional Development

KEY TERMS

Match each of the following key terms to its proper definition.

_____ 1. Compromise

_____ 2. Laissez-faire

_____ 3. Autocratic

_____ 4. Democratic

_____ 5. Delegation

A. Using decision making that allows input from all team members

B. Making unilateral decisions while dominating team members

C. The distribution of tasks in a way that prioritizes activities and available resources

D. Strategy in which there is negotiation or tradeoffs

E. Organizational structure in which the leader exercises little control over the group

---

_____ 6. Conflict

_____ 7. Accommodation

_____ 8. Leadership

A. Strategy in which both parties meet the problem on an even playing field with equal concern for the issues, allowing everyone to win by identifying areas of agreement and differences

B. A process used to move a group toward setting and achievement of goals

C. One side denies that a problem exists or withdraws, so there is no active resolution

_____ 9. Collaboration

D. Strategy in which one person or a group is willing to yield to the other

_____ 10. Avoidance

E. A disagreement or antagonism between groups, individuals, or ideas

LEARNING OUTCOMES

1. What are the factors that govern licensure and standards of care?

2. What is the purpose of and terminology used in nurse practice acts?

3. What are the important aspects of the LPN/LVN code of ethics?

4. Name and describe each of the different leadership styles and explain the important attributes of effective leaders.

5. List and describe the tasks involved in being a team leader.

6. What are the key concepts and expectations when delegating tasks?

7. What are the different reporting techniques, and how do they differ?

8. How does the SBAR technique for handoff procedures function?

9. What are the different types of paperwork that may be involved as team leader or nurse?

10. What are the stages of conflict and conflict resolution strategies?

11. What are the advantages of each method of nursing care delivery?

12. What are the Joint Commission safety goals for healthcare clients?

APPLY WHAT YOU LEARNED

The LPN/LVN is functioning as the charge nurse on the evening shift in a skilled nursing facility. The unit has been very busy because one of the staff nurses called in sick and couldn't be covered by another nurse. The charge nurse arranges the schedule so everyone can get away for a 30-minute dinner. It is 8 p.m. and the charge nurse has just assisted several different staff members with transferring their assigned clients back to bed and answers a call bell. The client says they haven't seen the nurse taking care of them for more than an hour and they would like to get back to bed. The charge nurse helps the client back into bed and goes to look for the client's assigned nurse. The nurse is finally found in the staff lounge. The charge nurse asks, "Are you okay?" The nurse responds, "Yes, I'm fine. I'm just tired and needed a break so I came in here to prop my feet up." The charge nurse feels angry because everyone is tired and has been working hard to care for all of the clients, and doesn't understand why this nurse feels it is okay just to take a break and leave assigned clients uncared for.

1. What role might this charge nurse have played that led to this situation?

2. How and when should the charge nurse deal with this situation?

3. Should the nurse report this situation to the unit manager? Why or why not? If it is reported, how would it be reported?

MULTIPLE CHOICE QUESTIONS

Circle the answer that best completes each of the following statements.

1. What are the minimum requirements an applicant must have to take the examination to obtain a nursing license? (Select all that apply.)
   A. High school diploma or equivalent
   B. Completion of an approved practical/vocational nursing program
   C. A current visa or U.S. citizenship
   D. Established residence in the state where the test is taken
   E. Pass the NCLEX-PN

2. The LPN/LVN is asked by the RN to suction a client's tracheostomy. The nurse practice act classifies this action as a:
   A. Delegated medical act
   B. Direct supervision
   C. Complex nursing situation
   D. Delegated nursing act

3. The nurse is caring for a client who may benefit from a new type of treatment the nurse just learned about in a continuing education course. The nurse approaches the physician with the suggestion this treatment be considered. The nurse has demonstrated which of the following?
   A. Good team leading skills
   B. Nursing Code of Ethics
   C. Working outside the scope of practice
   D. Delegation

4. The charge nurse assigns the LPN/LVN a specific task, tells the nurse how to perform the task, and says they will be back in 10 minutes to make sure the task was done properly. This charge nurse is what type of leader?
   A. Autocratic
   B. Democratic
   C. Laissez-faire
   D. Collaborating

5. The nurse has more to do than can be done autonomously. To provide timely client care, the nurse may do which of the following?
   A. Handoff procedures
   B. Conflict resolution
   C. Delegation
   D. Standards of care

6. The nurse responsible for making rounds, for making assignments, and for facilitating group conferences would be an example of which of the following?
   A. Laissez-faire leader
   B. Unit manager
   C. Autocratic leader
   D. Team leader

7. A disadvantage of this type of report is that questions must be tabled till the end to be addressed by a nurse who may be anxious to go off duty.
   A. Shift report
   B. Taped report
   C. An oral report
   D. Written report

8. What type of report is completed and filed with the risk management department?
   A. Transcription of orders
   B. SBAR
   C. Incident report
   D. Conflict resolution report

9. Nurse A needs to have Friday off to attend her son's graduation; Nurse B agrees to work for Nurse A on Friday if Nurse A works for Nurse B on Sunday so Nurse B can have a three-day weekend. What type of conflict resolution strategy is this?
   A. Compromise
   B. Collaboration
   C. Accommodation
   D. Avoidance

10. What type of nursing care method could create fragmented delivery of care for the client?
    A. Case method
    B. Primary nursing
    C. Functional nursing system
    D. Team nursing

Chapter 64

Preparing to Take the Licensure Exam

KEY TERMS

Match each of the following key terms to its proper definition.

_____ 1. Mnemonics

A. Agreement among several states that a nurse can practice in another state that is part of the compact, as long as he or she follows the nurse practice act and the rules and regulations pertaining to the act

_____ 2. Computer adaptive testing

B. A level of concern about testing that ranges from a normal, mild level of uneasiness that is motivating to a level of uneasiness and fear that immobilizes the test taker

_____ 3. Test anxiety

C. Document that aids candidates in determining areas of relative strength and weakness based on the NCLEX-PN test plan and in focusing their study prior to retaking the exam

_____ 4. Multistate compact

D. Method of examination that provides each student a unique computerized examination, selecting the test questions as the student takes the examination

_____ 5. Diagnostic profile

E. Techniques for developing memory

LEARNING OUTCOMES

1. What is the purpose of the NCLEX-PN examination, and when should you begin to study for it?

Purpose	When to Study For It

2. How does the National Council of State Boards of Nursing develop the test plan and the test? Where is the NCLEX-PN test available in your area? How does the multistate compact apply to it?

Test Plan and Test	Where Available	Multistate Compact

3. What are the different levels of NCLEX-PN questions, and what is the central concept on which the test is based?

Levels	Concept

4. What are the four categories of client needs and their subcategories?

5. How does computer adaptive testing create an individualized test for each student?

6. What is your individualized plan for preparing and reviewing for the NCLEX-PN?

7. How will you know when you are ready to take the examination?

8. How will you apply to take the examination?

9. What strategies can you use to overcome test anxiety?

10. What should you do the day before, the day of, and during the examination to increase your chances of success on the examination?

Day Before Examination	Day Of Examination	During Examination

11. What should you do with your time after the exam, and how should you use the results of your test?

APPLY WHAT YOU LEARNED

Using the table of contents at the front of your textbook, place each chapter title in one of the columns below based on how well you know the material. If a chapter contains information that you feel you know well, place it in the Strength column. If you know you are weak on material in a chapter, place it in the Weakness column. Those subjects that you feel you know but not well can be placed in the Neutral column. Use this self-evaluation to create your study plan, beginning with areas of weakness and then moving on to areas of neutrality. If there are topics within a chapter you feel differently about, list the specific topics in the area where they belong.

Weakness	Neutral	Strength

When answering questions in the NCLEX-PN, what strategies have you learned throughout your program that will help you to choose the right answer when you aren't sure what answer to choose?

MULTIPLE CHOICE QUESTIONS

Circle the answer that best completes each of the following statements.

1. How often does the National Council of State Boards of Nursing conduct a vocational nursing job analysis study to aid in the development of the framework for the NCLEX-PN examination?
   A. Semiannually
   B. Annually
   C. Every two years
   D. Every three years

2. The student nurse preparing for the NCLEX examination can expect the majority of test questions to be at which of the following cognitive levels or higher?
   A. Knowledge
   B. Comprehension
   C. Application
   D. Analysis

3. Which category of the client needs, as it relates to the NCLEX-PN test plan, would pharmacological therapies be associated with?
   A. Psychosocial integrity
   B. Physiological integrity
   C. Health promotion and maintenance
   D. Safe, effective care environment

4. At what point during the NCLEX-PN examination will the computer adaptive testing automatically end your examination?
   A. At five hours, including a tutorial, sample questions, and breaks
   B. On the 200th question
   C. The computer calculates with a 90% degree of confidence you are or are not a safe/competent practitioner
   D. On the 84th question

5. Which type of study aid would give the nurse an explanation, the rationales, and the distracters for each incorrect answer in a computerized format?
   A. Professional review courses
   B. Mock NCLEX-PN examinations
   C. NCLEX-PN review books
   D. Study groups

6. What are the two types of review classes a graduate nursing student might take if there is an indication they might not do well on the NCLEX examination?
   A. Orientation class
   B. Course work review class
   C. NCLEX-PN examination
   D. NCLEX preparedness class

7. Which entity provides the student nurse preparing to take the NCLEX examination with the Authorization to Test document?
   A. Your class nursing instructor
   B. The test administrating agency
   C. The Director of Nursing at your school
   D. The National Council of State Boards of Nursing

8. The nursing student might benefit from some relaxation techniques to relieve:
   A. Catatonic behavior
   B. Avolition
   C. Test anxiety
   D. Comprehension

9. What should the nurse do the day before, the day of, or during the examination to increase their chances of success? (Select all that apply.)
   A. Cram for the exam the night before.
   B. Avoid using stimulants or depressants the evening before examination.
   C. Get sufficient sleep the night before the examination.
   D. Eat a large meal packed with protein and carbohydrates before the examination.
   E. Join friends at a comedy club the night before the examination.

10. The nurse who fails the examination might benefit from which of the following? (Select all that apply.)
    A. A diagnostic profile
    B. Getting a tutor
    C. Worrying about what to do next
    D. Talking to the director of their nursing program
    E. Using the test results to prove they are a failure

Chapter 65

Finding That First Job

KEY TERMS

Match each of the following key terms to its proper definition.

_____ 1. Performance evaluation

A. Working jointly with other healthcare professionals, including physicians, in the performance of nursing roles within the scope of practice

_____ 2. Résumé

B. Program or time for newly hired individuals to prepare themselves to take on responsibilities of a new job

_____ 3. Collaborative

C. Review of work attendance, teamwork, and skills by an employer

_____ 4. Professionalism

D. Time during which an immediate supervisor evaluates the performance of a newly hired employee

_____ 5. Probationary period

E. Behavior showing dedication to a vocation that requires knowledge of some department of learning or science

_____ 6. Orientation

F. Concise, systematic summary of professional experience and educational background

_____ 7. Networking

A. An itemized visual account of skills and best practices that are related to the position being sought

_____ 8. Career ladder

B. A vocation requiring knowledge of some department of learning or science

_____ 9. Portfolio

C. Brief document containing essential information about oneself that is often provided with a résumé to a potential employer

_____ 10. Cover letter

D. The deliberate attempt to make connections among people for a variety of interests, including employment opportunities

_____ 11. Profession

E. Progression from one level in a profession to another through educational pursuits and professional experience

LEARNING OUTCOMES

1. What are the components of a portfolio?

2. What information should be included when developing a cover letter?

3. What are the steps involved in preparing a résumé?

4. How does the interview process work, and what steps could be taken to improve the success of the interview?

5. What are the important aspects of the job search process?

6. What are the concepts of orientation, probationary period, and performance evaluation as they apply to the hiring process?

Orientation	Probationary Period	Performance Evaluation

7. What strategies can you use to succeed and prove yourself on your first job?

8. What strategies can you implement in order to continue moving up the career ladder in the nursing profession?

APPLY WHAT YOU LEARNED

Write a sample cover letter, résumé, and thank-you letter to be used when you begin job searching. After having it reviewed and correcting it, place these in your portfolio.

MULTIPLE CHOICE QUESTIONS

Circle the answer that best completes each of the following statements.

1. The best time for the LPN/LVN to start their portfolio for their first job is:
   A. After successfully passing the licensure examination.
   B. On the first day of the nursing program.
   C. Halfway into the nursing program.
   D. While waiting for the results of your licensure examination.

2. In which part of a cover letter would share your enthusiasm for the job you are applying?
   A. The introductory paragraph
   B. The second paragraph
   C. The closing paragraph
   D. After your signature at the bottom of the page

3. Which type of document would be used more frequently by a professionals further along in their careers to apply for a position?
   A. Curriculum vitae
   B. Chronological résumé
   C. Functional résumé
   D. Combination of chronological and functional résumé

4. Which of the following is a helpful tip for having a successful interview?
   A. Admit your shortcomings.
   B. Avoid direct eye contact.
   C. Arrive 30 minutes before the interview.
   D. Articulate why you have chosen this facility for application.

5. What document is customary when leaving one position for another?
   A. A referral
   B. A letter of resignation
   C. A thank-you letter
   D. No document needed

6. The nurse might expect a small salary increase after the completion of which of the following?
   A. First six weeks on the job
   B. Orientation
   C. Interview
   D. Probationary period

7. The nurse employs what types of strategies to succeed during their first year on the job?
   A. Point out errors in the way things are done.
   B. Be a teacher, showing others how to perform tasks.
   C. Be a stress buster.
   D. Work independently.

8. The nurse, volunteering for a hospital-wide committee on client care and unit operations, would be participating in what type of nursing practice?
   A. Collaborative
   B. Adaptive
   C. Cognitive
   D. Networking

9. The nurse interviewing for a position is asked, "Are you single?" by the interviewer. What act made these types of questions illegal to ask?
   A. The Multi-State Compact
   B. The Federal Civil Rights Act
   C. The Nurse Practice Act
   D. The Scope of Practice Act

10. Which of the following should *not* be included in your portfolio?
    A. Case studies
    B. Community service
    C. CPR card
    D. Your hobbies and interests

Answer Key

Chapter 1 Succeeding as a Nursing Student

Matching

1. D
2. A
3. B
4. C

Learning Outcomes

1. See section entitled "Nursing Values and Characteristics."
   Learning Outcome: 1-1
2. See section entitled "Studying Effectively."
   Learning Outcome: 1-2
3. See section entitled "Managing Time."
   Learning Outcome: 1-3
4. See section entitled "Managing Time."
   Learning Outcome: 1-4
5. See section entitled "Taking Tests."
   Learning Outcome: 1-5
6. See section entitled "Participating in Clinical Experiences."
   Learning Outcome: 1-6
7. See section entitled "Prioritizing in the Clinical Setting."
   Learning Outcome: 1-7

Multiple Choice Questions

1. D
   Rationale: Nursing, at its core, is a profession of caring. Providing safe, effective care requires good hygiene, critical thinking and precision.
   Learning Outcome: 1-1
2. C
   Rationale: While group study can be very helpful, group mates should be chosen with care to assure compatibility in approach, motivation, and organization.
   Learning Outcome: 1-2
3. D
   Rationale: You certainly can document your schedule however you choose, but a calendar is most helpful because you can see what is required of you on a daily basis. Calendars make it easy to add entries as new demands on your time arise.
   Learning Outcome: 1-3
4. B

Rationale: Although financial aid may help you to pay for nursing school, and is essential to being able to continue in school, it does not contribute to academic success. Rather, it provides the opportunity for you to succeed. To take advantage of that opportunity, it is important for you to maintain your current responsibilities (care of children, basic daily needs, etc.), participate in group study sessions, and maintain a well-planned calendar to stay ahead of obligations.

Learning Outcome: 1-4

5. A

   Rationale: When a question asks you to contrast something, it is asking for the differences between the two items.

   Learning Outcome: 1-5

6. C

   Rationale: You must never do something you *think* is *probably* right. You must be sure that what you are doing is absolutely correct in order to prevent client injury or error. If you are not certain of how to proceed, talk with your nursing instructor to verify the correctness of your planned actions. No matter how long you practice as a nurse, situations will always arise that require peer consultation.

   Learning Outcome: 1-6

7. A

   Rationale: To prioritize care as a nurse, you first must have information about what is being prioritized. Gathering information begins by reviewing pertinent client information, often performed by nursing students the day before actually being assigned to provide care. After reviewing pertinent information and listening to the report, you will visit each client to introduce yourself, determine which client to begin with (when you are assigned more than one client), and perform an examination of the client. Medications should never be prepared before seeing the client.

   Learning Outcome: 1-7

8. B

   Rationale: Aiming for perfection is a goal that is almost always unsuccessfully met. Nurses are human beings, and as such cannot do everything perfectly. However, caring, precision, and timeliness are reasonable goals you are expected to aim for because people's lives depend on it.

   Learning Outcome: 1-6

9. D

   Rationale: Knowledge questions require you to restate something you memorized; comprehension questions require you to understand information you learned; application questions ask you to apply the knowledge you gained; analysis questions require you to assess how various factors will affect a situation.

   Learning Outcome: 1-5

10. C

    Rationale: Although flexibility, prioritizing, and participating in required activities are all very important, first and foremost in importance is safety. Delivering care safely, maintaining both the client's and your own safety, and looking out for the safety of your coworkers is of greatest importance.

    Learning Outcome: 1-7

Chapter 2 History of Nursing

Matching

1. D
2. F
3. A
4. G

5. H
6. B
7. E
8. C

Learning Outcomes

1. See section entitled "Influences on the Development of Nursing."
   Learning Outcome: 2-1
2. See section entitled "Leading Nurses of History."
   Learning Outcome: 2-2
3. See section entitled "Male Nurses in History."
   Learning Outcome: 2-3
4. See section entitled "Practical and Vocational Nursing Today."
   Learning Outcome: 2-4
5. See section entitled "History of LPNs/LVNs."
   Learning Outcome: 2-5
6. See section entitled "Practical and Vocational Nursing Today."
   Learning Outcome: 2-6
7. See section entitled "Professional Organizations for LPN/LVN Students and Graduates."
   Learning Outcome: 2-7

Multiple Choice Questions

1. C
   Rationale: Marcella was one of the matrons.
   Learning Outcome: 2-1
2. B
   Rationale: Clara Barton is noted for having created the American Red Cross.
   Learning Outcome: 2-2
3. C
   Rationale: St. Camillus de Lellis started the first ambulance service.
   Learning Outcome: 2-3
4. D
   Rationale: The nurse is promoting health and wellness in this scenario by promoting a healthier lifestyle and teaching people about the dangers of abusing substance. Activities that prevent the occurrence of an illness such as immunizations or hand washing would be preventing illness. Restoring health indicates someone is sick and requires treatment. Caring for the dying usually involves palliative care or comfort care.
   Learning Outcome: 2-4

5. A

   Rationale: The American Nurses Association published a position paper that clearly defined the differences and similarities as well as the scope of practice for LPN/LVNs and RNs.

   Learning Outcome: 2-5

6. A

   Rationale: Nurse practice acts exist with the primary purpose of protecting the public by requiring that minimum standards are met when authorizing nurses to provide care.

   Learning Outcome: 2-6

7. B

   Rationale: NFLPN is the central organization for LPN/LVNs that describes current trends and changes in practice.

   Learning Outcome: 2-7

8. C

   Rationale: Expertise takes time to develop, so a minimum of one year is required. This time period enables the nurse to learn new skills and gather more experiences for improved decision making.

   Learning Outcome: 2-6

9. C

   Rationale: New York was the first state to require licensure for practical nurses. Prior to this, practical nursing had been seen as a homemaking service that delivered the most basic care.

   Learning Outcome: 2-5

10. D

   Rationale: Sister Elizabeth Kenny worked extensively with polio clients. Unfortunately, she died before Dr. Jonas Salk's vaccine was discovered.

   Learning Outcome: 2-2

Chapter 3 Promoting Culturally Proficient Care

Matching

1. Prejudice: C
2. Stereotypes: D
3. Ethnocentrism: B
4. Discrimination: E
5. Acculturation: A

1. Cultural awareness: D
2. Cultural competence: C
3. Cultural empathy: A
4. Cultural sensitivity: B

1. Biocultural ecology: A
2. Domains: D
3. Intercultural communication: B
4. Segregation: C

Learning Outcomes

1. See section entitled "Development of Transcultural Nursing."
   Learning Outcome: 3-1
2. See section entitled "Theoretical Basis of Transcultural Nursing."
   Learning Outcome: 3-2
3. See section entitled "Racial and Ethnic Disparities in Health Care."
   Learning Outcome: 3-3
4. See section entitled "Culturally Based Communication."
   Learning Outcome: 3-4
5. See section entitled "Transcultural Communication and Client Concerns."
   Learning Outcome: 3-5
6. See section entitled "Conducting the Cultural Assessment."
   Learning Outcome: 3-6
7. See section entitled "Subculture of Health Care."
   Learning Outcome: 3-7

Multiple Choice Questions

1. A
   Rationale: Dr. Leininger's work on cultural nursing care continues to be the most extensive work on the subject, although current researchers are expanding upon her work.
   Learning Outcome: 3-1
2. C
   Rationale: Ethnocentrism describes our tendency to define other's behaviors by what we see as right or wrong, and can introduce cultural bias and prejudice if not recognized.
   Learning Outcome: 3-2
3. B
   Rationale: Finances are not a domain of culture. Communication, workforce issues, and death rituals are all influenced by culture.
   Learning Outcome: 3-3
4. D
   Rationale: To learn about culture, it is important for the nurse to examine cultural attitudes, learn more about other cultures, and develop skills to provide culturally competent care.
   Learning Outcome: 3-4
5. D
   Rationale: In Asian cultures, touching an infant's head may be perceived as placing a curse on the infant and should be avoided by the nurse.
   Learning Outcome: 3-4
6. B
   Rationale: HIPAA mandates the client provide informed consent for treatment.
   Learning Outcome: 3-5
7. C

Rationale: Learning the client's preferred language is important, even when the client speaks proficient English, because during times of stress it may be easier for the client to speak in their preferred language. Asking this question helps the nurse learn more about the client's cultural identity.
Learning Outcome: 3-6

8. B
    Rationale: Cultural empathy helps the nurse experience an event as the client experiences it, and requires knowledge of the client.
    Learning Outcome: 3-7

9. A
    Rationale: Asian Pacific culture teaches that a member of the family who does something shameful brings shame to the entire family.
    Learning Outcome: 3-1

10. D
    Rationale: Personal space is part of the communication domain.
    Learning Outcome: 3-3

Chapter 4 Legal and Ethical Issues of Nursing

Matching

1.	C	6.	F	11.	E
2.	D	7.	J	12.	H
3.	G	8.	A	13.	M
4.	I	9.	K		
5.	B	10.	L		

Learning Outcomes

1. See section entitled "Kinds of Legal Actions."
    Learning Outcome: 4-1
2. See section entitled "Regulation of Nursing Practice."
    Learning Outcome: 4-2
3. See section entitled "Legal Roles of Nurses."
    Learning Outcome: 4-3
4. See section entitled "Legal Protection for Nurses."
    Learning Outcome: 4-4
5. See section entitled "Legal Protection for Nurses."
    Learning Outcome: 4-5
6. See section entitled "Legal Protection for Nurses."
    Learning Outcome: 4-6
7. See section entitled "Selected Legal Aspects of Nursing Practice."
    Learning Outcome: 4-7
8. See section entitled "Selected Legal Aspects of Nursing Practice."
    Learning Outcome: 4-8
9. See section entitled "Understanding Ethical Issues."
    Learning Outcome: 4-9

10. See section entitled "Client Advocacy."
    Learning Outcome: 4-10
11. See section entitled "Nursing Ethics."
    Learning Outcome: 4-11
12. See section entitled "Specific Ethical Issues."
    Learning Outcome: 4-12

Apply What You Learned

Suggested Answers

1. The nurse must complete an incident report but does not place it in the client's medical record or make any notation in the record about the completion of the report.
2. Left arm above the wrist is edematous and red. Fluid leaking from IV insertion site. IV discontinued and restarted in right hand. Warm soak applied to left forearm. Physician notified and orders received to maintain warm soaks for 20 minutes every four hours. Nursing supervisor notified.
3. The nurse is not responsible or liable for the event because it was noted at the beginning of the shift. The nurse caring for the client on the previous shift could be liable for neglect if there is nothing documented about the IV within the last hour. Many times no one is liable because an IV can infiltrate minutes after assessing the site and phlebitis develops by the next hourly check. Clients who are alert and able should be taught to notify the nurse if they have any discomfort at the insertion site.

Multiple Choice Questions

1. B
   Rationale: A civil wrong is defined as a tort. Although negligence is a type of tort, there are other types as well, such as invasion of privacy. Assault and battery is a criminal wrong.
   Learning Outcome: 4-1
2. A
   Rationale: Invasion of privacy is pursued if the nurse shares private information that affects the client's feelings (embarrassment, etc.) and/or standing in the community even if the information shared is truthful. Slander is saying something untrue and harmful about another person. Defamation is a false accusation, and libel is a false and malicious statement made in writing.
   Learning Outcome: 4-2
3. C
   Rationale: Permissive licensure allows the nurse to perform nursing duties without a license. It is not allowed anywhere in the U.S. or in most of Canada.
   Learning Outcome: 4-3
4. C
   Rationale: The Good Samaritan Act was initiated to encourage people to provide first aid at the site of an emergency without concern about being sued for their actions. Note, however, that nurses have additional training

and skills, and are expected to act as a prudent nurse would in the same situation. Americans with Disabilities Act protects people with handicaps from being treated differently than those who are not disabled. Auto insurance has no coverage for helping someone at the scene of an accident or emergency.

Learning Outcome: 4-4

5. A

    Rationale: Nurses and other professionals are liable for the actions they perform or fail to perform. Liability extends beyond the nurse's responsibility at work and is important to consider whenever you give medical advice or care, whether to a neighbor, family member, or to a charitable organization. Ethics are beliefs about what is right or wrong. Scope of practice is the permissible actions, procedures, and processes a professional, such as a nurse, is allowed and expected to perform. Laws are rules imposed by society.

    Learning Outcome: 4-5

6. D

    Rationale: The best strategy to avoid liability is to always ask for assistance when you are unsure of how to proceed in order to prevent errors. Being polite and friendly should be an approach used on all clients and not just a means of reducing liability. Practice procedures in the clinical laboratory, not on clients. Proper documentation should be done before leaving work.

    Learning Outcome: 4-6

7. B

    Rationale: The nurse wants to avoid sharing privileged communication about the client without the client's permission.

    Learning Outcome: 4-7

8. D

    Rationale: The nurse finding the error is responsible for completing the incident report. Completion of an incident report does not indicate responsibility for the event.

    Learning Outcome: 4-8

9. A, B

    Rationale: The nurse might call the client's spiritual advisor (priest, minister, rabbi), or could involve the ethics committee to help the client's family come to a resolution about the plan of care. Social services and the board of nursing would not be appropriate referrals. A healthcare team conference may provide information, but after the family is informed of treatment options they would not be the best choice to help families resolve internal conflicts.

    Learning Outcome: 4-9

10. A

    Rationale: The nurse is acting as a client advocate to help the client make their wishes understood by the physician.

    Learning Outcome: 4-10

Matching

1.	E	5.	B
2.	G	6.	D
3.	A	7.	C
4.	F		

Learning Outcomes

1. See section entitled "Critical Thinking."
   Learning Outcome: 5-1
2. See section entitled "Critical Thinking."
   Learning Outcome: 5-2
3. See section entitled "Theories and Models."
   Learning Outcome: 5-3
4. See section entitled "Theories and Models."
   Learning Outcome: 5-4
5. See section entitled "Theories and Models."
   Learning Outcome: 5-5
6. See section entitled "Evidence-Based Practice."
   Learning Outcome: 5-6

Multiple Choice Questions

1. C
   Rationale: The word *assumes* indicates that the nurse did not gather information to determine the accuracy of the belief upon which the nurse is basing actions. Instead of assuming, the nurse using critical thinking would have questioned the client and gathered data to determine exactly what happened.
   Learning Outcome: 5-1
2. C
   Rationale: The nurse does not discard solutions that were not chosen because they may be needed later if the chosen solution is not effective in resolving the situation.
   Learning Outcome: 5-2
3. C
   Rationale: Central to all nursing theories is the environment (of the client, the nurse, and/or the facility), the role of the nurse, the needs of the client, and the desire to improve health. Time, ethics, values, bioethics, and attitudes may play a role in some theories, but they are not central to all theories of nursing.
   Learning Outcome: 5-3
4. C
   Rationale: Betty Neuman's systems model explored the role of various stressors on individual responses.
   Learning Outcome: 5-4

5. D

    Rationale: Use of critical thinking requires the nurse to gather as many facts about the event as possible before choosing a course of action. Eventually the linen will need to be changed and the physician may need to be notified, but it is possible the blood is the result of a spilled blood transfusion, which would require a totally different action plan than if the client had a bleeding wound.

    Learning Outcome: 5-5

6. D

    Rationale: Although the newspaper article may be interesting, there is no proof of the validity of the information. Before doing anything else, the nurse should consult nursing or healthcare literature to learn more about the study and ongoing research being conducted to control for questions that arose during the initial study. Not all things in print are reliable.

    Learning Outcome: 5-6

7. A, B, D, E

    Rationale: Evidence-based practice requires the nurse to stay current with changes in nursing and base their nursing practice on methods that have been shown by research to be most effective. To do this, reading current literature, collecting accurate data, collaborating with the RN, and participating in continuing education are all important steps. This will improve the type of care provided to clients.

    Learning Outcome: 5-6

8. B

    Rationale: Governing the thoughts that govern us means not reflexively reacting to a situation, but rather thinking through the various components of the situation to determine exactly what is going on. We can analyze our own thinking, but not the thinking of others. We subject our egocentric thoughts to close scrutiny, not our altruistic roots, and instead of embracing all standards we must examine standards and choose those that we consider best.

    Learning Outcome: 5-1

9. C

    Rationale: Inference allows us to take the information we know and predict other things. For example, if it is known that salt causes water retention, which can result in an increase in blood pressure, and a client is seen eating potato chips, we can infer that his blood pressure is likely to be higher when next measured.

    Learning Outcome: 5-1

10. A

    Rationale: When diagnosing, the nurse takes the data and analyzes it to determine client problems or needs. Misinterpretation of the meaning of the data could result in inaccurate nursing diagnosing. Assessment is collecting data; implementing is putting the nursing plan into action; and evaluating is a reassessment to determine the effectiveness of the plan.

    Learning Outcome: 5-1

Matching

1.	B	6.	C	11.	D
2.	E	7.	A	12.	C
3.	D	8.	D	13.	B
4.	A	9.	E	14.	E
5.	C	10.	B	15.	A

Learning Outcomes

1. See section entitled "The Nursing Process."
   Learning Outcome: 6-1
2. See section entitled "The Nursing Process."
   Learning Outcome: 6-2
3. See section entitled "The Nursing Process."
   Learning Outcome: 6-3
4. See section entitled "Assessment."
   Learning Outcome: 6-4
5. See section entitled "Assessment."
   Learning Outcome: 6-5
6. See section entitled "Assessment."
   Learning Outcome: 6-6
7. See section entitled "Diagnosis."
   Learning Outcome: 6-7
8. See section entitled "Planning."
   Learning Outcome: 6-8
9. See section entitled "Implementation."
   Learning Outcome: 6-9
10. See section entitled "Evaluation."
    Learning Outcome: 6-10

Multiple Choice Questions

1. C
   Rationale: During the planning stage, the nurse looks at the data that has been gathered and determines what can be done to help the client prevent, reduce, or resolve the problem identified.
   Learning Outcome: 6-1
2. D
   Rationale: During the evaluation phase, the nurse reassesses the client to determine if the actions that were done during the intervention phase resolved, reduced, or prevented the problem. If so, nothing further is needed. However, if only partial resolution of goals is achieved, further assessment, planning, and implementation is required and the nursing plan of care is evaluated to see if it can be improved upon.
   Learning Outcome: 6-2

3. **C**

   Rationale: During the assessment phase, the LPN/LVN contributes by assisting with collection of data through observation of the client, measuring vital signs, reporting changes in status, and learning more about the client. The initial admission assessment is the responsibility of the RN, although the LPN/LVN may assist with gathering data. Reviewing and revising the plan of care is done in the evaluation phase. Identifying strengths and health problems that can be prevented is done in the planning and diagnosing stages.

   Learning Outcome: 6-3

4. **B**

   Rationale: This is objective data because it was observed by the nurse. Had the nurse documented that the client was "sad," that would be subjective data because only the client knows how they are feeling. Secondary data comes from sources other than the client. There is no such thing as manifestation data.

   Learning Outcome: 6-4

5. **D**

   Rationale: When documenting subjective data, the nurse writes exactly what the client says in their own words, and places it in quotes to indicate it is an exact quotation from the client.

   Learning Outcome: 6-5

6. **C**

   Rationale: The nurse is interviewing the client. An intervention is an action, an observation is what is seen, and an examination would review objective data.

   Learning Outcome: 6-6

7. **D**

   Rationale: Nursing diagnoses are created by the RN. The LPN/LVN should be familiar with nursing diagnosis to determine the appropriateness. It also influences the interventions to be performed.

   Learning Outcome: 6-7

8. **A**

   Rationale: During the planning phase, the nurse sets priorities for care to be delivered.

   Learning Outcome: 6-8

9. **A**

   Rationale: Assessment is the first step in the nursing process, and the nurse's first action would be to attempt to arouse the client, assess to determine if they are breathing, and assess for a pulse. Only after collecting this information would the nurse plan what to do next.

   Learning Outcome: 6-9

10. **A**

    Rationale: Before performing any procedure, it is very important the nurse always assess the client's continuing need for that procedure. A client who requires straight catheterization postoperatively may no longer require the procedure as effects of analgesia subside, as healing takes place, or for a variety of reason. Procedures should never be performed routinely.

    Learning Outcome: 6-10

Matching

1.	B	6.	C
2.	C	7.	E
3.	D	8.	B
4.	A	9.	A
5.	D		

Learning Outcomes

1. See section entitled "Levels of Health Care."
   Learning Outcome: 7-1
2. See section entitled "Types of Healthcare Settings."
   Learning Outcome: 7-2
3. See section entitled "Types of Healthcare Settings."
   Learning Outcome: 7-3
4. See section entitled "Rights and Health Care."
   Learning Outcome: 7-4
5. See section entitled "Providers of Health Care."
   Learning Outcome: 7-5
6. See section entitled "Factors Affecting Healthcare Delivery."
   Learning Outcome: 7-6
7. See section entitled "Models of Care."
   Learning Outcome: 7-7
8. See section entitled "Healthcare Economics."
   Learning Outcome: 7-8

Multiple Choice Questions

1. B
   Rationale: Secondary care is involved with treating existing illness. Primary care prevents illness; tertiary care helps to prevent disability from existing conditions. Ambulatory care is delivered in the outpatient setting.
   Learning Outcome: 7-1
2. A
   Rationale: Caring for clients in the home allows the nurse to better assess the client's cultural beliefs and the role they play in the client's life.
   Learning Outcome: 7-2
3. D
   Rationale: Extended care facilities provide care for those who are unable to care for themselves independently, and can range from skilled nursing care for those requiring complex procedures to assisted living facilities where clients require assistance with ADLs.
   Learning Outcome: 7-3

4. C

Rationale: Clients have the right to self-determination whether they choose not to participate in a research study or they choose not to accept a treatment plan.

Learning Outcome: 7-4

5. B

Rationale: Social workers help to find placement for clients being discharged from an acute care facility who cannot go home and need rehabilitation or extended care.

Learning Outcome: 7-5

6. D

Rationale: Rural areas often have problems with adequate healthcare providers to meet residents' needs due to uneven distribution of services. It is common to find more physicians, nurses, and other members of the healthcare team in urban versus rural areas.

Learning Outcome: 7-6

7. C

Rationale: Client-focused care is a delivery model that brings all services and care providers to the client to decrease the number of personnel involved as well as the steps to get work done. In this model of care, cross-training of personnel is an essential component.

Learning Outcome: 7-7

8. D

Rationale: Social Security supplemental income is paid to disabled clients, and is often used to purchase medicines or cover costs of extended health care.

Learning Outcome: 7-8

9. B

Rationale: Homeopathy is a form of alternative care based on the belief that exposing the body to small amounts of a substance, like medications, will help the body form its own response to illness.

Learning Outcome: 7-5

10. C

Rationale: The Patient's Bill of Rights was adopted by the AHA in 1973 to protect hospitalized clients and ensure that their rights were maintained.

Learning Outcome: 7-4

Chapter 8 Complementary and Alternative Medicine in Health Care

Matching

1.	C	4.	E
2.	F	5.	B
3.	A	6.	D

Learning Outcomes

1. See chapter introduction.
   Learning Outcome: 8-1

2. See section entitled "Defining Terms Related to Complementary and Alternative Medicine."
   Learning Outcome: 8-2
3. See section entitled "Use of CAM Therapies."
   Learning Outcome: 8-3
4. See section entitled "Defining Terms Related to Complementary and Alternative Medicine."
   Learning Outcome: 8-4
5. See section entitled "CAM Therapies and Nursing Practice."
   Learning Outcome: 8-5
6. See section entitled "CAM Therapies and Nursing Practice."
   Learning Outcome: 8-6

Apply What You Learned

Suggested Answers

1. The client might have feared ridicule or was embarrassed to mention the complementary and alternative therapies utilized. The client may also not have realized what was meant when the nurse referred to "supplements."
2. The nurse should list all of the supplements taken by the client, and also question the client about any other CAM therapies the client might be using. The information should be documented in the client's chart and the physician should be made aware of the therapies used because they may impact the medical treatment regimen.
3. It is important to use a nonjudgmental and unbiased approach to the client, explaining the importance of notifying the physician of all therapies used as they may impact or interact with medical treatment.

Multiple Choice Questions

1. D
   Rationale: The FDA does not examine products for purity, efficacy, or safety, but does regulate that false claims are not made about the effects of the product. The label may not claim to cure, treat, or resolve any issue, but they may list recommended uses on the label if they choose to.
   Learning Outcome: 8-1
2. C
   Rationale: Conventional, or Western, medicine is the term used to describe traditional medical treatment delivered by most physicians in the United States.
   Learning Outcome: 8-2
3. A
   Rationale: Naturopathy believes in the power of nature to maintain health and promotes exposure to sun, air and water as part of the therapy.
   Learning Outcome: 8-3
4. B
   Rationale: Chiropractic medicine requires the intervention of a trained chiropractor who is not a physician but is trained in chiropractic technique. The other therapies can be delivered by a trained professional or self-performed.
   Learning Outcome: 8-4

5. B, C, E

   Rationale: Herbal medications may be prescribed by the physician for the inpatient, and it is important that the nurse know potential drug interactions of any supplement administered. In addition, if the client is using a specific CAM therapy, the nurse must understand what is involved in order to support the purpose of the therapy.

   Learning Outcome: 8-5

6. D

   Rationale: It is recommended the client discontinue this herb at least two weeks before therapy to reduce the risk of intraoperative bleeding.

   Learning Outcome: 8-6

7. A

   Rationale: Harpagophytum procumbens is believed to have analgesic, anti-inflammatory, and antidiabetic properties and may be useful for clients with osteoarthritis.

   Learning Outcome: 8-6

8. C

   Rationale: Magnet therapy is often used to relieve pain, and is believed to act by increasing endorphins, promoting blood flow, and relieving pain.

   Learning Outcome: 8-3

9. A

   Rationale: Garlic, commonly taken to reduce serum cholesterol levels, has potential side effects of headache, sweating, and hypoglycemia. Clients who take garlic daily may have a garlic odor to the skin.

   Learning Outcome: 8-1

10. C

    Rationale: CAM therapists individualize the diagnosis and treatment of clients, may use multiple botanical products, emphasize disease prevention instead of disease treatment, believe in maximizing the body's inherent healing ability, and treat the whole client.

    Learning Outcome: 8-1

Chapter 9 Safety

Matching

1. B
2. C
3. E
4. A
5. D

Learning Outcomes

1. See section entitled "Factors that Affect Safety."
   Learning Outcome: 9-1
2. See section entitled "Factors that Affect Safety."
   Learning Outcome: 9-2

3. See section entitled "Preventing Specific Hazards."
   Learning Outcome: 9-3
4. See section entitled "Hospital and Institutional Safety."
   Learning Outcome: 9-4
5. See section entitled "Hospital and Institutional Safety."
   Learning Outcome: 9-5
6. See section entitled "Restraining Clients."
   Learning Outcome: 9-6
7. See section entitled "Restraining Clients."
   Learning Outcome: 9-7
8. See section entitled "Restraining Clients."
   Learning Outcome: 9-8
9. See section entitled "Protection from Violence in the Healthcare Setting."
   Learning Outcome: 9-9

Apply What You Learned

Suggested Answers

1. Chemicals (medications, cleaning supplies, insecticides, etc.) should be placed in upper, locked cabinets, and poison control phone numbers should be placed on all of the telephones in the house. The mother needs to understand that children do not have fully mature taste buds, and are not bothered by the strong odors and tastes of chemicals in the same way adults are. The mother can start teaching her child to never put anything in his mouth that isn't food and to check with her before putting anything in his mouth.
2. Locks can be placed on stove handles to prevent fires, throw rugs should be removed to prevent slipping and sliding, stairs and other dark areas should be kept well lit, and locks requiring the use of a key should be used on all doors leading outside.
3. The child's mother may be experiencing caregiver role strain and should be cautioned to obtain adequate nutrition and sleep. Care must be taken during times of stress because there is increased risk of injuries. She may consider arranging for times when other family members can provide care so she can attend a gym, go to a movie, or do something she would find pleasant. The nurse can provide referrals to Alzheimer support groups or day care to help in providing care for the great-grandmother.

Multiple Choice Questions

1. A, C
   Rationale: Narcotics can affect how the client perceives the environment and reduce sensory perception of pain, which places the client at risk for injury. Narcotics also put the client at risk for mobility alterations because their balance may be adversely affected by the narcotic. Cognition, emotion, and environment are normally not affected by narcotics.
   Learning Outcome: 9-1

2. B

Rationale: It is unlikely that a child will cross the street or walk alone at night before reaching school age, and they should already have been taught this information by the time they reach adolescence.

Learning Outcome: 9-2

3. C

Rationale: Clients with orthostatic hypotension become dizzy when they stand and that places them at risk for falls.

Learning Outcome: 9-3

4. A, B, C

Rationale: The MSDS provides information about the product name, the relevant physical and chemical characteristics, the relevant physical hazards, and the permissible exposure limit. It also provides information about how to treat overdose or overexposure.

Learning Outcome: 9-4

5. D

Rationale: Code orange is used for a hazardous spill or release. Code red is used for fire, code yellow for a bomb threat, and code black is nonexistent.

Learning Outcome: 9-5

6. C

Rationale: Physicians must order restraints before they are placed. The other actions are not legal uses of restraints.

Learning Outcome: 9-6

7. D

Rationale: Assisting the confused client to use a bedside commode is a reasonable alternative to restraints to reduce the risk of falls. Although use of a safety belt is a reasonable caution, it is considered a restraint and should not be applied without the client's permission. Full-length side rails are a form of restraint, limiting the client's freedom of movements. Sedatives are a form of chemical restraints.

Learning Outcome: 9-7

8. A

Rationale: A mummy restraint may be used to restrict arm movement and prevent the child from reaching its eye. All of the other restraints would not limit this movement.

Learning Outcome: 9-8

9. D

Rationale: Deescalation techniques will enable the nurse to lower the emotions of an angry person and reduce the risk of violence.

Learning Outcome: 9-9

10. B

Rationale: Native American teens and young adults are twice as likely to die from alcohol use. The nurse must be aware of this risk in order to direct safety teaching to lower this risk.

Learning Outcome: 9-1

Matching

1.	C	6.	B	11.	D	16.	A	21.	B
2.	E	7.	C	12.	C	17.	E	22.	E
3.	A	8.	E	13.	D	18.	C	23.	D
4.	F	9.	A	14.	E	19.	D	24.	A
5.	D	10.	B	15.	B	20.	A	25.	C
								26.	B

Learning Outcomes

1. See section entitled "Microorganisms."
    Learning Outcome: 10-1
2. See section entitled "Microorganisms."
    Learning Outcome: 10-2
3. See section entitled "Infection."
    Learning Outcome: 10-3
4. See section entitled "Factors in the Chain of Infection."
    Learning Outcome: 10-4
5. See section entitled "Factors that Reduce Host Resistance."
    Learning Outcome: 10-5
6. See section entitled "Defenses against Infection."
    Learning Outcome: 10-6
7. See section entitled "Drug-Resistant Organisms."
    Learning Outcome: 10-7
8. See section entitled "Controlling Microorganisms in the Environment."
    Learning Outcome: 10-8
9. See section entitled "Controlling Microorganisms in the Environment."
    Learning Outcome: 10-9
10. See section entitled "Equipment For Infection Control."
    Learning Outcome: 10-10
11. See section entitled "Nursing Care."
    Learning Outcome: 10-11

Apply What You Learned

1.	C	6.	E
2.	A	7.	F
3.	B	8.	E
4.	D	9.	B
5.	D	10.	B

Multiple Choice Questions

1. C

   Rationale: The term *pathogen* is applied to disease-carrying microorganisms. Not all microorganisms are harmful, and some are essential to life. Resident flora can cause disease if they migrate from the area where they are normally found to an area where they do not belong. Pathogens are not helpful but are disease-carrying microorganisms.

   Learning Outcome: 10-1

2. B

   Rationale: Blood may contain any number of microorganisms and must be cleaned in a way that prevents contamination of others. Cover the blood spill first because direct spraying of bleach onto the blood could cause the blood to become airborne. Spray with bleach and wait 20 minutes, because the bleach will kill any pathogens, and then wipe up the stain while wearing gloves.

   Learning Outcome: 10-2

3. C

   Rationale: Septicemia is a bloodborne infection that causes systemic symptoms and can be fatal if not treated promptly. Sepsis is the presence of infection but does not indicate it exists throughout the body.

   Learning Outcome: 10-3

4. A

   Rationale: West Nile virus is a vector-borne infection that is spread by mosquitoes that have come in contact with an infected bird's feces.

   Learning Outcome: 10-4

5. B

   Rationale: Stress increases the production of cortisol that enters the bloodstream and reduces the immune response, thereby increasing the host's susceptibility to pathogens.

   Learning Outcome: 10-5

6. B

   Rationale: B cells are part of the antibody-mediated defense system, which is a specific immune response that originates in the bone marrow from stem cells.

   Learning Outcome: 10-6

7. A

   Rationale: Hand hygiene is the single best way to reduce the spread of infection, whether you are working or at home caring for sick children. Although the occurrence of drug-resistant organisms is on the rise, largely due to improper use of antibiotics, handwashing would reduce the spread of these organisms.

   Learning Outcome: 10-7

8. C

   Rationale: The bladder is a sterile area and the nurse would use surgical asepsis in order to prevent introduction of a pathogen into the area, resulting in a urinary tract infection.

   Learning Outcome: 10-8

9. A

Rationale: There is a wide variety of different types of infectious agents and not all agents work against all pathogens. It is important to know what type of infectious organism is present to allow the nurse to choose the proper disinfectant.

Learning Outcome: 10-9

10. D

Rationale: When dressed in sterile gown, anything below the waist is considered contaminated and care is taken to keep the hands above the level of the waist.

Learning Outcome: 10-11

Chapter 11 Client Communication

Matching

1.	E	6.	E
2.	D	7.	A
3.	A	8.	D
4.	B	9.	C
5.	C	10.	B

Learning Outcomes

1. See chapter introduction.
   Learning Outcome: 11-1
2. See section entitled "Factors Influencing Communication."
   Learning Outcome: 11-2
3. See section entitled "Modes of Communication."
   Learning Outcome: 11-3
4. See section entitled "Therapeutic Communication."
   Learning Outcome: 11-4
5. See section entitled "Principles of Communication."
   Learning Outcome: 11-5
6. See section entitled "Principles of Communication for the Clinical Setting."
   Learning Outcome: 11-6
7. See section entitled "Interviewing."
   Learning Outcome: 11-7
8. See section entitled "Interviewing."
   Learning Outcome: 11-8
9. See section entitled "Interviewing."
   Learning Outcome: 11-9
10. See section entitled "Interviewing."
    Learning Outcome: 11-10
11. See section entitled "Interviewing."
    Learning Outcome: 11-11

Apply What You Learned

Suggested Answers

1. It is important to ask the client questions to determine if she plans to attempt suicide again, if she would like anyone notified of her admission, if she has need to talk with a spiritual counselor, and how she feels about her failed attempt at suicide. Other questions related to her current physical condition include a pain assessment and questions to determine if she is having any other symptoms.
2. Open-ended questions, reflecting her feeling back to her, offering self, providing leads, and using touch are several therapeutic techniques that may be useful in helping the client share her thoughts, feelings, and concerns.
3. You must examine your own feelings about these things to determine if you have any biases or judgments against or sympathetic to the client's lifestyle. It is equally nontherapeutic to overly identify with this client as it is to judge or condemn her.

Multiple Choice Questions

1. C
   Rationale: After the message is received, the receiver sends feedback in response.
   Learning Outcome: 11-1
2. A
   Rationale: Personal space is the area around you that, when someone invades, makes you feel uncomfortable. How well you know a person often determines how much personal space you require. It might be acceptable for someone you love to come within a few inches of you, but if your instructor got that close it would be more likely to make you feel uncomfortable. Culture influences how much personal space we require.
   Learning Outcome: 11-2
3. D
   Rationale: Although nonverbal communication can provide clues to client feelings, they can be easily misinterpreted or misunderstood, so it is important to validate the meaning of the nonverbal behavior to prevent acting on a misconception.
   Learning Outcome: 11-3
4. B
   Rationale: This method is used to clarify the meaning of what the client is saying. For example, if a client said, "My husband will kill me if I don't get to the store today," the nurse could clarify by asking, "Your husband threatened you?" This allows the nurse to determine if the nurse's perception of the client's words matches the meaning the client attaches to them and helps the client think more about what they are saying.
   Learning Outcome: 11-4

5. C

   Rationale: The primary form of communication used by staff nurses is the shift report that can be conducted in a variety of different ways with the goal of providing continuity of care by assuring the oncoming nurse knows how the client's care and status have changed.

   Learning Outcome: 11-5

6. D

   Rationale: When the nurse gives opinions to the client it fosters dependence because the client is not assisted to make the best choice for themselves, but rather to do what the nurse thinks is best for them.

   Learning Outcome: 11-6

7. A

   Rationale: The nondirective interview allows the client control over the interview and the client can share information with the nurse, thus building rapport.

   Learning Outcome: 11-7

8. B

   Rationale: Trust is created when the nurse communicates in a consistent, dependable, and honest manner in all communications with the client. Use of medical terminology should be avoided because it leads to client misunderstandings due to lack of ability to translate words. Humor can destroy the nurse/client relationship if used inappropriately and should never substitute for dealing honestly with uncomfortable issues.

   Learning Outcome: 11-8

9. B

   Rationale: Leading questions tell the person what answer the questioner is looking for, such as, "You aren't having any pain, are you?" which may result in the client giving the answer suggested to please the nurse.

   Learning Outcome: 11-9

10. D

   Rationale: The nurse should sit so the client can see them and be close enough to interpret nonverbal communication, but not so close as to invade personal space.

   Learning Outcome: 11-10

Chapter 12 Client Teaching

Matching

1. E	6. B	11. D
2. D	7. D	12. C
3. B	8. E	13. A
4. A	9. C	14. B
5. C	10. A	

Learning Outcomes

1. See section entitled "Client Education."

   Learning Outcome: 12-1

2. See section entitled "Learning Theories."
   Learning Outcome: 12-2
3. See section entitled "Learning Theories."
   Learning Outcome: 12-3
4. See sections entitled "Factors that Facilitate Learning" and "Factors that Inhibit Learning."
   Learning Outcome: 12-4
5. See section entitled "Teaching."
   Learning Outcome: 12-5
6. See section entitled "Role of LPNs/LVNs in Teaching."
   Learning Outcome: 12-6
7. See section entitled "Nursing Care."
   Learning Outcome: 12-7
8. See section entitled "Nursing Care."
   Learning Outcome: 12-8
9. See section entitled "Nursing Care."
   Learning Outcome: 12-9

Apply What You Learned

Suggested Answers

1. There are numerous barriers and special considerations in this situation. The client is elderly.
   - The client speaks little English (natural communication barrier). The client is scheduled to undergo a procedure that involves bodily functions that may cause embarrassment. Cultural values may impact the client's comfort level and compliance with the preparation and procedure. Western medicine may conflict with the client's native healing beliefs and cultural practices. The client's family, out of state, will not be available to provide translation.

2. You can obtain information: Hospitals may have translators available for non-English-speaking clients. Reaching into the Laotian community will provide necessary information.

3. These are some of the necessary transcultural teaching guidelines for this situation:
   - Obtain foreign language teaching materials. Use visual aids. Use clear, simple language. Avoid slang or colloquialisms. Present only one idea at a time.
   - Phrase questions positively. Validate verbal communication in writing. Use humor very cautiously.
   - Confirm nonverbal cues. Identify cultural gender issues.
   - When available, include the family in planning and teaching. Consider the client's time orientation.
   - Identify cultural health practices and beliefs.

4. These are some ways to communicate clearly and effectively:
   - Communicate respect and sensitivity. Become knowledgeable about the specific culture. Be clear and concise.
   - Address conflict directly. Be honest and open.
   - Utilize support persons such as a translator or other members of the community.

Multiple Choice Questions

1. C

   Rationale: The nurse is teaching about restoration of health because the child requiring health promotion or illness prevention would not require an IV. Adapting to altered health and function would indicate the problem is chronic, and that is not indicated by the question.

   Learning Outcome: 12-1

2. D

   Rationale: Think of behaviorism as teaching a behavior, such as modeling and imitating healthy behavior. Cognitivism is thinking and learning about a disease; humanism involves emotions; and motivation is finding ways to get a client to want to learn.

   Learning Outcome: 12-2

3. A

   Rationale: This teaching involves helping the client to understand the risk that previously used needles present to her family and the community, so this is a cognitive domain. Affective domain would involve feelings; psychomotor would involve a manual skill; and motivation is finding a means to encourage the client to want to learn.

   Learning Outcome: 12-3

4. B

   Rationale: The client learned how to use the inhaler but doesn't remember what to do when the need to use it weeks later arises, so the client is having trouble with retaining knowledge. Relevance involves understanding why it is important to know; repetition is the ability to repeat what was taught; and active learning is involving the client in the learning process.

   Learning Outcome: 12-4

5. A

   Rationale: Objectives for resolving the problem of knowledge deficit is teaching related because the nurse wants the client to have more knowledge.

   Learning Outcome: 12-5

6. A, B, E

   Rationale: The LPN may act as a preceptor for a new graduate LPN/LVN, teach CPR, or contribute to the creation of a teaching plan. Teaching the clients transitioning from one level of care to another or initiating discharge teaching should be done by the RN, and the LPN/LVN can reinforce or answer questions after initial teaching is begun.

   Learning Outcome: 12-6

7. D

Rationale: Role playing requires the learner to think and feel what is required in that role.

Learning Outcome: 12-7

8. D

Rationale: Gestural cues can have many different meanings in different cultures, so it is important for the nurse to confirm the meaning with that client. Family should be included, medical terminology should be excluded to avoid misunderstandings, and humor must be used very cautiously in transcultural nursing because different cultures view humor in different ways.

Learning Outcome: 12-8

9. B

Rationale: Affective learning involves feelings and emotions, and can be very difficult to evaluate because it is based on interpreting behavior and cues indication what is felt.

Learning Outcome: 12-9

10. C

Rationale: When teaching a client, the words chosen by the nurse should be specific, and explicitly understood by the client. Redundancy becomes boring to the client and reduces motivation. Involving the client in planning increases desire to learn. Rapport is developed between the client and the teacher, and teaching should involve multiple senses to enhance learning.

Learning Outcome: 12-7

Chapter 13 Documentation

Matching

1.	C	5.	F	9.	F
2.	A	6.	E	10.	B
3.	D	7.	D	11.	C
4.	B	8.	E	12.	A

Learning Outcomes

1. See section entitled "Purposes of Client Records."
   Learning Outcome: 13-1
2. See section entitled "Guidelines for Recording."
   Learning Outcome: 13-2
3. See section entitled "Guidelines for Recording."
   Learning Outcome: 13-3
4. See section entitled "Guidelines for Recording."
   Learning Outcome: 13-4
5. See section entitled "Confidentiality of Client Records."
   Learning Outcome: 13-5
6. See section entitled "Documentation Systems."
   Learning Outcome: 13-6

7. See section entitled "Reporting."
    Learning Outcome: 13-7
8. See section entitled "Nursing Care."
    Learning Outcome: 13-8

Apply What You Learned

Suggested Answers

1. *Date:*
    Time:

    S: States, "I need something for pain." "How will I get over this in time for my daughter's graduation?"

    O: BP 140/86, P 92, R 18, T 99F. Alert and oriented 3. Grimacing and clenching jaw. Rates pain at 7 on a scale of 0–10. Dressing dry and intact. 20 mL light pink clear drainage in JP collection container. Up in chair 2 this shift and ambulated in hall 1 with assist. Drank 250 mL of various clear liquids for breakfast and tolerating well. Faint bowel sounds heard in all four quadrants. Indwelling urinary catheter draining clear amber urine. Demerol 75 mg IM given at 0800 and 1200.

    A: Reports relief from pain meds—rated pain at 3 on a scale of 0–10.

    Signature:

Multiple Choice Questions

1. D
    Rationale: Although the chart is a legal document, avoiding lawsuits is not a purpose for documenting. Thorough documentation helps to explain the client's care and can prove that proper care was delivered in a court of law, but the best way to avoid lawsuits is by providing safe nursing care. All of the other options are purposes of nursing documentation.
    Learning Outcome: 13-1

2. B
    Rationale: Although it is important to be timely in documenting on the client, the safety and needs of the client take precedence over the documentation of the change in condition. After the client is stabilized or transferred to a higher acuity area, the nurse should document immediately. The physician will be notified in most cases before the client stabilizes and although orders received will immediately be entered in the record, nursing documentation comes after carrying out those orders needed to stabilize the client's condition. An incident report isn't required unless the change in the client's condition was secondary to an unexpected event or error.
    Learning Outcome: 13-2

3. C
    Rationale: DAT stands for *diet as tolerated,* meaning the nurse can order the tray best tolerated by the client such as liquid, soft, or pureed.
    Learning Outcome: 13-3

4. D

Rationale: The nurse would treat this error the same as any other type of error, putting a line through the error without occluding the words, writing her initials above the line, and begin writing the note again in the correct location. The page cannot be discarded because prior notes would be eliminated. There is no need to notify the nursing supervisor or complete an incident report. The note should be continued in the wrong location.

Learning Outcome: 13-4

5. A

Rationale: The nurse should minimize the screen to prevent the family from reading any information about a client, but should not unplug the computer because this can cause damage to the computer and the data it contains. The family member should be instructed not to enter the nurse's station, but that is not the first priority action. An incident report may need to be completed, depending on facility policy, but that is not the first priority.

Learning Outcome: 13-5

6. A

Rationale: D stands for data in the focus charting system, so data gathered from the assessment would be charted in this area. A is for Action; R for response.

Learning Outcome: 13-6

7. A

Rationale: Each nurse should establish a system for administering report that is comfortable, either system by system or head to toe. Reviewing physician's orders would not include nursing orders or nursing actions that the client requires. The Kardex, if used by the facility, does not provide a comprehensive review of the client's status. Writing everything down ahead of time would take a great deal of time the nurse most likely doesn't have.

Learning Outcome: 13-7

8. C

Rationale: The client's medical record will be kept in the home so the family caregiver can record care provided between nursing visits.

Learning Outcome: 13-8

9. C

Rationale: Teaching is documented on the teaching record, which allows the nurse to document what was taught and the client's response to teaching. Some facilities may not use a teaching record, in which case the information would be documented in the progress notes, but it is always best to use the teaching record if available.

Learning Outcome: 13-6

10. D

Rationale: Although it would be best to look further for a black ink pen, of the choices provided the black marker would be the best choice because it is black permanent ink. Gel ink tends to fade with time and is not a good choice. Legal documentation cannot be written with anything erasable, so the pencil and the erasable ink would not be a legally prudent choice.

Learning Outcome: 13-4

Matching

1. B
2. G
3. F
4. E

5. C
6. A
7. D

Learning Outcomes

1. See section entitled "Admitting a Client."
   Learning Outcome: 14-1
2. See section entitled "Admitting a Client."
   Learning Outcome: 14-2
3. See section entitled "Admitting a Client."
   Learning Outcome: 14-3
4. See section entitled "Admitting a Client."
   Learning Outcome: 14-4
5. See section entitled "Admitting a Client."
   Learning Outcome: 14-5
6. See section entitled "Transferring a Client."
   Learning Outcome: 14-6
7. See section entitled "Transferring a Client."
   Learning Outcome: 14-7
8. See section entitled "Discharging a Client."
   Learning Outcome: 14-8
9. See section entitled "Discharging a Client."
   Learning Outcome: 14-9

Apply What You Learned

Suggested Answers

1. The healthcare environment promotes dehumanization or the removal of unique human qualities by asking clients to surrender their belongings, privacy, and independence. A loss of self-identity occurs when individuals are referred to as a number, a diagnosis, or a nickname or when they are called by their first name without having given permission. Prior to admission to the long-term facility, Mrs. Levy enjoyed power and control in her life. Like all of us, she values her independence and now perceives herself as powerless and helpless. Her behavior indicates some unmet need.
2. Culture is a set of learned attitudes and behaviors associated with particular values, ethnic traditions, and religious beliefs. Clients such as Mrs. Levy come from many different cultures, and so have a variety of attitudes and beliefs related to illness and medical treatment. Clients' views about health care and their behavior during hospitalization or institutionalization may be expressions of their cultural beliefs. Often, the client's view is different from the

nurse's view. Regardless of the cultural differences between the nurse and the client, it is the nurse's obligation to provide culturally sensitive care.

3. It is the nurse's responsibility to help protect the client from feeling dehumanized by anticipating and avoiding situations that are likely to provoke these feelings. In addition, the nurse must strive to help reduce the specific fears and anxieties of each client. The client's integrity and personal dignity must always be maintained. Determining the reasons behind Mrs. Levy's behavior will assist with understanding and planning.

4. Including Mrs. Levy in making decisions about her plan of care, allowing her choices as appropriate, and fostering independence will decrease her feeling of powerlessness. Spending time with Mrs. Levy and helping her to explore her feelings will convey respect, empathy, and caring.

Multiple Choice Questions

1. A
   Rationale: The goal of nursing care is to ensure continuity of individualized client care during admission, transfer, and discharge. Although options 2, 3, and 4 are used as parts of admission, transfer, and discharge, on their own these options are not the goal.
   Learning Outcome: N/A

2. A
   Rationale: It is important to make a positive first impression on the client. Each individual client deserves to be greeted in a caring manner that demonstrates concern and respect.
   Learning Outcome: 14-2

3. B
   Rationale: Clients' responses to hospitalization are influenced by their particular gender, age, culture, religion, and coping behaviors. The client's responses are also related to needs identified by Maslow.
   Learning Outcome: 14-2

4. D
   Rationale: Dehumanization includes such things as asking clients to surrender their belongings, privacy, and independence.
   Learning Outcome: 14-2

5. D
   Rationale: Calling a client by a nickname is an example of dehumanization of the client. It is best to ask the client what he or she would like to be called.
   Learning Outcome: 14-2

6. B
   Rationale: Each hospital has written policies for transferring a client. The procedure usually requires the following: receiving a physician order, informing the client and family about the reason for the transfer, assisting the client to gather all belongings, and completing the required documentation.
   Learning Outcome: 14-6

7. 4
   Rationale: The client's level of care would be the primary consideration for where they are placed within the hospital.
   Learning Outcome: 14-6

8. D

    Rationale: Part of discharge planning for a nurse is to explain referral agencies and provide information about people or groups to contact.

    Learning Outcome: 14-9

9. A

    Rationale: Two of the most common nursing diagnoses that are identified when discharging clients are self-care deficit and deficient knowledge because clients are typically concerned about how they will care for themselves upon discharge and how to follow discharge instructions properly.

    Learning Outcome: 14-9

10. B

    Rationale: Clients are typically concerned about how they will care for themselves upon discharge and how to follow discharge instructions properly. Therefore, it is important that the nurse provide the opportunity for clients to ask questions.

    Learning Outcome: 14-9

11. C

    Rationale: Children are likely to express separation anxiety from their parents during the admission process.

    Learning Outcome: 14-1

12. A

    Rationale: Hospital admission is usually a very stressful time for clients. The nurses who initially provide assistance with admission and orientation will influence the client's reaction to hospitalization and treatment.

    Learning Outcome: 14-2

13. A

    Rationale: The Joint Commission requires that an RN perform the admission assessment. Subjective and objective data are collected throughout the interview, medical history, and physical assessment. The RN may delegate parts (not the entire) of the assessment to the LPN/LVN.

    Learning Outcome: 14-2

14. A

    Rationale: If the client is rational and a court order does not exist to detain the client, he or she cannot be forcibly detained.

    Learning Outcome: 14-8

15. B

    Rationale: Valuables should always be given to a family member when possible. If not possible, security should be involved to inventory, document, and secure the property.

    Learning Outcome: 14-6

Matching

1.	E	6.	D
2.	D	7.	A
3.	A	8.	E
4.	C	9.	B
5.	B	10.	C

Learning Outcomes

1. See section entitled "Erikson's Psychosocial Development Theory."
   Learning Outcome: 15-1
2. See section entitled "Theorists And Their Theories."
   Learning Outcome: 15-2
3. See section entitled "Kohlberg's Moral Development Theory."
   Learning Outcome: 15-3
4. See section entitled "Piaget's Cognitive Development Theory."
   Learning Outcome: 15-4
5. See section entitled "Maslow's Hierarchy of Basic Human Needs."
   Learning Outcome: 15-5
6. See section entitled "Therapies."
   Learning Outcome: 15-6
7. See section entitled "Therapies."
   Learning Outcome: 15-7

Apply What You Learned

1. Stages of Erikson's psychosocial developmental theory:
   - 17-Year-Old - identity versus role confusion
   - 87-Year-Old - ego integrity versus despair
   - 56-Year-Old - generativity versus stagnation
   - 34-Year-Old - intimacy versus isolation
2. Maslow's hierarchy of needs:
   - 17-Year-Old - physiologic; social
   - 87-Year-Old - physiologic; safety
   - 56-Year-Old - physiologic; social; esteem
   - 34-Year-Old - physiologic; social; esteem
3. Rogers's theory focuses on the client–therapist (nurse) relationship. He suggested that all individuals have the ability to guide their own lives in a manner that is personally satisfying and socially constructive. In a therapeutic helping relationship, individuals are free to find their inner wisdom and confidence, and they will make increasingly healthy and more constructive choices. Rogers believed that each individual is capable of developing deeper self-understanding. According to Rogers, a person must be fully accepted for who he or she is.

Characteristics necessary for a supportive environment include:
- Genuineness
- Unconditional positive regard
- Empathetic understanding
- Active listening
- Use of silence
- Reflection

These characteristics are key to the nurse–client relationship. To have credibility with our clients, we must be genuine, honest, and trustworthy. Our clients deserve respect, unconditional positive regard, and empathetic understanding. Listening actively and attentively to our clients not only helps to build rapport, it also provides an opportunity to target those areas the client perceives as problematic. Rather than providing advice and false reassurance, nurses guide clients as they work through these areas.

4. Hildegard Peplau described nursing as a therapeutic interpersonal process. Peplau identified communication growth and development, and roles as major concepts of her theory. Following her theory, the nurse would identify the client's developmental stage to provide appropriate, holistic care.

Multiple Choice Questions

1. A
   Rationale: The id is part of the unconscious. It is the biological and psychologic drives with which an individual enters this world. It is self-centered and concerned with immediate gratification, such as the baby who needs to be fed or changed.
   Learning Outcome: 15-6

2. C
   Rationale: The subconscious mind is also called the preconscious and consists of the individual's memory. Moral behavior is part of the superego. The conscious mind is aware of reality and perceptions in the moment. The unconscious mind is made of repressed memories and experiences such as early experiences in infancy.
   Learning Outcome: 15-6

3. D
   Rationale: The anal stage coincides with control of urination and defecation.
   Learning Outcome: 15-6

4. C
   Rationale: The genital stage is the final stage of psychosexual development where the goal is to develop satisfying relationships with the opposite sex. Option A refers to the phallic stage, Option B refers to the oral stage, Option D refers to the anal stage.
   Learning Outcome: 15-6

5. C
   Rationale: A toddler whose development is frustrated will develop shame versus doubt.
   Learning Outcome: 15-1

6. A
   Rationale: Kohlberg believed that individuals could only progress through stages one at a time and they could only understand the moral rationale one stage above their own.
   Learning Outcome: 15-3

7. B
   Rationale: The safety level of Maslow's Hierarchy of Needs consists of security and protection from physical and emotional harm.
   Learning Outcome: 15-5

8. A
   Rationale: Skinner believed that behavior could be controlled by rewards and punishment. Desired behaviors are reinforced so they continue.
   Learning Outcome: 15-6

9. C
   Rationale: Cognitive therapy looks at distortion of thought as the cause of psychologic distress.
   Learning Outcome: 15-7

10. A
    Rationale: Rogers believed that if a person had self-understanding and was fully accepted for who he or she was, he or she could not help but change. The maturing process leads to positive choices and increased capacity for problem solving.
    Learning Outcome: 15-7

11. D
    Rationale: Rogers believed that three characteristics were necessary to a supportive climage: genuineness, unconditional positive regard, empathetic understanding.
    Learning Outcome: 15-6

12. C
    Rationale: According to Piaget, a 10-year-old child is in the concrete operations phase where the child solves concrete problems and begins to understand relationships such as size and direction.
    Learning Outcome: 15-4

Chapter 16 Life Span, Health Promotion, and Family Systems

Matching

1.	F	5.	C	9.	B
2.	E	6.	D	10.	A
3.	A	7.	C	11.	F
4.	B	8.	D	12.	E

Learning Outcomes

1. See section entitled "Growth and Development."
   Learning Outcome: 16-1

2. See section entitled "Growth and Development."
   Learning Outcome: 16-2

3. See section entitled "Growth and Development."
   Learning Outcome: 16-3
4. See section entitled "Life Stages."
   Learning Outcome: 16-4
5. See section entitled "Family Systems."
   Learning Outcome: 16-5
6. See section entitled "Nursing Care."
   Learning Outcome: 16-6

Apply What You Learned

1. The classic definition of *family* is two or more people related by blood or marriage who reside together. In recent years, the definition has been broadened to two or more individuals who come together for the purpose of nurturing.

2. There are four family types:
   - **Nuclear family**—A family consisting of parents and biological offspring.
   - **Extended family**—An egocentric network of relatives such as grandparents, aunts, uncles, and cousins.
   - **Blended family**—A situation in which one or both spouses have had a previous marriage and children from that marriage.
   - **Communal family**—A family that includes adults and children who may or may not be related; family decision making and responsibilities are shared.

3. Functions of the family are as follows:
   - Provide economic support for other family members.
   - Satisfy emotional needs for love and security.
   - Provide a sense of place and position in society.

4. There are two important factors to consider when analyzing parenting styles:
   - **Demandingness**—relates to the demands that parents make on the children, their expectations for mature behavior, the discipline and supervision they provide, and their willingness to confront behavioral problems.
   - **Responsiveness**—relates to how much they foster individuality, self-assertion, and self-regulation, and how responsive they are to special needs and demands.

Multiple Choice Questions

1. A, B, C, E
   Rationale: Factors that influence growth and development are genetic and environmental. Genetics includes sex, physical stature, and race. Environmental factors include family, religion, climate, culture, school, community, and nutrition.
   Learning Outcome: 16-1
2. A
   Rationale: Poorly nourished children are more likely to have infections than are well-fed children, and they may not attain their full height potential. Appropriate growth and development depends on appropriate nutrition.
   Learning Outcome: 16-1

3. A

   Rationale: Growth and development follow a predictable sequence and all humans follow the same pattern. Standard norms have been developed that are part of an assessment of a child.

   Learning Outcome: 16-1

4. A

   Rationale: An infant at this stage is exploring his environment. Feeding, language and fine motor skills all develop at a later stage.

   Learning Outcome: 16-3

5. A

   Rationale: Toddlers are usually chubby, with relatively short legs and a large head. Average weight gain is five pounds in the first two years and two to five pounds in the next year. Average height gain is between four to five inches. Toddlers are developing their sense of autonomy by liberal use of the word "no."

   Learning Outcome: 16-3

6. C

   Rationale: School-aged children are at Kohlberg's stage 1 (punishment and obedience) or stage 2 (instrumental-relativist). As such, these children are able to reason and understand cause and effect and reversibility.

   Learning Outcome: 16-3

7. A

   Rationale: Preschoolers' vocabulary is increasing but they are not old enough to cut deciduous teeth or work independently.

   Learning Outcome: 16-3

8. C

   Rationale: Slowed metabolism will mean less calories are burned and more are retained. This leads to a potential increase in weight.

   Learning Outcome: 16-3

9. D

   Rationale: During this phase of the child's life the parents should be helped to recognize the importance of promoting their child's school achievement as a way of promoting healthy development for the child. Encouraging the child to explore their environment occurs with preschool children, reestablishing the roles of wife or husband occurs when the children begin leaving the home, and developing a stable family unit occurs when newborns are entering the family.

   Learning Outcome: 16-4

10. B

    Rationale: The parents allow the child to make decisions indicating they are permissive, and this results in children who are encouraged to make decisions before they are mature enough to make good choices. Authoritarian parents would value obedience and be highly directive, while authoritative parents would allow give-and-take communication.

    Learning Outcome: 16-5

11. A, B, D, E

    Rationale: The child's development impacts almost the entire plan of care. Medication dosage is ordered by the physician, not the nurse, and is based on the child's weight, which is growth related more than development. The

child's diet must take into consideration the ability to feed oneself, which is the result of development. Teaching should be directed toward the child's development, both psychological and cognitive. Diversional activities work best if they are developmentally appropriate. Both the performance of the procedure and the choice of equipment is based on growth and development.
Learning Outcome: 16-6

Chapter 17 Psychosocial Nursing of the Physically Ill Client

Matching

1.	C	5.	F	9.	F
2.	D	6.	A	10.	E
3.	B	7.	D	11.	C
4.	E	8.	A	12.	B

Learning Outcomes

1. See section entitled "Psychosocial Assessment."
   Learning Outcome: 17-1
2. See section entitled "Psychosocial Assessment."
   Learning Outcome: 17-2
3. See section entitled "Psychological Responses to Serious Medical Illness."
   Learning Outcome: 17-3
4. See section entitled "Psychological Responses to Serious Medical Illness."
   Learning Outcome: 17-4
5. See section entitled "Psychological Responses to Serious Medical Illness."
   Learning Outcome: 17-5
6. See section entitled "Coping."
   Learning Outcome: 17-6
7. See section entitled "Coping."
   Learning Outcome: 17-7
8. See section entitled "Other Psychosocial Factors in Medical Illness."
   Learning Outcome: 17-8
9. See section entitled "Meeting Psychosocial Needs of the Seriously Ill or Dying Child."
   Learning Outcome: 17-9
10. See section entitled "Nursing Care."
    Learning Outcome: 17-10

Apply What You Learned

1. The client is drinking large amounts of alcohol daily to relax and unwind. The use of this amount of alcohol presents a variety of physiologic, psychologic, and social risks. Though he sees this as a positive coping strategy, in the short and long term it is clearly an ineffective way for him to cope with stress.

2. The client is using denial and rationalization. He is denying the fact that the alcohol abuse is impacting his life. He rationalizes his use as a means to relax and unwind. This justification of his behavior underscores his faulty logic and his ascription of his motives, making them socially acceptable. He is making an attempt to ignore unacceptable reality by refusing to acknowledge them.

3. Minorities are just as likely as nonminorities to experience severe mental disorders. Because of lack of access to services, cultural and language barriers, and limited research concerning mental health and minorities, these individuals are far less likely to receive treatment. Approximately 20% of African Americans do not have a primary health care provider. Cultural beliefs about mental health strongly affect whether or not some people seek treatment, persons' coping styles and social supports, and the stigma they attach to mental illness. Many people from different cultures see mental illness as shameful and delay treatment until symptoms reach crisis proportions.

Multiple Choice Questions

1. D
   Rationale: Common responses to physical illness are depression, anxiety, stress, grief, denial, and fear of dependency.
   Learning Outcome: 17-3

2. B
   Rationale: Good listening skills are critical in obtaining an accurate history and assessment.
   Learning Outcome: 17-1

3. A
   Rationale: Symptoms of major depression vary by age group and it is important to understand what constitutes "normal" development in infants, children, and adolescents.
   Learning Outcome: 17-4

4. A
   Rationale: Unpredictable reactions are also known as idiosyncratic reactions.
   Learning Outcome: 17-4

5. A
   Rationale: ECT may be used for people with severe depression who have not responded well to other treatments. Some people have indicated that it has helped them, while it has not helped other clients.
   Learning Outcome: 17-4

6. C
   Rationale: PTSD can develop after exposure to one or more terrifying events in which grave physical harm occurred or was threatened.
   Learning Outcome: 17-6

7. B
   Rationale: The client is projecting her anger at becoming increasingly dependent. Her frustration is manifesting as anger toward the nurse.
   Learning Outcome: 17-7

8. A

Rationale: The fight-or-flight response is a reaction to stress. With this reaction comes an increase in blood pressure and heart rate.

Learning Outcome: 17-6

9. C

Rationale: These are symptoms of possible depression. It is important to talk with someone about them before the symptoms escalate.

Learning Outcome: 17-4

10. B

Rationale: A dual diagnosis is the presence of substance abuse along with a concurrent psychiatric disorder.

Learning Outcome: 17-8

11. B

Rationale: Smoking a cigarette is a maladaptive behavior that actually will lead to increased stress and the increased need for coping.

Learning Outcome: 17-7

12. B

Rationale: ICU psychosis is a disorder during which clients in the ICU become temporarily psychotic. Although the exact causes are not known, factors that contribute are sensory deprivation, sensory overload, pain, sleep deprivation, disruption of normal rhythm of night and day, and the loss of control of their lives.

Learning Outcome: 17-9

13. D

Rationale: You should never ignore the threat of suicide. It is crucial to respond in a nonjudgmental manner addressing the situation.

Learning Outcome: 17-5

14. D

Rationale: Almost everyone who commits or attempts to commit suicide has given some clue or warning. Do not ignore suicide threats.

Learning Outcome: 17-5

Chapter 18 Loss, Grief, and Death

Matching

1.	E	5.	C	9.	A
2.	D	6.	A	10.	B
3.	F	7.	E	11.	F
4.	B	8.	C	12.	D

Learning Outcomes

1. See section entitled "Loss, Grief, and Dying."
   Learning Outcome: 18-1
2. See section entitled "Factors Influencing Loss and Grief Responses."
   Learning Outcome: 18-2

3. See section entitled "Factors Influencing Loss and Grief Responses."
   Learning Outcome: 18-3
4. See section entitled "Stages and Manifestations of Grief."
   Learning Outcome: 18-4
5. See section entitled "Tasks, Rights, and Needs of the Grieving Person."
   Learning Outcome: 18-5
6. See section entitled "Tasks, Rights, and Needs of the Grieving Person."
   Learning Outcome: 18-6
7. See section entitled "Legal Issues."
   Learning Outcome: 18-7
8. See section entitled "Nursing Care."
   Learning Outcome: 18-8
9. See section entitled "Nurse's Self-Care in Relation to Death."
   Learning Outcome: 18-9

Apply What You Learned

1. The Kübler-Ross stages of grieving being demonstrated by this client are:
   - **Denial**—This client is unable to believe that the loss has happened and is unready to deal with the practical problems.
   - **Depression**—The client is grieving over what has happened and what cannot be.
2. Potential factors affecting this client's grieving response:
   - Age
   - Culture
   - Spiritual beliefs
   - Gender
   - Socioeconomic status
   - Support systems
   - Cause of loss or death
3. Four important questions are:
   - Are you having trouble sleeping? Eating? Concentrating? Breathing?
   - Do you have any pain or other new physical problems?
   - Are you taking any drugs or medications or using alcohol to help you cope with this loss?
   - What are you doing to help deal with this loss?
4. Various nursing interventions that could be used to help this client work through her grief include:
   - Provide opportunities for the client to participate in decision making about daily activities. *Involvement in decision making is empowering and helps the client begin to organize the experience.*
   - Encourage the client to share loss with significant others. *This will assist with acceptance of loss.*
   - Encourage the client to become increasingly involved in her usual activities. *This will help the client establish a routine and help with closure.*
   - Encourage the client to get enough sleep and adequate nutrition. *This will help keep the client from becoming ill.*
   - Encourage the client to seek out support services and resources available to assist during difficult episodes. *This will help promote healthy grieving.*

An objective listener can sometimes help a person get past an emotional barrier.

- Encourage the client to verbalize positive expectations for the future. *This will help promote a positive focus.*

Multiple Choice Questions

1. D
   Rationale: Unresolved grief can lead to continued physical and emotional problems. To achieve mental and physical health, survivors must work through and resolve their grief.
   Learning Outcome: 18-2

2. B
   Rationale: The client is bargaining – feeling guilt about past sins and indicating promises if she could have him back
   Learning Outcome: 18-4

3. C
   Rationale: The client has come to terms with loss by her statement acknowledging their great, long life together. Option 1 represents anger. Option 2 represents depression. Option 3 represents denial.
   Learning Outcome: 18-4

4. D
   Rationale: The nurse would expect to see slowing of the circulation, which would manifest as dusky or bluish nail beds. Changes in respirations would occur, but not increased respirations. The extremities do not stiffen until after death. Before death there would be loss of muscle tone. There is an impairment of sense, not heightened senses.
   Learning Outcome: 18-9

5. B
   Rationale: The client is grieving an event that will occur tomorrow as part of the preparatory process of coping with the anticipated surgery.
   Learning Outcome: 18-2

6. C
   Rationale: It is best to explain simply that the loved one has died, and it may be appropriate (depending on family's beliefs) to tell them what happens after death based on their spiritual beliefs. Children interpret things very literally so it is important to ask questions to determine how they interpreted what they were told. They should not be told she went to sleep because it can cause fear that they will go to sleep and not wake up.
   Learning Outcome: 18-3

7. B
   Rationale: Tearing of the clothing is often done by Orthodox Jews to show they are in mourning for someone who has died. There is no security risk here.
   Learning Outcome: 18-2

8. D

Rationale: Grief is the internal process of working through the effects of loss while mourning is the outward expression. Grieving is the client's depression while mourning is going to church and lighting a candle in memory of her lost husband.

Learning Outcome: 18-6

9. C

Rationale: The behavior described by the daughter is normal and to be expected from someone who is mourning the loss of a loved one who died recently. However, the daughter should be told when to call the doctor, including signs of illness, confusion, or mourning that lasts longer than is healthy.

Learning Outcome: 18-4

10. C

Rationale: The client has expressed their wishes through the advance directive and legally those wishes are the ones to be respected. The ethics committee may be called to help the family understand the need to carry out advance directives.

Learning Outcome: 18-7

11. B

Rationale: Nurses may grieve for clients with whom they've bonded. This is a normal response to the loss of a client with whom the nurse has bonded. Recognizing what is going on and allowing time to grieve is all that is necessary.

Learning Outcome: 18-9

12. D

Rationale: The statement that the cell type is slow-growing indicates the client is denying the risk of death in order to cope with the diagnosis. The other statements are the client's attempt to indicate her wishes regarding the plan of care or asking for help in talking with her husband.

Learning Outcome: 18-4

13. C

Rationale: Many clients and families worry about drug addiction when receiving frequent narcotic analgesics. It's important to explain the difference between addiction and dependence and that dependence can be reversed when the client is no longer in pain.

Learning Outcome: 18-8

14. A

Rationale: The client does not yet have the results of the testing so it is closed awareness. Although the client may suspect the worst, or worry that there has been a return and metastasis of cancer, it has not yet been confirmed. There is no such thing as partial awareness.

Learning Outcome: 18-8

15. C

Rationale: The nurse is legally allowed to witness the consent.

Learning Outcome: 18-8

Matching

1.	A	6.	G
2.	E	7.	C
3.	F	8.	H
4.	I	9.	D
5.	B	10.	J

Learning Outcomes

1. See section entitled "Physical Health Assessment."
   Learning Outcome: 19-1
2. See section entitled "Physical Health Assessment."
   Learning Outcome: 19-2
3. See section entitled "Preparation for Assessment."
   Learning Outcome: 19-3
4. See section entitled "Physical Health Assessment."
   Learning Outcome: 19-4
5. See section entitled "Methods of Examination.,"
   Learning Outcome: 19-5
6. See section entitled "Terminology for Documenting Data."
   Learning Outcome: 19-6
7. See section entitled "Nursing Care."
   Learning Outcome: 19-7
8. See section entitled "Terminology for Documenting Data.,"
   Learning Outcome: 19-8
9. See section entitled "Physical Health Assessment."
   Learning Outcome: 19-9

Apply What You Learned

1. Level of consciousness (LOC) can lie anywhere along a continuum from a state of alertness to coma. A fully alert client responds to questions spontaneously; a comatose client may not respond at all to verbal stimuli.
2. A focused assessment may be conducted by the LPN/LVN at the beginning and end of the shift. It may be conducted in several ways. One efficient method is by starting at the head and proceeding in a systematic manner downward to the toes. The procedure can vary according to the age of the individual, the severity of the illness, the method preferences of the nurse, the location of the examination, and the agency's priorities and required procedures. Regardless of what type of procedure is used, the client's energy and time need to be considered. The physical health assessment is always conducted in a systematic and efficient manner that requires the fewest position changes for the client.

3. Components of a neurologic check and description:
   - LOC (level of consciousness)
     - A/O (alert and oriented to name, time, and place)
   - Verbal response
     - Clear
     - Incoherent, rambling, slurred, stuttering
     - Dysphasia, aphasia
   - Motor response (bilaterally)
     - Grips (note strength)
     - Obeys commands, localizes pain, withdrawal, flexion, extension, none
     - Pain—sharp, burning, intense, sudden, agonizing, throbbing, stabbing
     - Pain level 1–10
   - Assess pupils
     - Note shape
     - Pupils equal, react to light, and accommodation (PERRLA)
       - 1 mm after surgery
       - 2–3 mm normal
       - 6–9 mm blown; if permanent, possible herniation
4. The Glasgow Coma Scale was originally developed to predict recovery from a head injury; however, it is used by many professionals to assess LOC. It tests in three major areas: eye response, motor response, and verbal response. An assessment totaling 15 points indicates that the client is alert and completely oriented. A comatose client scores 7 or less.

Multiple Choice Questions

1. C

   Rationale: Part of assessing LOC is assessing the client's orientation to time, place, and person. Of the options, option 3 assesses orientation.
   Learning Outcome: 19-2

2. A

   Rationale: To auscultate the anterior chest, the nurse should begin just above the clavicle starting on the client's right side.
   Learning Outcome: 19-2

3. D

   Rationale: For accurate measurements of height and weight, the client should be measured at the same time every day, using the same scale, with the client wearing the same kind of clothing and no shoes. Measurements of weight should not occur directly after eating a meal.
   Learning Outcome: 19-2

4. A

   Rationale: When there is too little circulating blood or hemoglobin, it results in reduced amounts of oxygen being carried to body tissues, causing a change in the coloration.
   Learning Outcome: 19-2

5. C
   Rationale: The characteristic "pot belly" appearance of toddlers persists until about age 5.
   Learning Outcome: 19-4
6. D
   Rationale: Asymmetric gluteal folds, asymmetric abduction of the legs, or apparent shortening of the femur suggests developmental dysplasia of the hip (congenital dislocation).
   Learning Outcome: 19-4
7. B
   Rationale: If the client grimaces and clenches his jaw, it should be seen as an indicator of pain or tenderness. The other options could have other explanations.
   Learning Outcome: 19-7
8. A
   Rationale: The nurse should assess skin turgor over the sternum in older adults. Loss of subcutaneous tissue in aging makes the skin of the arms a less reliable indicator of fluid status.
   Learning Outcome: 19-7
9. D
   Rationale: Bluish hue, freckled brown pigmentation in dark-skinned clients, and a uniform pink color in light-skinned clients are all normal findings. A yellowish discoloration indicates jaundice, which is an abnormal finding.
   Learning Outcome: 19-2
10. D
    Rationale: Purple striae are associated with Cushing's disease.
    Learning Outcome: 19-2
11. C
    Rationale: If the nurse suspects that bowel sounds are absent, she or he should continue to listen for up to five minutes.
    Learning Outcome: 19-2
12. D
    Rationale: Pronation (in-turning) of the feet is common between 12 and 30 months of age.
    Learning Outcome: 19-4
13. A
    Rationale: Taste sensations diminish due to atrophy of the taste buds and a decreased sense of smell.
    Learning Outcome: 19-4

Chapter 20 Hygiene

Matching

1. C
2. D
3. B
4. E
5. A

6. C
7. D
8. A
9. B

Learning Outcomes

1. See chapter introduction.
   Learning Outcome: 20-1
2. See chapter introduction.
   Learning Outcome: 20-2
3. See section entitled "Skin, Foot, and Nail Care."
   Learning Outcome: 20-3
4. See section entitled "Skin, Foot, and Nail Care."
   Learning Outcome: 20-4
5. See section entitled "Skin, Foot, and Nail Care."
   Learning Outcome: 20-5
6. See section entitled "Hair Care."
   Learning Outcome: 20-6
7. See section entitled "Mouth Care, Eye Care, Ear Care, Nose Care."
   Learning Outcome: 20-7
8. See section entitled "Supporting a Hygienic Environment."
   Learning Outcome: 20-8
9. See section entitled "Supporting a Hygienic Environment."
   Learning Outcome: 20-9
10. See section entitled "Supporting a Hygienic Environment."
    Learning Outcome: 20-10

Apply What You Learned

1. Factors influencing individual hygienic practices include:
   - Culture
   - Religion
   - Economics
   - Environment
   - Developmental level
   - Health and energy
   - Personal preferences
2. Personal hygiene is a sociocultural issue. The client may follow religious or cultural practices that prohibit bathing during the menstrual cycle or following childbirth. Ceremonial washings at the end of the menstrual cycles are practiced by some religions.
3. Each of us is unique, with unique values, beliefs, and experiences. We (the dominant North American culture) seem to have an obsession with minimizing natural body odors. Daily bathing with use of a deodorant, mouthwash, and perfumes is the norm for us. With so many cultures represented in the United States and Canada today, nurses may be called upon to care for clients from cultures that are not bothered by body odor and do not cover up natural smells. It is important not to prejudge the person because of values and beliefs that differ from our own.
4. LPNs/LVNs must know exactly how much assistance a client needs for hygienic care. Caring for our clients provides a great opportunity to learn about others and expand our worldview. As nurses, we are obligated to incorporate

and integrate the client's practices into the care plan as much as possible. We must be respectful and nonjudgmental. In planning care, the LPN/LVN identifies nursing interventions that will assist the client to maintain or improve skin cleanliness, maintain circulation to the skin, and improve or maintain a sense of well-being. When planning to assist a client with personal hygiene, the nurse considers the client's personal preference, health, and limitations; the best time to give the care; and the equipment, facilities, and personnel available. A client's personal preferences about when and how to bathe should be followed as long as they are compatible with the client's health.

Multiple Choice Questions

1. A
   Rationale: Mineral oil is contraindicated because aspiration could cause an infection. Hydrogen peroxide is not recommended because if not diluted properly, it can irritate the oral mucosa. The alcohol in mouthwash could lead to further dryness of the mucosa. Normal saline solution is recommended for oral hygiene of the dependent client.
   Learning Outcome: 20-7

2. B
   Rationale: A footboard for the feet is the most appropriate answer.
   Learning Outcome: 20-5

3. C
   Rationale: Nothing should be placed into the ear to remove cerumen, as it could push the wax in further or injury the ear canal. The best method is to retract the auricle downward to loosen and remove visible wax.
   Learning Outcome: 20-7

4. D
   Rationale: As one ages hair generally becomes thinner, grows more slowly, and loses its color. There is generally no change in the oiliness of the hair.
   Learning Outcome: 20-6

5. A
   Rationale: Trimming the nail straight across prevents ingrown toenails (not digging into the lateral corners). Nails should be filed rather than cut with a diabetes client to avoid injury to tissues.
   Learning Outcome: 20-3

6. D
   Rationale: Scabies is a contagious skin infestation by the itch mite. Hirsutism is a condition of excessive hair growth, pediculus capitis is a scalp infection, and tularemia is a plague-like infectious disease.
   Learning Outcome: 20-3

7. A
   Rationale: Hygiene is a personal matter that is determined by individual values and practices. Culture plays a large role in determining how often a person bathes and how much privacy a person needs when bathing.
   Learning Outcome: 20-2

8. C
   Rationale: Disposing of soiled materials will help prevent microorganisms and the overall smell of the room.
   Learning Outcome: 20-2
9. B
   Rationale: The appropriate way to remove an artificial eye is to use clean gloves and use the dominant thumb to pull the client's lower eyelid down over the infraorbital bone.
   Learning Outcome: 20-7
10. C
   Rationale: Not having regular and easy access to things like a restroom, a shower, clean towels and clothes, etc. would be the greatest challenge that would influence a homeless person's hygiene.
   Learning Outcome: 20-2
11. B
   Rationale: For dry skin, it is recommended to bathe less frequently, use no soap, use alcohol-free moisturizer, and to increase fluid intake.
   Learning Outcome: 20-3
12. D
   Rationale: It is important to check the client's record to determine if he is receiving any anticoagulants in case a facial nick occurs and bleeding starts when shaving.
   Learning Outcome: 20-6
13. C
   Rationale: Cheilosis refers to cracking of the lips. The best intervention is to lubricate the lips with an antimicrobial ointment to avoid infection.
   Learning Outcome: 20-3

Chapter 21 Vital Signs

Matching

1. E	6. D	11. A	16. E	21. F	26. A
2. A	7. C	12. B	17. A	22. B	27. E
3. B	8. E	13. F	18. D	23. A	28. C
4. C	9. D	14. C	19. D	24. C	29. D
5. F	10. F	15. B	20. E	25. B	

Learning Outcomes

1. See chapter introduction.
   Learning Outcome: 21-1
2. See chapter introduction.
   Learning Outcome: 21-2
3. See section entitled "Body Temperature."
   Learning Outcome: 21-3
4. See section entitled "Pulse."
   Learning Outcome: 21-4

5. See section entitled "Pulse."
   Learning Outcome: 21-5
6. See section entitled "Pulse."
   Learning Outcome: 21-6
7. See section entitled "Respirations."
   Learning Outcome: 21-7
8. See section entitled "Respirations."
   Learning Outcome: 21-8
9. See section entitled "Blood Pressure."
   Learning Outcome: 21-9
10. See section entitled "Blood Pressure."
    Learning Outcome: 21-10

Apply What You Learned

1. Nurses should be aware of the factors that can affect a client's body temperature. They should recognize normal temperature variations and understand the significance of body temperature measurements that deviate from normal.

   Among the factors that affect body temperature are:
   - Age
   - Diurnal variations (circadian rhythms)
   - Exercise
   - Hormones
   - Stress
   - Environment

2. During an *intermittent fever,* the body temperature alternates at regular intervals between periods of fever and periods of normal or subnormal temperature.

3. When the skin over the entire body becomes chilled, or when cold sensors in the brain are stimulated, three physiological processes take place to increase body temperature:
   - *Shivering* increases heat production.
   - *Sweating* is inhibited to decrease heat loss.
   - *Vasoconstriction* decreases heat loss.

4. Physiological processes at work are:
   - *Sweating,* which increases evaporation and cooling
   - *Peripheral* vasodilatation, which facilitates cooling

Multiple Choice Questions

1. D
   Rationale: The most appropriate answer is that older adults lose subcutaneous body fat and are more susceptible to temperature changes.
   Learning Outcome: 21-3
2. C
   Rationale: Tachypnea is a faster than normal respiratory rate.
   Learning Outcome: 21-2

3. A

Rationale: Hyperventilation is characterized by prolonged, deep breaths and may be associated with anxiety.

Learning Outcome: 21-7

4. D

Rationale: Hypothermia would be manifested by decreased vital signs, pale, cool, waxy skin, and hypotension (not hypertension).

Learning Outcome: 21-3

5. B

Rationale: Providing adequate nutrition and fluids helps meet the increased metabolic demands of fever and prevents dehydration.

Learning Outcome: 21-3

6. D

Rationale: The temporal pulse site is located where the temporal artery passes over the temporal bone of the head. Because the radial, femoral, and carotid arteries are inaccessible because of burns, the temporal site is the most appropriate.

Learning Outcome: 21-4

7. A

Rationale: Typically if blood pressure is between 140/90 and 159/99, the protocol is to recheck within two months to confirm hypertension.

Learning Outcome: 21-9

8. D

Rationale: It is important when documenting to not make assumptions and describe things in standard terms. In this case, it should be noted as rust-tinged sputum.

Learning Outcome: 21-7

9. C

Rationale: Cheyne-Stokes breathing is a rhythmic waxing and waning of respirations from very deep to very shallow with periods of apnea in between.

Learning Outcome: 21-8

10. B

Rationale: When measuring the blood pressure of a client who has orthostatic hypotension, it is important to place the client in a supine position for 2 to 3 minutes to stabilize blood pressure. The blood pressure is then taken. Then the client should be assisted to a sitting or standing position for one minute and the blood pressure taken again from the same site.

Learning Outcome: 21-9

11. D

Rationale: Axillary temperature is one taken under the armpit. It is the only site listed that does not involve putting the thermometer into a body orifice to obtain a reading; therefore, it is the most noninvasive.

Learning Outcome: 21-3

12. D

Rationale: The pedal pulse is in the foot, the femoral pulse is in the inner thigh, the brachial pulse is in the arm, and the popliteal pulse is behind the knee.

Learning Outcome: 21-4

13. B
   Rationale: Because physical activity increases cardiac output and blood pressure, the nurse should ask the client to rest for 20 to 30 minutes to allow blood pressure to stabilize and return to his normal before the reading is obtained.
   Learning Outcome: 21-9
14. A
   Rationale: Many medications can affect heart rate. Digitalis is a medication that lowers the heart rate.
   Learning Outcome: 21-4

Chapter 22 Pain: The Fifth Vital Sign

Matching

1. E
2. F
3. A
4. B
5. C

6. D
7. B
8. F
9. A
10. E

11. D
12. C

Learning Outcomes

1. See section entitled "Types of Pain."
   Learning Outcome: 22-1
2. See section entitled "Concepts Associated with Pain."
   Learning Outcome: 22-2
3. See section entitled "Physiology of Pain."
   Learning Outcome: 22-3
4. See section entitled "Physiology of Pain."
   Learning Outcome: 22-4
5. See section entitled "Physiology of Pain."
   Learning Outcome: 22-5
6. See section entitled "Management of Pain."
   Learning Outcome: 22-6
7. See section entitled "Management of Pain."
   Learning Outcome: 22-7
8. See section entitled "Management of Pain."
   Learning Outcome: 22-8
9. See section entitled "Key Factors in Effective Pain Management."
   Learning Outcome: 22-9
10. See section entitled "Administering Pain Medication."
    Learning Outcome: 22-10
11. See section entitled "Barriers to Pain Management."
    Learning Outcome: 22-11
12. See section entitled "Nursing Care."
    Learning Outcome: 22-12

13. See section entitled "Nursing Care."
   Learning Outcome: 22-13
14. See section entitled "Nursing Care."
   Learning Outcome: 22-14

Apply What You Learned

1. Some clients may accept pain more readily than others, depending on the circumstances and the client's interpretation of its significance. Clients respond to pain experiences based on their culture, personal experiences, and the meaning the pain has for them. For many people, pain is expected and accepted as a normal aspect of illness or aging. Clients may not report pain because they expect nothing can be done, or they think it is not severe enough. Moreover, the client may have a high pain threshold and tolerance. Pain tolerance may increase with age. Furthermore, clients may not report pain to the physician or nurse because they feel it would distract or prejudice the healthcare provider. Healthcare professionals need to be aware of their own values and perceptions, as they affect how they evaluate the patient's response to pain and ultimately how pain is treated. Even subtle cultural and individual differences can impact care.

2. Reducing a client's misconceptions about the pain and its treatment will often avoid intensifying the pain. Clients and families may lack knowledge of the adverse effects of pain and may have misinformation regarding the use of analgesics. The client may believe that pain is to be expected as part of the recovery or aging process and a necessary part of life. These beliefs about how pain is to be managed may be different between family members. Clients may fear the risks associated with opioid drugs.

3. This client is probably experiencing chronic pain. Chronic pain is debilitating and frustrating and remains at least three to six months after an episode of acute pain. It is important for the nurse to understand that clients with unrelenting chronic pain may suffer more intensely. They may respond with despair, anxiety, and depression because they cannot attach a positive significance or purpose to the pain. Unlike acute pain, chronic pain elicits a parasympathetic nervous system response, leaving the vital signs normal, skin warm and dry, and pupils normal or dilated. Persons with chronic pain often don't mention the pain unless asked and generally don't exhibit behavior indicative of pain.

4. I'd like you to think about how often during the day your pain interferes with your ability to take care of yourself, for example, bathing, eating, dressing, and going to the toilet. Does it interfere with your ability to take care of your home-related chores, such as going grocery shopping and preparing meals?

5.
   - Establish a trusting relationship with the client.
   - Believe that the client is experiencing pain.
   - Acknowledge that the client is the real authority about the pain.
   - Maintain an unbiased attitude.
   - Educate the client and support people about pain.
   - Spend time with the client.

- Listen carefully.
- Clarify misconceptions.
- Encourage independence.

Multiple Choice Questions

1. C
   Rationale: Mild to moderate pain would be treated with something like acetaminophen, not an opioid or a antimigraine drug.
   Learning Outcome: 22-7

2. A
   Rationale: Anxiety, depression, and hopelessness often accompany chronic pain. Chronic pain is not self-limiting and typically does not respond to usual interventions. Fatigue can increase a person's perception of pain and ability to cope.
   Learning Outcome: 22-1

3. D
   Rationale: Cutaneous pain originates in the skin or subcutaneous tissue, such as a superficial burn. Somatic pain arises from ligaments, tendons, bones, blood vessels, and nerves. Visceral pain results from pain in the abdominal cavity, cranium, and thorax. Neuropathic pain is the result of a disturbance of the nerve pathways.
   Learning Outcome: 22-1

4. D
   Rationale: The initial response to acute pain would be a stimulation of the sympathetic nervous system, resulting in the "fight-or-flight" response. This response would increase vital signs and cause diaphoresis.
   Learning Outcome: 22-3

5. B
   Rationale: Morphine can cause respiratory depression. Therefore, it is critical that the nurse assess for bradypnea prior to administering.
   Learning Outcome: 22-12

6. B
   Rationale: Mild to moderate pain should initially be treated with nonopioid analgesics such as NSAIDs.
   Learning Outcome: 22-7

7. D
   Rationale: Pain is a very personal sensation. Having therapeutic communication with the client about the pain and listening to the patient's response is the most appropriate response. It is not appropriate to make assumptions about anyone's pain.
   Learning Outcome: 22-12

8. A
   Rationale: Because pain is a highly personal sensation, the most reliable indicator is the client's self-report of pain.
   Learning Outcome: 22-9

9. D
   Rationale: Constipation is a common side effect of Demerol. Increasing fluids is the most appropriate preventive measure the nurse can take.
   Learning Outcome: 22-12

10. C

Rationale: The most effective reversal agent of morphine for a potential morphine overdose is Narcan.

Learning Outcome: 22-9

11. C

Rationale: Preventing pain before it occurs or becomes severe is a key factor in pain management. Fear of addiction is a common response in clients and the nurse should address that when used to treat acute pain, individuals are unlikely to become addicted.

Learning Outcome: 22-9

12. D

Rationale: The IM route is the least desirable route for opioids because of variable absorption, pain involved in administration, and the need to repeat administration every 3 to 4 hours.

Learning Outcome: 22-10

13. B

Rationale: Quality of pain refers to what the pain feels like. Asking when the pain started is asking about the timing of pain. What causes or relieves the client's pain is the precipitation/palliation of pain.

Learning Outcome: 22-12

14. B

Rationale: Phantom pain refers to the pain felt when a limb is removed.

Learning Outcome: 22-1

15. A

Rationale: Nonpharmacologic approaches to pain can be important with severe types of pain, such as cancer pain, in addition to pharmacologic approaches.

Learning Outcome: 22-8

Chapter 23 Activity, Rest, and Sleep

Matching

1.	E	6.	D
2.	D	7.	C
3.	A	8.	E
4.	C	9.	A
5.	B	10.	B

Learning Outcomes

1. See section entitled "Normal Movement."
   Learning Outcome: 23-1
2. See section entitled "Factors Affecting Body Alignment and Activity."
   Learning Outcome: 23-2
3. See section entitled "Effects of Immobility."
   Learning Outcome: 23-3

4. See section entitled "Assistive Devices."
   Learning Outcome: 23-4
5. See section entitled "Nursing Care."
   Learning Outcome: 23-5
6. See section entitled "Nursing Care."
   Learning Outcome: 23-6
7. See section entitled "Nursing Care."
   Learning Outcome: 23-7
8. See section entitled "Nursing Care."
   Learning Outcome: 23-8
9. See section entitled "Rest and Sleep."
   Learning Outcome: 23-9
10. See section entitled "Factors Affecting Sleep."
    Learning Outcome: 23-10
11. See section entitled "Common Sleep Disorders."
    Learning Outcome: 23-11
12. See section entitled "Diagnostic Studies for Sleep Disorders."
    Learning Outcome: 23-12

Apply What You Learned

1. When the body is aligned, organs are properly supported. This allows them to function at their best, while also maintaining balance. Numerous factors affect an individual's body alignment and mobility. These include growth and development, physical health, mental health, nutrition, personal values, and attitudes.
2. Mobility is directly affected by any disorder of the musculoskeletal or nervous systems. Musculoskeletal trauma limiting mobility includes strains, sprains, fractures, joint dislocations, amputations, and joint replacement. A sedentary lifestyle or history of inactivity due to injury or illness increases the risk of major disease. The level of risk depends on the duration of inactivity, the client's general health, and sensory awareness. Nurses must understand these risks and encourage client mobility. Early ambulation after illness or surgery is an essential preventive measure. Signs of prolonged immobility are most often manifested in the musculoskeletal system. Muscular strength decreases in the absence of physical activity. Common musculoskeletal problems resulting from prolonged immobility include:
   - Disuse osteoporosis
   - Disuse atrophy
   - Contractures
   - Joint pain and stiffness
3. Nursing strategies you will implement:
   - Position the client in good body alignment at least every two hours.
   - Move and turn the client in bed at least every two hours.
   - Provide passive ROM exercises.
   - Transfer the client from bed to chair.
   - Assess the skin and provide skin care before and after a position change.

- Initiate pain control measures before beginning positioning or joint exercise.
- Collaborate with a physical therapist in developing and providing passive ROM exercises.

4. When the body is well aligned, there is little strain on the joints, muscles, tendons, or ligaments, as well as proper support of the organs.
   - Assess the amount of assistance needed—size up your load.
   - If possible, ask for the client's help in lessening your workload.
   - Raise the bed to the height of your center of gravity, with the head of the bed as low as the client can tolerate.
   - Lock the wheels on the bed and raise the rail on the side of the bed opposite you.
   - Face the direction of movement.
   - Assume a broad stance, with the foot nearest the bed behind the forward foot and weight on the forward foot.
   - Incline your trunk forward from the hips.
   - Flex your hips, knees, and ankles.
   - Tighten your gluteal, abdominal, leg, and arm muscles, and rock from the back leg to the front leg and back again.

Multiple Choice Questions

1. A
   Rationale: Performing passive ROM exercises on an immobile client prevents the effects of immobility.
   Learning Outcome: 23-7

2. C
   Rationale: Telling the client that moving is critical to recovery is the best response. Although the client may still refuse to cooperate, the nurse must attempt to educate the client on why this order has been written.
   Learning Outcome: 23-7

3. A
   Rationale: Buildup of carbon dioxide in the blood results in respiratory acidosis.
   Learning Outcome: 23-3

4. D
   Rationale: The hips and knees are classified as joints and are responsible for carrying the weight of a person.
   Learning Outcome: 23-1

5. B
   Rationale: Osteoporosis is caused by the depletion of calcium in bone.
   Learning Outcome: 23-2

6. C
   Rationale: Drinking alcohol, raising the room temperature, and exercise are all things that contribute to difficulty falling asleep. The most appropriate answer is to wear loose-fitting nightwear and to be comfortable when trying to fall asleep.
   Learning Outcome: 23-10

7. D

Rationale: Adduction refers to movement of the bone toward the midline of the body.

Learning Outcome: 23-1

8. C

Rationale: Placing a trochanter roll lateral to the femur will help prevent rotation of the hips when the client is in low Fowler's position. A footboard prevents foot drop. A small pillow under the lumbar curvature prevents posterior flexion of lumbar curvature. A pillow under the lower legs at the knees prevents hyperextension of the knees.

Learning Outcome: 23-6

9. B

Rationale: REM sleep deprivation causes clinical signs such as excitability, restlessness, irritability, confusion, and emotional lability. Hyporesponsiveness, apathy, and withdrawal are signs of NREM deprivation.

Learning Outcome: 23-9

10. D

Rationale: Raising the head of the bed as far as it will go will decrease the distance that the client needs to move to sit up on the side of the bed.

Learning Outcome: 23-8

11. B

Rationale: NREM sleep is a deep, restful sleep that is represented by slowed heart and respiratory rates as well as other body processes.

Learning Outcome: 23-9

12. D

Rationale: It is always the best thing to pace activities based on the client's tolerance.

Learning Outcome: 23-7

13. B

Rationale: Sims' position is a semiprone position that is halfway between the lateral and prone positions.

Learning Outcome: 23-6

14. A

Rationale: When the body is well aligned, there is little strain on the joints, muscles, tendons, or ligaments.

Learning Outcome: 23-1

15. D

Rationale: Wearing elastic stockings at night will inhibit venous pooling in the legs. All other options will increase the chance of postural hypotension, not decrease it.

Learning Outcome: 23-4

Matching

1. D	6. B	11. D	16. D
2. A	7. D	12. A	17. F
3. E	8. E	13. B	18. A
4. B	9. A	14. E	19. C
5. C	10. C	15. C	20. B
			21. E

Learning Outcomes

1. See section entitled "Skin Integrity."
   Learning Outcome: 24-1
2. See section entitled "Wound Terminology."
   Learning Outcome: 24-2
3. See section entitled "Wound Healing."
   Learning Outcome: 24-3
4. See section entitled "Wounds."
   Learning Outcome: 24-4
5. See section entitled "Caring for Wounds."
   Learning Outcome: 24-5
6. See section entitled "Caring for Wounds."
   Learning Outcome: 24-6
7. See section entitled "Caring for Wounds."
   Learning Outcome: 24-7
8. See section entitled "Nursing Care."
   Learning Outcome: 24-8
9. See section entitled "Pressure Ulcers."
   Learning Outcome: 24-9
10. See section entitled "Pressure Ulcers."
    Learning Outcome: 24-10
11. See section entitled "Skin Integrity."
    Learning Outcome: 24-11

Apply What You Learned

1. Assessing common pressure sites:
   - Be sure there is good lighting.
   - Regulate the environment before beginning so that the room is neither too hot nor too cold.
   - Inspect pressure areas for any whitish or reddened spots; discoloration can be caused by impaired blood circulation to the area.
   - Inspect pressure areas for abrasions and excoriations.
   - Palpate the surface temperature of the skin over the pressure areas. Normally, the temperature is the same as that of the surrounding skin. Increased temperature is abnormal and may be due to inflammation or blood trapped in the area.

- Palpate over bony prominences and dependent body areas for the presence of edema, which feels spongy.

2. Specific tasks to prevent the formation of pressure ulcers:
   - Turn the client at least every two hours.
   - Keep the client clean, dry, and free of irritation from urine.
   - Use a mild cleansing agent sparingly, and apply a moisturizing lotion after each cleansing.
   - Assist the client with each meal to ensure adequate nutritional intake.
   - Provide the client with a smooth, firm, wrinkle-free area to sit or lie down.
   - Use supportive devices as needed.

3. Rationales for the delegated tasks:
   - At least every two hours, reposition any at-risk client who is confined to bed, even when a special support mattress is used. Immobility often causes a reduction in the amount of movement. Pressure ulcers are lesions caused by unrelieved pressure that results in damage to underlying tissue and prevents blood from circulating freely through the area. When blood cannot reach the tissue, the cells are deprived of oxygen and nutrients, and waste products accumulate in the cells.

     Prolonged, unrelieved pressure damages the small blood vessels, and the tissue eventually dies.
   - Moisture from incontinence promotes skin maceration, or softening of tissue, by prolonged wetting and making the epidermis susceptible to injury. Any accumulation of secretions or excretions is irritating to the skin, harbors microorganisms, and makes an individual prone to skin breakdown and infection.
   - When bathing the client, avoid using hot water and apply minimal force and friction. Mild cleansing agents and moisturizers can help maintain the skin's natural barriers. Minimize dryness by not exposing the client to cold and low humidity.
   - Nutritional factors are crucial in the development of pressure ulcers. Generally, prolonged, inadequate nutrition causes weight loss, muscle atrophy, and the loss of subcutaneous tissue. Less padding between the skin and the bones increases the risk of pressure sore development. Inadequate intake of protein, carbohydrates, fluids, and vitamin C contributes to pressure sore formation. Providing adequate meals and nutritional supplements for nutritionally compromised clients is a vital nursing intervention in the prevention of pressure ulcers.
   - Sheets rubbing against skin create friction. Friction can remove the superficial layers of the skin, making it more prone to breakdown. Wrinkles in the sheets, blankets, or underpads cause uneven pressure and contribute to skin breakdown. Providing a smooth, firm, wrinkle-free area will reduce the chance of damage by friction or shearing.
   - When lifting a client to change his or her position, use a lifting device such as a trapeze rather than dragging the client across or up in bed. The friction that results from dragging the skin against a sheet can cause blisters and abrasions, which may contribute to more extensive tissue damage. Supportive devices such as a lift will help relieve pressure on bony prominences.

4. In addition to providing the nursing assistant with the above rationale for appropriate interventions, two comments she made need to be addressed. Her comments were as follows:

"I know what to do. I'll turn her when I get to it, do a two-person transfer to the chair, try to feed her breakfast and lunch, [1] order a doughnut for her to sit on when she is up, and [2] massage those areas that look red."

- Statement 1 reflects a lack of understanding by the nursing assistant and must be corrected. Doughnut-type cushion devices should not be used because they place uneven pressure on the skin and surrounding tissue, making it prone to breakdown.
- Statement 2 refers to a nursing intervention that nurses and nursing assistants have used for years to stimulate blood circulation with the intention of preventing pressure sores. However, scientific evidence does not support this belief. In fact, massage may lead to deep tissue trauma.

Multiple Choice Questions

1. B
   Rationale: Bright sanguineous exudate refers to fresh bleeding. Dark sanguineous exudate would be older bleeding. The presence of pus would be a purulent exudate. Dehiscence is the partial or total rupturing of a sutured wound.
   Learning Outcome: 24-2

2. A
   Rationale: Primary intention healing occurs where the tissue surfaces have been closed and there is minimal or no tissue loss. A closed surgical incision is an example of this type of healing.
   Learning Outcome: 24-3

3. A
   Rationale: A hypertrophic scar is a keloid scar. Eschar is dried plasma proteins and dead cells. Exudate is fluid that escapes. A scab is the combination of clots and dead or dying tissue on the surface of a wound.
   Learning Outcome: 24-3

4. C
   Rationale: Secondary intention healing differs from primary intention healing in three ways: the repair time is longer, the scarring is greater, and the risk of infection is greater.
   Learning Outcome: 24-3

5. A
   Rationale: Wound healing requires a diet rich in protein, carbohydrates, lipids, vitamins A and C, and minerals such as iron, zinc, and copper.
   Learning Outcome: 24-4

6. D
   Rationale: Wound healing is accelerated with people who exercise regularly and have good circulation. Blood brings oxygen and nourishment to the wound. Obese clients are likely to have less circulation to the wound.
   Learning Outcome: 24-4

7. D

Rationale: Gauze packing is placed in wounds to facilitate formation of granulation tissue and healing by secondary intention.

Learning Outcome: 24-6

8. A

Rationale: Disadvantages of hydrocolloid dressings include obscuring wound visibility, limited absorption, facilitating anaerobic bacterial growth, can soften and wrinkle at edges, and they can be difficult to remove.

Learning Outcome: 24-6

9. A

Rationale: White blood cells fight infection. With a lower leukocyte count, the client will be at risk for infection and it will delay healing.

Learning Outcome: 24-9

10. A

Rationale: Stage I pressure ulcers are characterized by nonblanchable erythema of intact skin.

Learning Outcome: 24-10

11. B

Rationale: Establishing a written schedule for turning and repositioning the client reminds nurses and holds nurses accountable for preventing pressure ulcers.

Learning Outcome: 24-11

12. A

Rationale: The nurse should keep the skin clean and dry. Transfer of clients should be done with a lifting device. The nurse should not massage over bony prominences. The client should have a smooth, firm, and wrinkle-free foundation to sit or lie down on.

Learning Outcome: 24-11

13. C

Rationale: Shearing force is a combination of friction and pressure that occurs commonly when a client assumes Fowler's position in bed. The body slides down toward the foot of the bed but the skin of the sacrum tends not to move. Keeping the client in a low Fowler's or lower position will avoid this from happening.

Learning Outcome: 24-9

14. C

Rationale: The appropriate outcome would be for the wound to be maintained and heal without infection.

Learning Outcome: 24-11

15. D

Rationale: Vascular changes such as atrophy of capillaries in the skin can inhibit or delay wound healing in older adults.

Learning Outcome: 24-1

Chapter 25 Nutrition and Diet Therapy

Matching

1. E
2. A
3. B
4. C
5. D

6. C
7. D
8. E
9. B
10. A

Learning Outcomes

1. See section entitled "Nutrients."
   Learning Outcome: 25-1
2. See section entitled "Standards for a Healthy Diet."
   Learning Outcome: 25-2
3. See section entitled "Standards for a Healthy Diet."
   Learning Outcome: 25-3
4. See section entitled "Specialized Diets."
   Learning Outcome: 25-4
5. See section entitled "Nursing Care."
   Learning Outcome: 25-5

Apply What You Learned

1. In preparation for medication administration, you must first determine if the client is allergic to any of the prescribed medications. In addition, it may be necessary to gather client data, such as pulse, blood pressure, and lab values.
2. The liquid medications may be safely administered through the tube. If they are thick or syrupy, a small amount of water may be added. If only a pill form is available, it will be necessary to crush the tablet and dissolve it in a small amount of warm water. Any medication that is enteric coated or time release may NOT be administered through an enteral tube. These medications may NEVER be crushed, or in the case of the capsule, opened. Crushing these types of tablets or opening the capsules alters their absorption and metabolism, resulting in unpredictable drug effects and sometimes producing a bolus dosing of the drug.
3. Before administering any medication through an enteral tube, you must ensure proper placement of the tube. If the client is receiving a continuous feeding, it may also be necessary to check for residual. After *separately* crushing and dissolving each medication, a 60-mL syringe is attached to the feeding tube. The syringe is held upright at a 90-degree angle, and 30 to 60 mL tap water is administered, allowing the fluid to *flow by gravity*. Each dissolved medication is then poured *separately* into the syringe and allowed to *flow by gravity*. A small amount of water may be run through the tube between each medication. Medications should NEVER be mixed together or with the enteral feeding. The plunger of the syringe should NEVER be used

to force liquids or medications through the enteral tube. After all medications have been administered, an additional 30 to 60 mL of water is added. If the client's intake and output are being measured, the amount of water used during the medication administration is added to the intake total.

4. Because the enteric-coated tablet and time-release capsule cannot be administered through the enteral tube, it may be necessary to contact the pharmacist to determine if alternate forms of the medications are available. The physician may need to be contacted for further direction or new medication orders.

Multiple Choice Questions

1. B
   Rationale: Refined or processed sugars include table sugar, molasses, and corn syrup. These have been added to soft drinks, cookies, candy, ice cream, and some cereals.
   Learning Outcome: 25-1

2. C
   Rationale: Glucose that cannot be stored as glycogen is converted by the body to fat to be stored.
   Learning Outcome: 25-2

3. C
   Rationale: A clear liquid diet is limited to water, tea, coffee, clear broths, ginger ale or other carbonated beverages, strained and clear juices, and plain gelatin.
   Learning Outcome: 25-4

4. B
   Rationale: Placement of the feeding tube should be checked at least once per shift and prior to administering any mediations through the tube.
   Learning Outcome: 25-5

5. C
   Rationale: When administering an intermittent enteral feeding, 30 minutes allows enough time for the feeding to infuse without causing stomach distention or discomfort. Allowing more time means the next feeding will be administered with inadequate time for the prior feeding to be absorbed.
   Learning Outcome: 25-5

6. B
   Rationale: Involving the client in setting goals for improving nutrition is important. The healthcare team members and the client should work together to establish goals.
   Learning Outcome: 25-5

7. D
   Rationale: Positioning the client in the high Fowler's position will facilitate passage of the tube into the esophagus.
   Learning Outcome: 25-5

8. B
   Rationale: The tube should be lubricated with a water-soluble lubricant. An oil-based lubricant, such as petroleum jelly, will not dissolve and could cause respiratory complications if it enters the lungs.
   Learning Outcome: 25-5

9. D

Rationale: The contents should be returned because they are rich in electrolytes. Only if the contents were curdled or harmful would they be discarded, which is not indicated by the question. There is no need to send the contents to the lab for analysis unless the provider has specifically ordered gastric content analysis. The pH will be impacted by the type of food eaten and how long ago it was ingested, but it is unlikely to have a pH of 6 or higher because stomach acids are far more acidic.

Learning Outcome: 25-5

10. A

Rationale: The stoma should be cleaned daily with soap and water and allowed to air dry. Do not apply a dressing over the PEG, as a dressing and tape may result in skin excoriation and breakdown.

Learning Outcome: 25-5

11. A

Rationale: Checking with the pharmacy is the best course of action to determine whether or not this drug can be used. The nurse should not go ahead and crush or try to dissolve the medication, or try to give it orally.

Learning Outcome: 25-5

12. C

Rationale: An older widower living alone is more at risk for not having adequate nutrition. He may not be able to prepare meals adequately or get out to get adequate groceries.

Learning Outcome: 25-5

13. C

Rationale: BMI is calculated by dividing the weight in kilograms by the height in meters squared. The client is 104.5 kg and is 1.92 meters. Therefore the BMI is 28.3, which corresponds to being overweight.

Learning Outcome: 25-5

14. B

Rationale: Complementary proteins are plant proteins and therefore can be, and should be, included in a vegetarian diet.

Learning Outcome: 25-4

15. C

Rationale: Saturated fats are found in animal products and are usually solid at room temperature. The hardness of the fat at room temperature indicates the amount of saturated fat.

Learning Outcome: 25-1

Chapter 26 Fluids, Electrolytes, and Acid-Base Balance

Matching

1.	E	6.	D	11.	A	16.	E
2.	A	7.	F	12.	D	17.	C
3.	B	8.	E	13.	D		
4.	F	9.	C	14.	A		
5.	C	10.	B	15.	B		

Learning Outcomes

1. See section entitled "Body Fluids and Electrolyte Balance."
   Learning Outcome: 26-1
2. See section entitled "Body Fluids and Electrolyte Balance."
   Learning Outcome: 26-2
3. See section entitled "Acid-Base Balance."
   Learning Outcome: 26-3
4. See section entitled "Acid-Base Imbalances."
   Learning Outcome: 26-4
5. See section entitled "Acid-Base Imbalances."
   Learning Outcome: 26-5
6. See section entitled "Nursing Care."
   Learning Outcome: 26-6
7. See section entitled "Nursing Care."
   Learning Outcome: 26-7

Apply What You Learned

1. Common strategies for prevention of fluid and electrolyte imbalance include:
   - If permitted, drink at least eight to ten 8-ounce glasses of water per day.
   - Limit consumption of fluids high in salt (sodium), sugar, caffeine, or alcohol.
   - Drink water before, during, and after strenuous exercise.
   - Avoid routine use of laxatives, antacids, weight-loss products, or enemas.
   - Take daily weights at the same time each day.
   - Contact your physician if you have sudden changes in weight, decreased urine output, swelling in your hands, legs, or feet, shortness of breath, or dizziness.
   - Contact your physician if you should experience prolonged vomiting, diarrhea, or an inability to eat solid foods or drink liquids.
   - Eat a well-balanced diet, including fresh fruits and vegetables, low-fat proteins, dairy products, and whole grains, nuts, and legumes.
   - Discuss medications prescribed for the client and how they may impact on fluid and electrolyte balance.
   - Instruct the client to follow through on physician visits and medication compliance.
2. Metabolic acidosis occurs when the bicarbonate is lost or acid is increased within the plasma. When the body cannot utilize the glucose from the foods eaten, such as is the case in uncontrolled diabetes mellitus, fat is burned for energy instead. When fat or fatty acids are catabolized or burned, they change to ketone bodies, which are acidic. When the level of carbon dioxide becomes too high, the body's acid–base balance is upset. Initially, the body's buffer system will respond. In addition, the respiratory system also triggers faster and deeper breaths that help to "blow" off the excess carbon dioxide.

Although this will correct the imbalance initially, it will not be enough compensation to correct the metabolic imbalance. Medical intervention may become necessary.

3. In addition to implementing the strategies in #1, a client with diabetes mellitus *must* adhere to the prescribed diet, faithfully monitor blood sugars, administer prescribed amounts of insulin, and maintain regular contact with the healthcare provider.

4. Cultural food preferences and practices can play a large role in contributing to adequate and inadequate intake of electrolytes. A preference for certain foods can also contribute to the development of an illness, such as diabetes. African Americans often eat diets high in sodium content, which contributes to hypertension and heart disease. The nurse needs to be aware of cultural differences and provide teaching when indicated.

Multiple Choice Questions

1. B
   Rationale: A cation is a positively charged ion and only potassium is positively charged. Chloride, phosphate, and fluoride are all anions or negatively charged ions.
   Learning Outcome: 26-1

2. B
   Rationale: Dietary calcium is highest in dairy products, such as nonfat yogurt. The other options are not good sources of calcium.
   Learning Outcome: 26-2

3. D
   Rationale: A pH higher than 7.45 is alkaline and 7.55 is the only option that meets this criterion. 7.35 and 7.45 are within normal limits and 7.15 is acidic.
   Learning Outcome: 26-3

4. A
   Rationale: The body has a strong tendency toward acidity because acids are continually produced, so the buffer system is the first line of defense because it is more alkaline than acid. If the buffer system cannot compensate, the respiratory system is the next line of defense, while the renal system takes longer to compensate. There is no carbonic regulation system.
   Learning Outcome: 26-3

5. B
   Rationale: The body attempts to lower the pH of the blood by blowing off carbon dioxide, causing both an increase in rate and depth of respirations because the deeper and faster the client breathes, the more carbon dioxide they remove. Pulse rate may increase, but strength would not.
   Learning Outcome: 26-5

6. A
   Rationale: The pH is low so it is acidic, the HCO_3^- is normal, while the PCO_2 is elevated, indicating the acidosis is respiratory in nature.
   Learning Outcome: 26-5

7. D

   Rationale: This blood gas indicates pH is greater than 7.45, demonstrating alkalosis. PCO_2 is normal, while HCO_3^- is elevated, indicating a metabolic, not respiratory, alkalosis.

   Learning Outcome: 26-5

8. B

   Rationale: A client with an elevated temperature is likely to breathe more quickly in an attempt to dissipate heat. As the client breathes faster, more carbon dioxide is blown off, which causes an increase in pH, resulting in a respiratory alkalosis.

   Learning Outcome: 26-7

9. D

   Rationale: Loss of stomach acids through the nasogastric tube to low suction means there is a loss of acid in the body, causing alkalosis to occur. Because the cause is not respiratory in nature, it is a metabolic alkalosis.

   Learning Outcome: 26-7

10. D

    Rationale: Antacids are alkaline and are used to neutralize the acidity of the stomach. The increased intake of antacids would result in alkalosis. Because the cause of the alkalosis is not respiratory in nature it is a metabolic alkalosis.

    Learning Outcome: 26-7

11. A

    Rationale: Kussmaul's respirations are slow and deep and normally result from diabetic ketoacidosis, a buildup of acidic ketones in the body. The loss of carbon dioxide from deep breathing combined with the buildup of acid from ketosis would result in an acidic pH, with low carbon dioxide and low bicarbonate levels as displayed in option 1.

    Learning Outcome: 26-7

12. C

    Rationale: This client's serum potassium levels will most likely reveal hyperkalemia, resulting in the symptoms described in the question. This is most likely due to too much oral potassium. The symptoms do not fit any of the other options.

    Learning Outcome: 26-4

13. A

    Rationale: The kidneys work to maintain acid base balance by controlling hydrogen ions, which combine with carbon and oxygen to form HCO.

    Learning Outcome: 26-3

14. B

    Rationale; Hyperventilation results in increased losses of carbon dioxide, leading to respiratory alkalosis.

    Learning Outcome: 26-3

15. C

    Rationale: Clients with anorexia are at increased risk for metabolic acidosis because the body will begin to break down protein sources, such as muscles, in order to provide nutrition for the cells. This results in an increase in circulating acids, ending in metabolic acidosis.

    Learning Outcome: 26-3

Chapter 27 Medications

Matching

1. E	6. A	11. A	16. B	21. B
2. D	7. E	12. B	17. A	22. E
3. F	8. F	13. F	18. C	23. A
4. C	9. D	14. D	19. C	
5. B	10. C	15. E	20. D	

Learning Outcomes

1. See introduction to chapter.
   Learning Outcome: 27-1
2. See section entitled "Drug Standards."
   Learning Outcome: 27-2
3. See section entitled "Effects of Drugs."
   Learning Outcome: 27-3
4. See section entitled "Medication Orders."
   Learning Outcome: 27-4
5. See section entitled "Systems of Measurement."
   Learning Outcome: 27-5
6. See section entitled "Equipment."
   Learning Outcome: 27-6
7. See section entitled "Routes of Administration and Drug Dispensing and Supply Systems."
   Learning Outcome: 27-7
8. See section entitled "Nursing Care."
   Learning Outcome: 27-8
9. See section entitled "Nursing Care."
   Learning Outcome: 27-9
10. See section entitled "Nursing Care."
    Learning Outcome: 27-10
11. See section entitled "Nursing Care."
    Learning Outcome: 27-11
12. See section entitled "Nursing Care."
    Learning Outcome: 27-12

Apply What You Learned

1. Nursing practice acts define limits on the nurse's responsibilities regarding medications. Under the law, nurses are responsible for their own actions, whether or not a written order exists. Nurses must question any order that appears unreasonable and refuse to give the medication until the order is clarified. The nurse should always question the physician about any order that is ambiguous or unclear, unusual, or contraindicated by the client's

condition. When the LPN/LVN judges that a physician-ordered medication is inappropriate, the following actions are required:

- Discuss the order with the RN and/or the nursing supervisor.
- Contact the physician and discuss the rationale for believing the medication or dosage to be inappropriate.
- Document in notes the following: time the physician was notified, by whom, information conveyed to the physician, and the physician's response (using the physician's words, if possible).
- If the physician cannot be reached, document all attempts to contact the physician and the reason for withholding the medication.
- If someone else gave the medication, document data about the client's condition before and after the medication was given.
- If an incident report is indicated, document factual information.

Another aspect of nursing practice governed by law is the use of controlled substances. Each facility is required to have a specific protocol governing the use of controlled substances, and nurses have a professional responsibility to follow this protocol to the letter. Finally, the nurse must follow all policies and procedures governing medication administration. By adhering to the standards set by the profession, nurses can and will practice safely and knowledgeably.

2. Medication orders must include the client's name, date and time the order is written, name of the medication, dosage, route, frequency of administration, and signature of the person writing the order.

3. Abbreviations:
   - mg: milligram
   - IM: intramuscular
   - gm: gram
   - PO: by mouth
   - tid: three times a day
   - mL: milliliter
   - mEq: millequivalent

4. Haloperidol answer: 0.2 mL
   Xanax answer: 2.5 mL
   KCL answer: 20 mL

5. Essential steps to follow when preparing and administering medications:
   - Verify the client's ability to take medication orally.
   - Verify the physician's order for accuracy.
   - Check the expiration date on the order or medications.
   - Obtain the appropriate medications.
   - Using the five rights (right client, right drug, right dosage, right route, and right time) and three checks, prepare the medication.
   - Compare the client's name on the MAR with the name band the client is wearing.
   - Make certain that the client has swallowed the medication.
   - Document appropriately.

6. The nurse should return to assess the client when the medication is expected to take effect—usually 30 minutes.

1. B

    Rationale: When a client points out a pill they are not familiar with, the nurse should ALWAYS stop and double-check the order, the medication, and the client to prevent making a medication error. It may be the right medication but from a different supplier, but that should not be assumed and the medication should be checked again before administering it.

    Learning Outcome: 27-4

2. A

    Rationale: The route determines the absorption rate, with IV administration being the fastest and intradermal administration having the slowest absorption rate. The medication is absorbed at the same rate regardless of the prescribed amount, the type of medication, and the time of day it is administered.

    Learning Outcome: 27-3

3. D

    Rationale: Before a dermatological preparation can be applied topically to the skin, the skin should be cleansed to allow for proper absorption and effects.

    Learning Outcome: 27-12.

4. C

    Rationale: IM is the abbreviation for intramuscular. Intravenous is IV, subcutaneous is subQ or SC, and intradermal is not usually abbreviated.

    Learning Outcome: 27-1.

5. B

    Rationale: The powder remaining in the vial is most likely unmixed medication. Many medications are damaged by vigorous shaking and that is not advised. There is no need to replace the vial but the medication should be properly mixed before administering it because the dosage will be incorrect if all the medication is not in solution form.

    Learning Outcome: 27-10.

6. B

    Rationale: The drug is to be given every day, so it is a standing order. PRN orders are to be given only when needed and single orders are only to be given once. STAT orders are to be given immediately.

    Learning Outcome: 27-4.

7. A

    Rationale: Because a total of 19 units are to be given (15 units of NPH and 4 units of regular) a low-dose syringe is indicated. Both insulin orders use U100, so a U100 syringe is indicated.

    Learning Outcome: 27-6.

8. D

    Rationale: Drowsiness is an anticipated side effect of the medication. An adverse effect is a more serious side effect, while an idiosyncratic effect is an unexpected and unusual effect of the medication not normally seen in most clients or perhaps never seen before. The desired effect is the antihistamine action for which the medication is administered.

    Learning Outcome: 27-3.

9. B

Rationale: Barbiturates have the potential to be habit forming and produce a drug tolerance if taken recurrently. The other medications do not create drug tolerance.
Learning Outcome: 27-3.

10. A

Rationale: Elixirs are medications dissolved in alcohol with sweetener added to make them more palatable. An aqueous solution is mixed in water. A liniment is applied to the skin and is not sweetened, while a syrup is sweetened but does not contain alcohol.
Learning Outcome: 27-1.

11. A

Rationale: It is the nurse's responsibility to evaluate the effectiveness of medications and the responsibility should not be delegated to the client or the unlicensed assistive personnel.
Learning Outcome: 27-3

12. A

Rationale: The medication will make the client feel better, thus a palliative response, but it will not cure the pain, restore tissues causing pain, or support the problem resulting in pain.
Learning Outcome: 27-3.

13. A

Rationale: When administering medication using a Z-track technique, the nurse pulls the skin laterally and down with the nondominant hand approximately 1 inch before inserting the needle. The skin is released at the same time the needle is removed, creating a track that is Z-shaped and reducing the likelihood of medication leaking from the site.
Learning Outcome: 27-11.

14. D

Rationale: Whenever an order is unclear it must be clarified with the physician, so the nurse should talk with the charge nurse of directly with the ordering provider for clarification.
Learning Outcome: 27-2. Describe drug standards and legal aspects of administering drugs.

15. D

Rationale: Whenever possible, handling the pills should be avoided, so it is best to introduce the medication from the cup one at a time and offer sips of water so each pill can be swallowed separately.
Learning Outcome: 27-8.

Chapter 28 IV Therapy

Matching

1.	D	6.	B	11.	C
2.	C	7.	F	12.	A
3.	E	8.	D		
4.	F	9.	B		
5.	A	10.	E		

Learning Outcomes

1. See section entitled "Legal Implications and Safety Issues with IV Therapy."
   Learning Outcome: 28-1
2. See section entitled "Purpose of Intravenous Therapy and IV Solutions."
   Learning Outcome: 28-2
3. See section entitled "Equipment Overview."
   Learning Outcome: 28-3
4. See section entitled "IV Rate Calculations."
   Learning Outcome: 28-4
5. See section entitled "Anatomy of Peripheral Veins."
   Learning Outcome: 28-5
6. See section entitled "Factors Affecting IV Site Selection."
   Learning Outcome: 28-6
7. See section entitled "Venipuncture Procedure."
   Learning Outcome: 28-7
8. See section entitled "Peripheral IV Therapy Complications."
   Learning Outcome: 28-8
9. See section entitled "Blood Transfusions."
   Learning Outcome: 28-9

Apply What You Learned

1. When selecting a cannula, it should be the smallest gauge and shortest length possible to accommodate the necessary therapy. The ONC is used for long-term peripheral infusion therapy. These catheters are easy to insert and are patent longer. Infiltration rate is lower and they are radiopaque.
2. The hand veins are the best place to begin IV therapy because they are the most distal, allowing any superior vein to be used when needed. This site allows for relatively easy movement of the hand and arm, though, depending on actual placement, wrist mobility could be limited.
   Factors affecting IV site selection:
   - Duration of IV therapy
   - Cannula size
   - Type of solution
   - Condition of the vein
   - Client's level of consciousness
   - Client activity
   - Client's age
   - Dominant hand
3. Assessment of possible complications at the IV insertion site includes:
   - Tenderness at the insertion site or tip of the catheter.
   - Redness at the tip of the catheter and along the vein.
   - Edema.
   - Vein or surrounding area hard on palpation.
   - Generalized discomfort, pain or burning at the site or surrounding area.
   - Tightness and blanching at the site.
   - Bruising around the site.
   - Temperature differences (warm vs. cool).

4. Areas to check when troubleshooting the source of the pump alarm:
   - Amount of fluid in the IV container
   - Level of fluid in the drip chamber
   - Placement of the eye on the drip chamber
   - The position of the IV
   - Kinks in the line
   - The rate and volume; verify accuracy
   - IV site patent and free-flowing
   - IV tubing slide/roller clamps are open
   - Alarm message on the pump
   - Air in the line

Multiple Choice Questions

1. A

   Rationale: A milliequivalent is used because it is a measure of chemical activity rather than weight of the ions involved in the mixture.
   Learning Outcome: 28-2

2. A

   Rationale: This client is demonstrating signs of pulmonary edema, indicating a fluid volume excess, and the assessment data should be reported to the provider if the symptoms are new or worsening because the IV rate may be too rapid for this client and new orders may be needed.
   Learning Outcome: 28-1

3. C

   Rationale: Blood is very viscous and requires a large-bore catheter so the best choice would be an 18 gauge. 14 gauge is too large and is generally only used when large volumes of blood need to be administered quickly. 22 and 24 gauge needles would not be used for blood transfusions unless the client's veins are too small to accept a larger bore needle, such as pediatric clients.
   Learning Outcome: 28-3

4. B

   Rationale: An inline filter must be used when administering blood and blood products to filter out microclots or other particulate matter. A burette or rubber bung is not needed and a microdrip is contraindicated because it is too small to drip the viscous blood solution.
   Learning Outcome: 28-9

5. A

   Rationale: 0.45% sodium chloride, or half-normal saline, is hypotonic and would cause water to move into the cells, resulting in swelling and bursting of the blood cell.
   Learning Outcome: 28-9

6. D

   Rationale: $D_5 0.45$ NS is hypertonic solution, which will pull fluid from the intracellular compartment, which is contraindicated in clients with diabetic ketoacidosis who are already experiencing cellular dehydration. As a result, this order should be questioned. Isotonic fluids, such as lactated Ringer's or

D_5 W, or hypotonic fluids, such as 0.45% NS, would be less dangerous and more appropriate.

Learning Outcome: 28-9

7. C

Rationale: Blood should be started within 30 minutes after removing it from the refrigerator in order to allow enough time for administration before the cells begin to degenerate.

Learning Outcome: 28-9

8. D

Rationale: A catheter should only remain in a peripheral vein for 72 hours before it is removed and placed in a different location in order to avoid complications.

Learning Outcome: 28-6

9. B

Rationale: A client with dehydration and fluid and electrolyte imbalance will display weight loss, low blood pressure if significant water loss has occurred, and an increased hematocrit, which is a measure of the percentage of cells to fluid in the blood.

Learning Outcome: 28-2

10. A

Rationale: The client's respiratory status should be carefully assessed for signs of fluid overload, which will include a productive cough, increased respiratory rate, and breath sounds revealing crackles.

Learning Outcome: 28-8

11. B

Rationale: The nurse should apply a tourniquet to the arm to prevent the remaining catheter from traveling through the bloodstream and potentially causing a myocardial infarction or cerebrovascular accident. However, once the tourniquet is in place, blood supply to the arm is blocked, so help must be obtained quickly. Notify the charge nurse and/or provider immediately.

Learning Outcome: 28-8

12. C

Rationale: Drip rate is calculated by determining first the amount of fluid to infuse per hour. 1000 mL is to infuse over 4 hours so 1000 ÷ 4 = 250 mL to infuse in one hour. Convert mL to infuse over one hour into drops to fall over one hour by multiplying fluid to infuse over one hour X drip rate or 250 mL × 10 = 2500. To calculate how many drops per minute, divide number of drops per hour by 60 minutes or 2500 ÷ 60 = 41.66 or 42 drops/minute.

Learning Outcome: 28-4

13. A

Rationale: The most likely fluid to be administered to this client would be normal saline because large amounts of isotonic fluids will be needed quickly to restore the client's fluid balance. Large quantities of dextrose-containing fluids would not be advisable and isotonic fluids are best.

Learning Outcome: 28-2

14. C
Rationale: It is always best to initiate IV therapy in the most distal vein, allowing for more IV sites as needed by moving proximally. As a result, the metacarpal veins would be the best first site. Larger veins should be saved for emergency use if needed.
Learning Outcome: 28-6

15. A
Rationale: Only lactated Ringer's is an isotonic fluid. Option 2 and 4 are hypertonic and option 3 is hypotonic.
Learning Outcome: 28-2

Chapter 29 Nursing Care of Clients Having Surgery

Matching

1.	E	6.	E
2.	A	7.	C
3.	D	8.	D
4.	B	9.	A
5.	C	10.	B

Learning Outcomes

1. See section entitled "Surgery."
   Learning Outcome: 29-1
2. See section entitled "Surgery."
   Learning Outcome: 29-2
3. See section entitled "Surgery."
   Learning Outcome: 29-3
4. See section entitled "Preoperative Phase."
   Learning Outcome: 29-4
5. See section entitled "Preoperative Phase."
   Learning Outcome: 29-5
6. See section entitled "Preoperative Phase."
   Learning Outcome: 29-6
7. See section entitled "Intraoperative Phase."
   Learning Outcome: 29-7
8. See section entitled "Postoperative Phase."
   Learning Outcome: 29-8
9. See section entitled "Postoperative Phase."
   Learning Outcome: 29-9
10. See section entitled "Nursing Care."
    Learning Outcome: 29-10
11. See section entitled "Nursing Care."
    Learning Outcome: 29-11

Apply What You Learned

1. Though this client will undergo elective surgery, total joint replacement is considered major surgery and involves a high degree of risk. The degree of risk involved in a surgical procedure is affected by the *client's age, general health, nutritional status, use of medications, and mental status*. The nurse must assess each of these factors in order to plan for safe, effective postoperative care.

2. Risk factors considered by the nurse when planning care for this client:

   Age: The client is 76 years old and, as a result, may heal more slowly because vascular changes associated with aging, such as atherosclerosis and atrophy of capillaries in the skin, can impair blood flow to the wound. Collagen tissue is less flexible, and scar tissue has decreased elasticity.

   General Health: Though the client perceives himself as in "pretty good shape," he does have underlying medical conditions or comorbidities that can have an impact on his recovery. Diabetes mellitus predisposes the client to wound infection and delayed healing. Hypertension and other cardiac conditions weaken the heart, thereby decreasing cardiac output and oxygen circulation. Smoking a pack of unfiltered cigarettes daily may also affect the client's respiratory status and impair breathing patterns and gas exchange following surgery.

   Nutritional Status: Malnutrition can lead to delayed wound healing, infection, and reduced energy. A diet high in fat, sugar, carbohydrates, and alcohol will contribute to hyperglycemia, uncontrolled diabetes mellitus, and delayed healing. Moreover, depending on the amount of alcohol this client is consuming each day, he may also need to be monitored for signs and symptoms of alcohol withdrawal postoperatively.

   Use of Medications: This client is not taking his medications as prescribed. The therapeutic action and response of each drug are dependent upon a regular medication regimen.

   Mental Status: Having recently lost his wife, this client has undergone significant loss and changes in his life over the past year. He admits being fearful of the surgery. Feelings of powerlessness and anxiety may be expressed, and the nurse must identify these problems and create an appropriate nursing care plan accordingly.

3. *Possible* nursing problem areas that may require a nursing diagnosis and care plan:
   (**Please note:** These problems are *not* listed in order of importance or priority)
   - Impaired Skin Integrity
   - Impaired Mobility
   - Imbalanced Nutrition
   - Ineffective Individual Coping
   - Impaired Social Interaction
   - Health Maintenance
   - Home Maintenance

- Ineffectual/Dysfunctional Grieving
- Risk for Injury
- Pain
- Ineffective Denial
- Anxiety
- Medication Compliance

4. Areas requiring client teaching prior to discharge:
   - Wound care
   - Use of assistive devices
   - Effectively managing diabetes and hypertension
   - Diet
   - Exercise
   - Health maintenance:
   - Smoking Cessation
   - Sobriety
   - Medication Compliance

Multiple Choice Questions

1. C
   Rationale: In order to reduce the risk of vomiting, histamine-receptor anti-histamines are frequently given to reduce gastric fluid volume. While they may also reduce oral secretions, that is not the indication for use. They have no effect on inducing calmness or reducing anxiety.
   Learning Outcome: 29-6

2. A
   Rationale: The purpose of sequential compression devices is to improve the return of blood from the legs and reduce the risk of postoperative throm-bophlebitis. They do not improve wound healing, secure abdominal dressings, or prevent hemorrhage postoperatively.
   Learning Outcome: 29-9

3. C
   Rationale: When wound edges of a smooth incision are closely approximated, it results in primary healing
   Learning Outcome: 3. List the types of wounds and their potential complications.

4. A
   Rationale: Observe for bleeding frequently by inspecting the dressing and checking beneath the client for pooling blood
   Learning Outcome: 29-3

5. C

   Rationale: Monitoring the client is essential to prevent infection.
   Learning Outcome: 29-4

6. A

   Rationale: Vitamins A and C are essential to wound healing. The other vitamins do not significantly contribute to wound healing.
   Learning Outcome: 29-8

7. A

   Rationale: Obese clients with generous amounts of fatty or adipose tissue are likely to have poor wound healing because of the poor blood supply found in adipose tissue.
   Learning Outcome: 29-9

8. C

   Rationale: A decrease in number of white cells (leukocytes) indicates a less than effective immune system, which could result in delayed wound healing and infection. It does not indicate the presence of an infection, so prophylactic antibiotics would not be required. It has no impact on clotting or nutrition.
   Learning Outcome: 29-4

9. A

   Rationale: Postoperative pain is usually most severe after intraoperative anesthesias are metabolized and last from 12 to 36 hours.
   Learning Outcome: 29-7

10. D

   Rationale: Coughing and deep breathing helps to offset the normal response of the respiratory system to general anesthetics and analgesics and prevent postoperative pneumonia.
   Learning Outcome: 29-7

Chapter 30 Clients with Integumentary System Disorders

Matching

1.	E	1.	B
2.	B	2.	D
3.	C	3.	A
4.	D	4.	G
5.	G	5.	C
6.	A	6.	F
7.	F	7.	E

Learning Outcomes

1. See section entitled "Structure and Function of the Integumentary System."
   Learning Outcome: 30-1
2. See section entitled "Skin Integrity."
   Learning Outcome: 30-2
3. See sections entitled "Skin Integrity" and "Bacterial Infections."
   Learning Outcome: 30-3
4. See section entitled "Viral Infections."
   Learning Outcome: 30-4
5. See section entitled "Fungal Infections."
   Learning Outcome: 30-5
6. See section entitled "Parasitic Infestations."
   Learning Outcome: 30-6
7. See section entitled "Chronic Skin Conditions."
   Learning Outcome: 30-7
8. See section entitled "Skin Cancer."
   Learning Outcome: 30-8
9. See section entitled "Plastic and Reconstructive Surgery."
   Learning Outcome: 30-9

Apply What You Learned

1. Specific tasks to prevent the formation of pressure ulcers:
   - Turn the client at least every 2 hours.
   - Keep the client clean, dry, and free of irritation from urine.
   - Use a mild cleansing agent sparingly, and apply a moisturizing lotion after each cleansing.
   - Assist the client with each meal.
   - Provide the client with a smooth, firm, wrinkle-free area to sit or lie down.
   - Use supportive devices as needed.
2. Rationales for the delegated tasks:
   - At least every 2 hours, reposition any at-risk client who is confined to bed, even when a special support mattress is used. Immobility often causes a reduction in the amount of movement. Pressure ulcers are lesions caused by unrelieved pressure that results in damage to underlying tissue and prevents blood from circulating freely through the area. When blood cannot reach the tissue, the cells are deprived of oxygen and nutrients, and waste products accumulate in the cells. Prolonged, unrelieved pressure damages the small blood vessels, and the tissue eventually dies.
   - Moisture from incontinence promotes skin maceration, or softening of tissue, by prolonged wetting and makes the epidermis susceptible to injury. Any accumulation of secretions or excretions is irritating to the skin, harbors microorganisms, and makes an individual prone to skin breakdown and infection.
   - When bathing the client, avoid using hot water and apply minimal force and friction. Mild cleansing agents and moisturizers can help maintain

the skin's natural barriers. Minimize dryness by not exposing the client to cold or low humidity.

- Nutritional factors are crucial in the development of pressure ulcers. Generally, prolonged, inadequate nutrition causes weight loss, muscle atrophy, and the loss of subcutaneous tissue. Less padding between the skin and the bones increases the risk of pressure sore development. Inadequate intake of protein, carbohydrates, fluids, and vitamin C contributes to pressure sore formation. Providing adequate meals and nutritional supplements for nutritionally compromised clients is a vital nursing intervention in the prevention of pressure ulcers.
- Sheets rubbing against skin create friction. Friction can remove the superficial layers of the skin, making it more prone to breakdown. Wrinkles in the sheets, blankets, or underpads cause uneven pressure and contribute to skin breakdown. Providing a smooth, firm, wrinkle-free area will reduce the chance of damage by friction or shearing.
- When lifting a client to change his or her position, use a lifting device such as a trapeze rather than dragging the client across or up in bed. The friction that results from dragging the skin against a sheet can cause blisters and abrasions, which may contribute to more extensive tissue damage. Supportive devices such as a lift will help relieve pressure on bony prominences.

3. In addition to providing the above rationale for appropriate interventions, two comments by the nursing assistant need to be addressed. Her comments were as follows:

"I know what to do. I'll turn her when I get to it, do a two-person transfer to the chair, try to feed her breakfast and lunch, [1] order a doughnut for her to sit on when she is up, and [2] massage those areas that look red."

- Statement 1 reflects a lack of understanding by the nursing assistant and must be corrected. Doughnut-type devices should not be used since they place uneven pressure on the skin and surrounding tissue, making it prone to breakdown.
- Statement 2 refers to a nursing intervention that nurses and nursing assistants have used for years to stimulate blood circulation with the intention of preventing pressure sores. However, scientific evidence does not support this belief. In fact, massage may lead to deep tissue trauma.

Multiple Choice Questions

1. A
   Rationale: The skin is the first line of defense against pathogen entry into the body, maintaining fluid homeostasis, and regulating temperature.
   Learning Outcome: 30-1.

2. B
   Rationale: As cells of the epidermis die, new cells push up from the dermal layer to replace the dead cells, and the epidermis replaces itself approximately once every 4 weeks.
   Learning Outcome: 30-1.

3. C

Rationale: Skin color is determined by the amount of melanin produced, with more melanin resulting in darker skin tones.

Learning Outcome: 30-1.

4. C

Rationale: This lesion would best be described as a wheal. Cysts are fluid-filled or semisolid sacs originating in the subcutaneous tissue or dermis. Erosions are a wearing away of superficial epidermis by friction or pressure. Pustules are small circumscribed elevations of the skin containing purulent material.

Learning Outcome: 30-2.

5. B

Rationale: Malnutrition is a significant contributor to skin breakdown and the nurse designs care to prevent this from occurring. The highest percentage of a healthy diet is made up of high-quality carbohydrates such as fruits and vegetables. Exercise and standing in place does not contribute to skin breakdown.

Learning Outcome: 30-3.

6. B

Rationale: A priority nursing measure to prevent skin breakdown is frequent repositioning, at least every 2 hours. Even when sitting in a chair, the client is prone to skin breakdown at pressure points. Adequate fluids and protein are important, but extra does not prevent skin breakdown.

Learning Outcome: 30-3.

7. B

Rationale: Impetigo is a highly contagious infection of the skin caused by staphylococcus and appears as a small red macule that develops into a thin-walled vesicle that ruptures and is loosely covered with a honey-yellow crust that is easily removed, but returns quickly.

Learning Outcome: 30-4.

8. D

Rationale: Onychomycosis is a fungal infection of the nails.

Learning Outcome: 30-5.

9. A

Rationale: Psoriasis is a genetic disorder believed to result from an autoimmune response, causing dry, flaky, highly vascular plaques, most commonly on the elbows, knees, scalp and lower back. It is not infectious or contagious. Option 2 describes acne, option 3 describes scabies, and option 4 describes warts.

Learning Outcome: 30-7.

10. D

Rationale: This is a test of skin turgor which indicates the client is dehydrated.

Learning Outcome: 30-7.

Chapter 31 Clients with Musculoskeletal System Disorders

Matching

1.	K	6.	B	11.	I
2.	F	7.	C	12.	D
3.	N	8.	E	13.	G
4.	J	9.	O	14.	H
5.	M	10.	A	15.	L

Learning Outcomes

1. See section entitled "Structure and Function of the Musculoskeletal System."
   Learning Outcome: 31-1
2. See Table 31-1, "Diagnostic Tests for Musculoskeletal Injuries."
   Learning Outcome: 31-2
3. See section entitled "Traumatic Bone Disorders."
   Learning Outcome: 31-3
4. See section entitled "Osteoporosis."
   Learning Outcome: 31-4
5. See section entitled "Traumatic Bone Disorders."
   Learning Outcome: 31-5
6. See Procedure 31-1.
   Learning Outcome: 31-7
7. See section entitled "Inflammatory Disorders."
   Learning Outcome: 31-7
8. See section entitled "Assisting Clients with Joint Replacements."
   Learning Outcome: 31-8
9. See section entitled "Spinal Disorders."
   Learning Outcome: 31-9
10. See section entitled "Joint and Muscle Disorders."
    Learning Outcome: 31-10
11. See Table 31-5 entitled "Advantages and Disadvantages of Heat and Cold Therapy."
    Learning Outcome: 31-11
12. See section entitled "Other Disorders."
    Learning Outcome: 31-12

Apply What You Learned

1. Dairy products, such as milk, cheese, or ice cream are high in calcium, but must be increased carefully because they are also high in fat. Clients can drink skim milk instead of whole milk and eat cheeses made from skin milk or that are lower in fat, such as cottage cheese. White beans, chickpeas, tofu, soybeans, cabbage, instant oats, and almonds are also high in calcium.
2. Vitamin D is found in foods such as cod liver oil, fish, tofu, soymilk, skim milk, and fortified orange juice, and is also supplemented in many cereals. The body makes vitamin D when exposed to sunlight. To prevent increased

risk of skin cancer from sun exposure, the client should spend no more than 20 minutes a day in the sun and avoid sun exposure during the height of the afternoon.

3. Assess Ms. Markum's stability when walking and consult the provider if she may benefit from the use of a cane or walker. If her strength and stability are adequate, recommend removal of all throw rugs, placing lights in stairways or dark areas of the home, avoiding electrical cords in walkways where the client could trip, leaving a light on at night in case she needs to get up to go to the bathroom, and avoiding clutter on the floor.

Multiple Choice Questions

1. B
   Rationale: Connectivity is not a basic property of skeletal muscles. Excitability is required for the muscle to respond to electrical stimulation, elasticity is required for muscles to contract and stretch, and extensibility is required for muscles to stretch.
   Learning Outcome: 31-1

2. D
   Rationale: The suffix *-centesis* indicates removal of fluid. Arthrocentesis indicates removal of fluid from the joint. This procedure can be done to test the fluid as well as to reduce edema caused by an excessive accumulation of fluid in the joint which causes pain and limits mobility.
   Learning Outcome: 31-2

3. A
   Rationale: A greenstick fracture can be seen on an x-ray as a crack that does not cause bone fragment separation and travels along the length of the bone, usually seen in infancy and childhood, which is still flexible and less brittle, and usually occurs as a result of a bending force.
   Learning Outcome: 31-3

4. C
   Rationale: Immune system modifiers are not indicated for use with a client diagnosed with osteoporosis. Vitamin supplements include vitamin D, which helps the body utilize calcium and has been found to reduce fractures in the elderly. Biphosphates are first-line treatment and include risedronate (Actonel), which helps to strengthen bone. Use of estrogen, a polypeptide hormone, is controversial, although it does help to prevent osteoporosis, but risk factors may outweigh benefits.
   Learning Outcome: 31-4

5. D
   Rationale: Lifting the weight removes the traction and can result in complications. Weights should never be placed on the bed or removed. The remaining options are good strategies for providing care for the client in traction.
   Learning Outcome: 31-6

6. A
   Rationale: Osteoarthritis is sometimes called a wear-and-tear disorder caused by overuse or injury to the joint, and is seen in older adults most commonly. Rheumatoid arthritis is believed to be an autoimmune disease;

osteomyelitis is caused by an infection; and osteomalacia is caused by insufficient vitamin D.
Learning Outcome: 31-7

7. C
    Rationale: Following a total hip replacement, flexion of the hip more than 90 degrees risks injury to the site.
    Learning Outcome: 31-8

8. B
    Rationale: CSF is high in glucose because the brain requires large quantities of glucose to function properly, which is why the client with a hypoglycemic reaction becomes confused and eventually will lose consciousness. If CSF fluid is suspected, testing for the presence of glucose can help to confirm the diagnosis.
    Learning Outcome: 31-9

9. D
    Rationale: The nerve passing through the carpal tunnel becomes inflamed due to impingement, creating these classic symptoms.
    Learning Outcome: 31-10

10. B
    Rationale: Cold therapy is generally applied to limit postinjury swelling and bleeding. Although it does cause vasoconstriction, this is considered a disadvantage that must be carefully monitored because excessive vasoconstriction could cause frostbite, leading to gangrene.
    Learning Outcome: 31-11

Chapter 32 Clients with Respiratory System Disorders

Matching

1. C	6. B	11. C
2. F	7. D	12. A
3. G	8. E	13. G
4. E	9. D	14. B
5. A	10. F	

Learning Outcomes

1. See section entitled "Structure and Function of the Respiratory System."
    Learning Outcome: 32-1
2. See section entitled "Structure and Function of the Respiratory System."
    Learning Outcome: 32-2
3. See section entitled "Factors that Influence Respiratory Function."
    Learning Outcome: 32-3
4. See section entitled "Factors that Affect Oxygenation."
    Learning Outcome: 32-4
5. See section entitled "Tests for Respiratory Disorders."
    Learning Outcome: 32-5

6. See section entitled "Respiratory Therapies."
   Learning Outcome: 32-6
7. See section entitled "Nursing Care."
   Learning Outcome: 32-7
8. See section entitled "Infections and Inflammations."
   Learning Outcome: 32-8
9. See section entitled "Trauma and Obstruction Tumors."
   Learning Outcome: 32-9
10. See section entitled "Lower Respiratory Disorders."
    Learning Outcome: 32-10
11. See section entitled "Infections and Inflammations."
    Learning Outcome: 32-11
12. See section entitled "Obstructive Disorders."
    Learning Outcome: 32-12
13. See section entitled "Lung Cancer" and "Interstitial Disorders."
    Learning Outcome: 32-13

Apply What You Learned

1. Tuberculosis is a chronic, infectious lung disease and is reportable to the Centers for Disease Control. Each year, approximately 8 million people worldwide develop active TB, and 3 million die from the disease. In the United States, 10 to 15 million people are infected and 1 in 10 of these will develop the active disease. Clients at greatest risk for developing TB include minorities, the elderly, intravenous drug abusers, the homeless and those living in poverty, the immunocompromised, cancer patients, those with diabetes mellitus, those in long-term care facilities, and those in prisons. The infecting agent for TB is *Mycobacterium tuberculosis*. It is spread via airborne droplets. Because TB is not highly contagious, repeated exposure is usually required to transmit the organism. In the primary stage of the disease, a lesion called a *tubercle* develops. This tubercle has a cheeselike center. Scar tissue then develops around the tubercle, and calcification occurs. Clients with effective immune systems will not develop the disease. However, the infection remains latent and may be reactivated if the client's immune system becomes compromised. At this time, secondary TB develops and clinical symptoms may appear.

2. Clinical manifestations of secondary TB are fatigue, anorexia, weight loss, fever, night sweats, and a dry cough that eventually produces purulent or blood-tinged sputum. Rupture of the tubercle may produce contamination of the pleural space, pleuritis, or produce air in the pleural space, called *pneumothorax*. TB may develop outside of the respiratory system. Areas of infestation include the blood, bone marrow, the urinary tract, the genitourinary tract, the subarachnoid space, and the bones and joints.

3. Because of the risk of spread of this disease, the nurse is involved in selective screening for the TB infection. This is accomplished via two methods. The multiple-puncture tine test injects into the client's forearm a small amount of purified protein derivative (PPD) through a small multipronged device. The Mantoux test uses 0.1 mL of PPD, also injected intradermally into the client's

forearm. Results can be read 48 to 72 hours following the test. The nurse assesses for an area of induration, a raised, reddened area that may become hard. This finding is considered positive, and further diagnostic tests such as repeated PPD, chest x-rays, and sputum smears and cultures may be necessary.

4. The nurse is responsible for obtaining a health history related to the lower respiratory disorder, including symptoms, especially dyspnea, cough, chest pain, weight loss, night sweats, current medications, immunization history, smoking history, and past medical and surgical history. Objective data obtained from a physical examination should include overall appearance and level of distress, vital signs, lung sounds, respiratory excursion, known allergies, and skin color.

5. Four common nursing diagnoses:
    *   Ineffective Airway Clearance
    *   Activity Intolerance
    *   Ineffective Therapeutic Regimen Management
    *   Altered Health Maintenance

6. *   The client will have effective airway clearance, as evidenced by a patent airway and arterial blood gas levels within normal limits.
    *   The client will tolerate activity, as evidenced by performing activities of daily living without fatigue.
    *   The client will verbalize understanding of the medication regimen, side effects, and the need for compliance.

7. Pertinent nursing actions/interventions:
    *   Position the client in the Fowler's or high Fowler's position, allowing him or her to expand the chest more effectively.
    *   Teach the client how to cough effectively, and to breathe deeply to help move secretions and clear the airway.
    *   Collaborate with the client to plan activities of daily living to reduce the drain on the client's energy.
    *   Educate the client on medications and the importance of compliance.

Multiple Choice Questions

1. D
    Rationale: The primary function of the respiratory system is to exchange gases. In the process of gas exchange, the respiratory system contributes to acid-base balance, but that is not the system's primary function. There are a number of factors within the respiratory system that protect the airway from infection, but this is not the respiratory system's primary function. The kidneys eliminate waste products.
    Learning Outcome: 32-1.

2. A
    Rationale: The upper respiratory system includes everything between the nose and the larynx. The trachea, bronchi, and alveoli are considered components of the lower respiratory tract.
    Learning Outcome: 32-1

3. B

Rationale: The pharynx comprises the throat and is divided into the nasal pharynx, the oral pharynx, and the laryngeal pharynx. The Adam's apple is the voice box or larynx and the esophagus is the tube connecting the pharynx to the stomach.

Learning Outcome: 32-1.

4. A

Rationale: The respiratory control center is found in the brainstem. The other options are incorrect.

Learning Outcome: 32-2

5. C

Rationale: When gases or other particulate matter attempts to equalize pressure or concentration from an area of high concentration to an area of lower concentration, it is called diffusion. Inhalation is the drawing in of gases into the respiratory system, expiration is the blowing out of gases, and perfusion is used to describe the circulation of blood to the tissues.

Learning Outcome: 32-3.

6. D

Rationale: Tidal volume is the amount of air, or tide of air, brought into the respiratory system during normal inhalation and is normally 500 mL. Peak pressure and inspiratory pressure measure the pressure under which air is inhaled, not the volume of air. Minute volume is the amount of air inhaled over 60 seconds.

Learning Outcome: 32-3

7. B

Rationale: When the amount of carbon dioxide in the blood increases, the body attempts to return homeostasis by increasing the rate and depth of respirations to blow off excessive amounts of carbon dioxide.

Learning Outcome: 32-3

8. A

Rationale: Clients with COPD have chronically high carbon dioxide levels, so this no longer serves as a stimulus for breathing. Instead, COPD clients breathe when their oxygenation levels lower. As a result, administration of high levels of oxygen can remove the COPD client's stimulus to breathe and result in apnea.

Learning Outcome: 32-3

9. B

Rationale: Care must be taken when administering narcotics and barbiturates because they depress the central nervous system and can depress respirations as well, causing a decrease in rate and depth of respirations leading to hypoxia or even death.

Learning Outcome: 32-3

10. A

Rationale: Clients with fever breathe faster in an attempt to expel heat and cool the body. Clients with metabolic acidosis breathe faster in order to expel carbon dioxide to reduce acidosis. Hypoxia causes an increase in respiratory rate to increase oxygen levels in the bloodstream, and clients in pain breathe more quickly as a result of central nervous system stimulation.

Learning Outcome: 32-3

11. A

Rationale: The pulse oximeter measures the amount of hemoglobin saturated with oxygen known as oxygen saturation. Hypercapnia, or high carbon dioxide levels, are measured with arterial blood gases or transcutaneous carbon monoxide monitoring devices. Expiratory tidal volume is determined by measuring the amount of air exhaled with a normal exhalation.

Learning Outcome: 32-5

12. B

Rationale: Oxygen will not spontaneously burn, but oxygen is needed for any fire to burn and the presence of oxygen facilitates combustion and burning.

Learning Outcome: 32-6

13. B

Rationale: When a new tracheotomy is performed, removal of the tracheostomy tube will result in closure of the tracheotomy and obstruction of the artificial airway. As a tracheotomy ages, this risk minimizes somewhat. An obturator is kept at the bedside to maintain the tracheotomy opening until a new tube can be inserted.

Learning Outcome: 32-12

14. C

Rationale: The question describes the use of pursed-lip breathing, which is frequently taught to clients with chronic obstructive pulmonary disease or at risk for atelectasis because it reduces the risk of airway collapse.

Learning Outcome: 32-12

15. A

Rationale: When suctioning the nasopharynx, the suction catheter is inserted and then suction is applied for 5-10 seconds while withdrawing the catheter. Applying suction while inserting the catheter would make catheter insertion difficult and traumatic. Applying suction for longer than 10 seconds is likely to result in the client becoming hypoxic.

Learning Outcome: 32-7

Chapter 33 Clients with Cardiovascular System Disorders

Matching

1. F	6. C	11. B	16. B	21. F	26. E
2. D	7. C	12. A	17. F	22. B	27. A
3. E	8. D	13. E	18. D	23. A	28. F
4. B	9. E	14. C	19. E	24. C	29. B
5. A	10. F	15. A	20. D	25. G	30. D
					31. C

Learning Outcomes

1. See section entitled "Structure and Function of the Cardiovascular System."
   Learning Outcome: 33-1

2. See section entitled "Factors that Affect Cardiovascular System Function."
   Learning Outcome: 33-2
3. See section entitled "Tests for Cardiovascular Disorders."
   Learning Outcome: 33-3
4. See section entitled "Heart Disorders."
   Learning Outcome: 33-4
5. See section entitled "Nursing Care."
   Learning Outcome: 33-5
6. See section entitled "Disorders Affecting the Heart and Lungs."
   Learning Outcome: 33-6
7. See section entitled "Other Heart Disorders."
   Learning Outcome: 33-7
8. See section entitled "Conduction Disorders."
   Learning Outcome: 33-8
9. See section entitled "Central Circulatory Disorders."
   Learning Outcome: 33-9
10. See section entitled "Peripheral Vascular Disorders."
    Learning Outcome: 33-10

Apply What You Learned

1. Congestive heart failure (CHF) is the inability of the heart to pump enough blood throughout the body with decreased cardiac output to maintain well-being. Blood that pools in the systemic venous circulation results in peripheral edema. CHF may be acute or chronic. The client experiences increasing dyspnea, or shortness of breath. Cardiac and respiratory rates also increase. This results in greater stress and anxiety.
2. The hallmark symptom is shortness of breath. In addition, the client may experience difficulty breathing, especially at night, pulmonary crackles, orthopnea, hemoptysis, and cough.
3. The outlook for clients with CHF depends on the cause of the syndrome and the response to treatment. Reduced cardiac output triggers compensatory mechanisms such as ventricular dilatation, hypertrophy, and increased sympathetic activity.
4. The treatment of CHF targets reduction of the workload of the heart in order to increase its efficiency.
5. Treatment includes (a) bed rest, (b) antiembolism stockings to prevent fluid pooling in the legs, and (c) medication to assist the heart. Medications are given to strengthen myocardial contractility and to increase cardiac output.
6. Lasix, HydroDiuril, Bumex
7. Lanoxin, Crystodigin
8. *Anxiety* related to change in health status; *decreased cardiac output* related to changes in the heart; *fluid volume excess* related to inability of the heart to pump effectively.
9. Nursing interventions for a client with CHF:
   • Weigh the client at the same time daily.
   • Check daily for peripheral edema.
   • Take vital signs frequently.
   • Check mental status.

- Apply antiembolism stockings.
- Check for calf pain and tenderness.
- Administer antianxiety/sedative agent as directed.
- Administer diuretics as ordered.
- Monitor intake and output every hour.
- Administer oxygen as needed.
- Check heart and breath sounds regularly.
- Monitor for diminished pulses, pallor, or cyanosis.
- Encourage bed rest and a quiet environment.
- Record and report any changes.

Multiple Choice Questions

1. B
   Rationales: The upper chambers are the atria while the lower chambers are the ventricles, both of which are divided by the septum into left and right. The tricuspid valve separate the right atrium from the right ventricle and the semilunar valve separates the left atrium from the left ventricle.
   Learning Outcome: 33-1

2. A
   Rationale: As the ventricle contracts, blood is ejected from the right ventricle into the pulmonary artery, where it travels to the lungs to receive oxygen. When the left ventricle contracts, blood enters the aorta to take oxygen to the tissues throughout the body.
   Learning Outcome: 33-1

3. B
   Rationale: Afterload describes how hard the heart must contract in order to overcome pressure in the blood vessels to push blood out of the ventricles and into the arteries. Hypertension increases pressure in the arterial system, thereby making the heart contract harder and increasing afterload.
   Learning Outcome: 33-1

4. B
   Rationale: The aorta carries blood from the left ventricle away from the heart and to the tissues of the body.
   Learning Outcome: 33-1

5. D
   Rationale: A cardiac catheterization allows for direct visualization of the heart, arteries, and valves. An echocardiogram displays an ultrasonic image but does not provide direct visualization. An electrocardiogram (ECG) displays the electrical activity of the heart in wave form. A thallium scan display's the heart's electrical response to stress or exercise.
   Learning Outcome: 33-3

6. A
   Rationale: As a result of blockage in the coronary arteries, oxygenated blood is unable to pass to the tissue and the tissue becomes ischemic (insufficient oxygen supply) and dies as a result (necrosis).
   Learning Outcome: 33-4

7. A

   Rationale: Pericarditis is inflammation of the pericardium, the sac that encloses and protects the heart.

   Learning Outcome: 33-4

8. D

   Rationale: A commissurotomy is the term used to describe surgery to separate the valve leaflets.

   Learning Outcome: 33-7

9. B

   Rationale: A heart rate lower than 60 beats per minute is called bradycardia while a rate faster than 100 beats per minute is called tachycardia.

   Learning Outcome: 33-8

10. D

    Rationale: Elevation of blood pressure that occurs rapidly and ends with a diastolic blood pressure greater than 120 mm Hg is called malignant hypertension. Primary hypertension describes blood pressure of unknown origin while secondary hypertension describes blood pressure caused by another problem. Orthostatic hypertension is an increase in blood pressure depending on position.

    Learning Outcome: 33-10

11. A

    Rationale: Fusiform aneurysms are tubular in appearance as the walls of the artery dilate equally.

    Learning Outcome: 33-9

12. D

    Rationale: Pain, tingling in the extremity, and absent pulses may be an indication of an emboli.

    Learning Outcome: 33-6

13. B

    Rationale: It is important to teach the client not to cross the legs at the knee or the ankle because this increases the risk of venous stasis and further emboli or thrombus formation.

    Learning Outcome: 33-7

14. D

    Rationale: The circulatory system includes the heart, lungs, and blood vessels.

    Learning Outcome: 33-1

15. A

    Rationale: Smoking, hypertension, and high blood cholesterol are all significant factors increasing the risk for cardiovascular disease.

    Learning Outcome: 33-2

Chapter 34 Clients with Hematologic and Lymphatic System Disorders

Matching

1. E
2. D
3. F
4. C

5. B
6. A
7. D
8. E

9. A
10. B
11. F
12. C

Learning Outcomes

1. See section entitled "Structure and Function of the Hematologic and Lymphatic Systems."
    Learning Outcome: 34-1
2. See section entitled "Laboratory Tests for Hematologic or Lymphatic Disorders."
    Learning Outcome: 34-2
3. See section entitled "Cross-Matching For Blood Product Transfusions."
    Learning Outcome: 34-3
4. See section entitled "Red Blood Cell Disorders."
    Learning Outcome: 34-4
5. See section entitled "Platelet and Coagulation Disorders."
    Learning Outcome: 34-5
6. See section entitled "White Blood Cell Disorders."
    Learning Outcome: 34-6
7. See section entitled "Lymphatic System Disorders."
    Learning Outcome: 34-7
8. See section entitled "Lymphatic System Disorders."
    Learning Outcome: 34-8

Apply What You Learned

1. Sickle cell anemia is a hereditary chronic condition in which some of the red blood cells assume a sickle shape when put under stress, such as infection, dehydration, cold temperatures, and vigorous exercise. Sickle cell disease has an autosomal dominant inheritance pattern. Both parents must have the sickle cell trait for a child to be born with the disease. The sickled red blood cells become lodged in the capillaries, occluding blood flow to the affected area. This situation is called a *sickle cell crisis*. This occlusion may lead to death of the involved tissues. Because sickle cells can occlude in any capillary, damage may occur in any body system. Some of the most common complications are chest pain, myocardial infarction, and stroke.
2. Red blood cells make up most of the cellular portion of the blood. Because red blood cells transport oxygen, when hypoxia occurs, the body sends the signal that more red blood cells are needed to compensate for the lowered oxygen content of the blood. The hemoglobin molecules transport the oxygen to all body tissues. Any disruption in the normal formation of red blood cells affects this oxygen transport and necessitates the administration

of oxygen via mask or cannula. Because the body is experiencing hypoxia and hypoxemia, the respiratory rate will increase as the body attempts to compensate and reestablish homeostasis. In addition, stress, pain, and anxiety can lead to shortness of breath. Moreover, as the sickled red blood cells become lodged in capillaries, they occlude blood flow to affected areas such as the lungs. This occlusion may interfere with oxygen transport and damage the tissues.

3. Impaired gas exchange related to abnormal red blood cell formation; pain

4. Client will maintain adequate gas exchange; client will report a decreased level or absence of pain.

5. Nursing actions/interventions for this client:
   - Assess pain and administer analgesics to increase the client's comfort.
   - Maintain a quiet, calm, temperature-controlled environment.
   - Administer oxygen by cannula or mask as ordered by the physician.
   - Provide at least 3000 mL/day of fluids.
   - Maintain bed rest for the client to decrease oxygen use.
   - Provide emotional support for the client and family.
   - Incorporate client preferences into the care plan.
   - Avoid caffeinated or alcoholic beverages.
   - Teach the client to avoid exposure to individuals with an illness.
   - Teach the client to avoid becoming chilled, anxious, or stressed.
   - Teach the client to avoid vigorous exercise.

6. Sickle cell anemia occurs most often among clients of African American descent. The sickle cell trait is present in about 8% of the African American population and occurs when a child inherits the gene from one parent. Both parents must have the sickle cell trait for a child to be born with the disease. If both parents are carriers of the trait, the child has a 25% chance of inheriting the gene from both parents and is likely to develop sickle cell anemia. This is a chronic, unpredictable disease. Genetic testing is particularly important for African American couples prior to deciding to start a family. Families need support, education, and a list of community resources—all of which the nurse can provide.

Multiple Choice Questions

1. C
   Rationale: Hemoglobin is a combination of protein and iron required for the transport of oxygen throughout the body.
   Learning Outcome: 34-1

2. C
   Rationale: Monocytes respond to foreign materials and play an important role in reducing pathogens in the body, but they do not promote a healthy immune system.
   Learning Outcome: 34-1

3. **A**

   Rationale: Platelets play an important role in blood clotting. Hemoglobin transports oxygen and eosinophils play a role in allergic reactions. Red blood cells live approximately 120 days and the liver stores products of the cells to contribute to formation of new red blood cells.

   Learning Outcome: 34-1

4. **B**

   Rationale: Elevation in white blood cells most likely indicate leukemia which is rapid production of immature cells that do not function as their mature counterparts would. Anemia is a deficiency in hemoglobin, sickle cell anemia is abnormally shaped hemoglobin, and polycythemia is an excess production of red blood cells.

   Learning Outcome: 34-6

5. **B**

   Rationale: Disseminated intravascular coagulation causes disruptions in clotting manifested by widespread clotting and bleeding. The other options are not part of the disease process of DIC.

   Learning Outcome: 34-5

6. **C**

   Rationale: Polycythemia results from elevated red blood cell count causing thicker, more viscous blood.

   Learning Outcome: 34-4

7. **A**

   Rationale: Stage I is the time when intensive and aggressive therapy is administered, often resulting in complications such as bone marrow suppression. In Stage 2, the dosage of treatment is reduced. Stage 3 is an even milder form of chemotherapy. There is no stage 4.

   Learning Outcome: 34-6

8. **D**

   Rationale: Lymph nodes are like the trash collectors of the body, collecting damaged cells or those that do not belong in the body. These cells may result from infection, inflammation or malignancy.

   Learning Outcome: 34-7

9. **C**

   Rationale: Lymphangitis is an inflammation of a lymphatic vessel and is usually caused by a bacterial infection manifested as a red streak along the course of the inflamed vessel. Lymphedema is swelling caused by the inability of the lymph system to remove all lymph fluid from the interstitial tissue. Lymphadenopathy is lymph node enlargement. Lymphoma is cancer of the lymphoid tissue.

   Learning Outcome: 34-7

10. **B**

    Rationale: Because of bone tissue destruction, the client is at risk for hypercalcemia and serum electrolyte levels must be carefully monitored.

    Learning Outcome: 34-8

11. **D**

    Rationale: All of these nursing diagnoses would be appropriate. Clients with disorders of either system are at risk for infection, injury, and fatigue.

    Learning Outcome: 34-8

12. A

Rationale: The client's activity tolerance must be considered when planning care for clients with hematopoietic and lymphatic disorders. Pain may or may not be a factor with these disorders. Loss of consciousness or alertness is not normally associated with lymphatic disorders unless other systems are involved.

Learning Outcome: 34-8

13. A

Rationale: A client with agranulocytosis has an absence of white blood cells and is prone to infection, so they should be placed in protective isolation.

Learning Outcome: 34-6

14. A

Rationale: Good hand washing is the best way of preventing the spread of infection, which is of primary concern when caring for a client with a low white blood cell count. A gown, gloves, and mask may be indicated if the count is low enough to require protective isolation, but is not always indicated and is not the best means of preventing infection. Repositioning and skin integrity are not high priority concerns for this client.

Learning Outcome: 34-6

15. D

Rationale: A hemolytic reaction is manifested as headache, nausea, flushing, and chest pain. An allergic reaction may be mild, manifesting as itching, hives, and fatigue, or severe, with hypertension, vomiting, and abdominal pain. Diplopia, dysuria, and polydipsia are not usually linked to blood reactions.

Learning Outcome: 34-3

Chapter 35 Caring for Clients with Immune System Disorders

Matching

1.	D	6.	A	11.	F
2.	F	7.	B	12.	A
3.	G	8.	C	13.	D
4.	E	9.	G	14.	E
5.	C	10.	B		

Learning Outcomes

1. See section entitled "Structure and Function of the Immune System."
   Learning Outcome: 35-1
2. See section entitled "Structure and Function of the Immune System."
   Learning Outcome: 35-2
3. See section entitled "Structure and Function of the Immune System."
   Learning Outcome: 35-3
4. See section entitled "Structure and Function of the Immune System."
   Learning Outcome: 35-4

5. See section entitled "Structure and Function of the Immune System."
   Learning Outcome: 35-5
6. See section entitled "Structure and Function of the Immune System."
   Learning Outcome: 35-6
7. See section entitled "Major Immune System Disorders."
   Learning Outcome: 35-7
8. See section entitled "Organ Transplantation."
   Learning Outcome: 35-8
9. See section entitled "Autoimmune Disorders."
   Learning Outcome: 35-9
10. See section entitled "Allergies."
    Learning Outcome: 35-10

Apply What You Learned

1. HIV/AIDS was first reported in the United States in 1981. According to the World Health Organization (WHO), it is estimated that 42 million people are living with HIV or AIDS worldwide, and in some African nations more than one-fourth of the population is infected. At the end of 2002, the Centers for Disease Control and Prevention reported that 886,575 people had the diagnosis of AIDS in the United States. Of that number, 159,271 were women and 9300 were children under 13.

2. HIV is transmitted through *blood, semen, vaginal secretions*, the *placenta, breast milk,* and *artificial insemination.* Intravenous drug use, prostitution, oral sex, anal sex, and vaginal intercourse increase the risk for passage of the infection through broken skin or mucous membranes. In addition, a person who received blood transfusions before effective screening was in place (between 1978 and 1985) is at risk. People who receive organ transplants or are artificially inseminated can also be at risk.

3. The client with HIV/AIDS often feels powerless over his or her situation. Because there is no cure for the disease and it is progressive in nature, the client sees the outlook for the future as bleak. Moreover, the client is frequently stigmatized by society and feels isolated, alone, and without support.

4. The nurse must deliver care with a nonjudgmental attitude. Confidentiality is the client's right and must be maintained. The client should be allowed to express feelings and verbalize fears and anxieties. The nurse *must* promote dignity and approach the client with respect. The client is a human being with an illness. The nurse should be available to listen attentively and provide support. The nurse must provide education on risk reduction behaviors and preventative measures for HIV infection. The nurse needs to be aware of the needs of all people in the community. It is the nurse's job to give accurate health information when people seek it and to present all options.

5. Originally, homosexuals were the primary population afflicted with HIV/AIDS, but current research, data, and documentation show that AIDS can affect persons of any age or nationality and both genders. It has become a major epidemic. Over 42 million people worldwide are infected with the disease, many of them women and children. It is important to realize that in addition to anal intercourse, HIV is spread through sexual contact with an infected person—male or female, injection with contaminated blood or

blood products, use of contaminated needles, and transmission from the mother to her fetus. As nurses, each of us has been issued a license to practice which requires that we provide nonjudgmental, effective care to all clients. Each person's value system may vary, but each nurse is obligated to provide safe, effective, competent, and compassionate care to all clients.

Multiple Choice Questions

1. B
   Rationale: The immunity is active because it is the body that produces the immunity, but it is artificial because it was not acquired by contracting the disease.
   Learning Outcome: 35-3.

2. A
   Rationale: An induration in the case of a PPD injection is a site of injection that the body's immune system reacts against, causing a hardened raised area. It is not fluid filled, it is not pinkish-blue, and it is not a cell-mediated response.
   Learning Outcome: 35-4.

3. D
   Rationale: An acute transplant rejection places stress on the liver, kidneys, and cardiac cells, impacting all of these lab values as the rejection becomes more severe.
   Learning Outcome: 35-8.

4. D
   Rationale: Following transplant surgery routine postoperative care is required, which includes assessment of the surgical wound, good aseptic technique, including hand washing and all clients receiving medication should be assessed and monitored for side effects.
   Learning Outcome: 35-8.

5. B
   Rationale: When helping a client to practice safer sex techniques in order to avoid contracting a sexually transmitted infection, the client should be taught to store condoms in a place where it is not excessively hot or cold, which can cause the latex to break or tear, reducing the effectiveness of the barrier technique. They should be discarded when past the expiration date, a spermicidal lubricant (not oil-based) should be used, and carrying the condom in the wallet or car exposes them to environmental hazards that damage the latex.
   Learning Outcome: 35-7.

6. C
   Rationale: Only Pneumocystis carinii pneumonia is an opportunistic disease related to HIV infection.
   Learning Outcome: 35-7.

7. A
   Rationale: A retrovirus is one that enters the host's body and begins to replicate within the cells of the host, not outside the host. HIV causes a decrease in CD4 and T-cell count and it replicates by changing the host's RNA.
   Learning Outcome: 35-7.

8. A

Rationale: The purpose of standard precautions and good hand hygiene is to reduce the risk of infection in both the client and the nurse, whether the infection be opportunistic or nosocomial in nature. It does not promote early detection of the disease, it is not a treatment for the disease, and it is not related to the body's response to the disease.

Learning Outcome: 35-7.

9. D

Rationale: The classic symptom of SLE is the butterfly rash that appears on the client's face across the nose and cheeks. The other symptoms are not commonly associated with SLE.

Learning Outcome: 35-9.

10. B

Rationale: These symptoms describe progressive systemic sclerosis and do not fit with any of the other options.

Learning Outcome: 35-9.

11. A

Rationale: Following organ transplant surgery, the client is put on immuno-suppressive medications to prevent organ rejection. This places the client at increased risk for infection because the immune system is suppressed or diminished.

Learning Outcome: 35-8.

12. C

Rationale: The question describes chronic rejection, which takes place over time, versus acute rejection, which occurs quickly and severely.

Learning Outcome: 35-8.

13. A

Rationale: Solu-Medrol is a commonly used immunosuppressive agent to prevent rejection. The other medications do not have common usage for preventing rejection.

Learning Outcome: 35-8.

14. D

Rationale: An autoimmune disorder is one in which the body sees its own tissues as foreign and develops autoantibodies to destroy the cells of the body. Most autoimmune disorders, such as systemic lupus erythematosus or rheumatoid arthritis, are most commonly diagnosed in women.

Learning Outcome: 35-9.

15. C

Rationale: Stress has been strongly linked to flare-ups of autoimmune disorders and stress can result from malnutrition. Proper nutrition and appropriate medications are also important to controlling the disease and preventing flare-ups. Past coping strategies would need to be assessed for their effectiveness and while diversions can help minimize pain, periods of rest are important and the client cannot be constantly kept busy.

Learning Outcome: 35-9.

Matching

1. D	6. B	11. C	16. C	21. G	26. C	31. B
2. F	7. D	12. B	17. D	22. A	27. E	32. D
3. E	8. E	13. B	18. A	23. B	28. F	
4. A	9. F	14. F	19. E	24. C	29. G	
5. C	10. A	15. E	20. D	25. F	30. A	

Learning Outcomes

1. See section entitled "Structure and Function of the Nervous System."
   Learning Outcome: 36-1
2. See section entitled "Neurologic Testing."
   Learning Outcome: 36-2
3. See section entitled "Neurologic Testing."
   Learning Outcome: 36-3
4. See section entitled "Neurologic Testing."
   Learning Outcome: 36-4
5. See section entitled "Increased Intracranial Pressure."
   Learning Outcome: 36-5
6. See section entitled "Nursing Care."
   Learning Outcome: 36-6
7. See section entitled "Cerebrovascular Disorders."
   Learning Outcome: 36-7
8. See section entitled "Seizure Disorders."
   Learning Outcome: 36-8
9. See section entitled "Infections of the Neurologic System."
   Learning Outcome: 36-9
10. See section entitled "Neurosensory Trauma and Tumors."
    Learning Outcome: 36-10
11. See section entitled "Neurosensory Trauma and Tumors."
    Learning Outcome: 36-11
12. See section entitled "Degenerative Neurologic Disorders."
    Learning Outcome: 36-12
13. See section entitled "Peripheral Nervous System Disorders" and "Cranial Nerve Disorders."
    Learning Outcome: 36-13
14. See section entitled "Disorders of Vision and Hearing."
    Learning Outcome: 36-14

Apply What You Learned

1. Meningitis is an inflammation of the meninges of the brain and spinal cord. The pia mater and arachnoid, the subarachnoid space, the ventricular system, and the cerebrospinal fluid (CSF) are infected. The CSF is thickened

with an exudate caused by neutrophils. The exudate may interfere with or obstruct CSF flow.

2. Three major organisms causing bacterial meningitis in children and adults are found in the nasopharynx; however, a predisposing factor, such as a prior upper respiratory infection, must be present before the bacteria become bloodborne. The three bacteria are:
   - Pneumococcal meningitis
   - *Haemophilus influenzae* meningitis
   - Meningococcal meningitis

3. The symptoms of meningitis are:
   - Headache
   - Fever
   - Nuchal rigidity (stiff neck)
   - Confusion
   - Irritability
   - Altered level of consciousness
   - Nausea and vomiting
   - Photophobia
   - Skin rash (with meningococcal meningitis)

   An early sign of meningeal irritation is a stiff neck. Active or passive flexion of the neck proves difficult and painful. Two additional signs of meningeal irritation are *Kernig's* and *Brudzinski's* signs. *Kernig's* sign is the inability to extend the leg when the hip is flexed at a 90-degree angle. In *Brudzinski's* sign, neck flexion causes the knees and hips to flex.

4. Treatment is based on the diagnosis, which is made after a complete history is taken. Specific treatment for the causative organism must be used. However, antibiotic treatment for infectious meningitis is started immediately to save the client's life and reduce complications. Some of the complications include sepsis, cranial nerve dysfunction, cerebral infarction, coma, and death. Residual effects of meningitis may be visual impairment, hearing loss or deafness, cranial nerve palsies, or paralysis.

5. Primary nursing considerations:
   - Elevate the head of the bed as ordered.
   - Instuct the client to avoid coughing or holding breath.
   - Monitor the level of consciousness and orientation.
   - Monitor the respiratory status and gag and swallowing reflexes.
   - Assess the location and severity of any discomfort.
   - Administer analgesics as ordered.
   - Keep the bed in a low position with side rails padded and raised.
   - Monitor intake and output.
   - Perform range-of-motion exercises as tolerated.
   - Maintain a quiet, calm environment.
   - Assist with hygiene as needed.
   - Provide skin care.
   - Provide emotional support.
   - Report any changes in the client's condition immediately.
   - Document all assessments, observations, interventions, and client responses.

Multiple Choice Questions

1. C

   Rationale: Amyotrophic lateral sclerosis (ALS), or Lou Gehrig's disease, is a rapidly progressive degenerative disease that causes progressive muscle weakness eventually affecting the respiratory muscles and leading to death usually within 2 to 5 years of diagnosis.

   Learning Outcome: 36-12

2. D

   Rationale: Myasthenia gravis is an autoimmune disease affecting the myelin coating of the nerve, leading to alterations in muscle function, mobility, and facial expressions. The other options do not match this clinical picture.

   Learning Outcome: 36-1

3. A

   Rationale: Trigeminal neuralgia is very painful and pain management is a primary focus when caring for clients with this disorder. Clients may not be able to eat and often require softer foods, so fluid, electrolyte, and nutrition should be monitored, but it is not the primary focus. Safety is always an important component of client care, but is not the primary focus for this client.

   Learning Outcome: 36-4

4. C

   Rationale: The client with Meniere's disease is unstable on their feet because their sense of balance is altered, so they are often placed on bed rest until the disease can be controlled to prevent falls.

   Learning Outcome: 36-4

5. A

   Rationale: Clients diagnosed with diabetes mellitus, especially those who do not have good control of their blood sugar, are at high risk for complications of the disease, including neuropathy, especially involving the lower extremities.

   Learning Outcome: 36-13

6. B

   Rationale: Migraines, especially severely painful migraines, can impact the client's quality of life to the point that some clients consider suicide to get relief from the pain. While other factors may be affected depending on the client, they are not the most commonly impacted factors.

   Learning Outcome: 36-3

7. C

   Rationale: Photophobia is defined as increased sensitivity to light and clients may find it difficult to be exposed to bright lights or sunshine.

   Learning Outcome: 36-3

8. B

   Rationale: The visual and auditory centers are located in the brainstem.

   Learning Outcome: 36-1

9. A

   Rationale: The dura mater is the outer layer of the brain. The middle layer is the arachnoid mater and the inner layer is the pia mater. Myelin is a coating over nerves that helps to speed impulse transmission.

   Learning Outcome: 36-1

10. A

Rationale: The cerebellum is responsible for muscle control and balance, so damage to this area would be manifested with lack of muscle control and difficulty with balance.

Learning Outcome: 36-1

11. B

Rationale: Following a myelogram, the client should sit with the head slightly elevated, approximately 16 to 30 degrees, for 12 hours following the test, at which time more normal positioning can be gradually assumed. This is done to avoid a severe headache following the test.

Learning Outcome: 36-2

12. C

Rationale: Level of consciousness is an important assessment to perform on all clients, but particularly during the neurological examination. While cranial nerve function may be necessary on some clients, it is not tested routinely on all neurological exams. Ability to understand and use language and reaction to sensory stimulation would be components of the test for level of consciousness.

Learning Outcome: 36-3

13. A

Rationale: Clients with a neurological deficit of any type from any cause are at risk for injury because the normal functioning of the neurological system is an important component of injury prevention.

Learning Outcome: 36-4

14. B

Rationale: Following a tonic-clonic seizure, clients will experience a postictal period when their level of consciousness is diminished and they are commonly very lethargic. During this phase, response to commands and level of consciousness will be diminished normally and will improve as they move beyond the postictal period. Only the pupil assessment will reveal any credible information.

Learning Outcome: 36-8

15. B

Rationale: The most important nursing priority is to keep the client free from injury and safe during the seizure. The seizure activity should be timed and the environment kept calm and quiet, but these are of lower priority than safety. Visitors need not be removed from the room unless they are a threat to a quiet environment.

Learning Outcome: 36-8. Name the types of seizures and describe nursing care for a client with seizures.

Matching

1. J	6. H	11. A	16. U	21. M	26. P
2. E	7. B	12. D	17. W	22. O	
3. K	8. C	13. T	18. X	23. Z	
4. I	9. F	14. R	19. N	24. Q	
5. G	10. L	15. V	20. Y	25. S	

Learning Outcomes

1. See section entitled "Structure and Function of the Gastrointestinal System."
   Learning Outcome: 37-1
2. See section entitled "Disorders of the Oral Cavity" and "Esophageal Disorders."
   Learning Outcome: 37-2
3. See section entitled "Stomach Disorders."
   Learning Outcome: 37-3
4. See section entitled "Upper GI Disorders"
   Learning Outcome: 37-4
5. See section entitled "Elimination Disorders."
   Learning Outcome: 37-5
6. See section entitled "Infectious or Inflammatory Disorders of the Intestines."
   Learning Outcome: 37-6
7. See section entitled "Structural Disorders."
   Learning Outcome: 37-7
8. See section entitled "Colorectal Cancer."
   Learning Outcome: 37-8
9. See section entitled "Accessory Organ Disorders."
   Learning Outcome: 37-9
10. See procedures at end of chapter.
    Learning Outcome: 37-10

Apply What You Learned

1. A bowel obstruction occurs when the intestinal contents are unable to flow normally along the intestinal tract due to some type of barrier. An obstruction can be partial or complete and can be found in any part of the intestine. A mechanical obstruction blocks intestinal flow. The most common reason is adhesions or scar tissue that can cause a kinking of the intestine. Other causes include strangulated hernia, tumors, fecal impaction, foreign bodies, volvulus, and intussusception. A functional or nonmechanical obstruction is found when the lumen remains open but peristalsis is absent. This is known as *paralytic ileus*. Gastrointestinal surgery, peritonitis, and narcotics can cause a functional obstruction.

2. Large bowel obstruction symptoms develop more slowly than small bowel obstruction symptoms. The colon traps gas and fecal material, resulting in abdominal distention; the intestinal loops may even be visible. The client complains of cramping abdominal pain. The bowel may empty for a short time to remove fecal contents distal to the obstruction. Fecal vomiting also occurs. Bowel sounds are absent in complete intestinal obstruction. If the condition is untreated, shock and death may result. When a bowel obstruction is complete, the client exhibits vomiting, abdominal pain, a distended abdomen, dehydration, and decreased blood pressure. X-rays of the abdomen confirm the obstruction, along with physical symptoms. Contrast medium such as barium may be used to enhance vision of the area.

3. The purpose of treatment is to relieve the obstruction.

4. A nasogastric tube may be inserted for gastric decompression. Stomach contents will be suctioned slowly through the tube and into a suction container.

5. When providing care for clients with structural disorders of the intestines, the primary nursing focus is on promoting bowel function and detecting lack of function. For clients with cancer of the lower gastrointestinal tract, the nursing focus is on providing physical and emotional support for the client during treatment.

6. *Pain* and *Anxiety* are two very important psychosocial nursing diagnoses for this client. The nurse must monitor pain and pain management by asking clients to rate their pain before and after pain medications are given. The nurse must evaluate the location and severity of the pain. Stress and anxiety can contribute to lower gastrointestinal disorders. Moreover, unmanaged pain increases stress and anxiety for the client.

7. Four specific nursing interventions:
   - Monitor and manage pain.
   - Inspect the abdomen and assess for distention, bowel sounds, or occult blood.
   - Assess for fluid volume deficit and monitor fluid replacement.
   - Provide emotional support and encourage the client to express feelings and to ask questions.

8. Purpose: A barium enema is used to diagnose colorectal cancer, inflammatory bowel disease, diverticulae, polyps, or lesions in the large bowel.

   Client Preparation: Because stool in the colon can obscure the clarity of the x-ray, laxatives and enemas until clear will usually be ordered. A low-residue diet may also be ordered 1 to 3 days prior to the test and clear liquids the day before the test. The client is NPO after midnight and until the procedure is completed. Barium sulfate is instilled by enema and retained while the x-ray is taken.

   Postdiagnostic Test Care: When the client returns from the test, the nurse should confirm that all testing has been completed. A routine laxative/cathartic is ordered because barium is very constipating. The client should be told to expect that stools will be light-colored for 24 to 48 hours as the barium is eliminated.

9. When preparing to administer an enema, the nurse must first explain to the client what is going to happen and why it is necessary. Encouraging the client to express concerns, ask questions, and share fears will assist the nurse to

provide emotional and physical support for the client. Because this procedure may cause embarrassment and discomfort, the nurse must provide privacy and appropriate draping for warmth and comfort. To minimize disruptions and undue additional stress, it is also paramount to have all necessary equipment and items ready prior to beginning. The nurse must assess the client often throughout the procedure and instill the liquid slowly to prevent cramping. Promoting client comfort during the procedure and following appropriate nursing procedure and facility policy is paramount.

Multiple Choice Questions

1. B
   Rationale: The projections within the small intestine that increase absorptive surface area are called villa.
   Learning Outcome: 37-1

2. C
   Rationale: The Valsalva maneuver is the action of straining to have a bowel movement accompanied by breath holding. It may be used to reduce heart rate due to vagal nerve stimulation during the activity.
   Learning Outcome: 37-5

3. D
   Rationale: Cathartics, or laxatives, are used to promote defecation.
   Learning Outcome: 37-5

4. A
   Rationale: As the bowel works harder to pass contents around an obstruction a high pitched sound is heard proximal (or above) the obstruction while bowel sounds are completely absent below and past the obstruction.
   Learning Outcome: 37-7

5. C
   Rationale: Colon cancer is often asymptomatic until adequate invasion occurs with one of the first symptoms being nonvisible, or occult, blood in the stool that can be found only through the use of guaiac testing kits or microscopic examination.
   Learning Outcome: 37-3

6. A
   Rationale: Pain relief is the initial priority nursing intervention. Dietary teaching can only occur once the client is comfortable enough to facilitate learning. Skin care and oral hygiene are generally not requirements of care unless the client has secondary problems.
   Learning Outcome: 37-9

7. D
   Rationale: Vitamin K plays an important role in blood clotting and is often deficient in clients diagnosed with cirrhosis of the liver.
   Learning Outcome: 37-9

8. B

   Rationale: A reduction in blood flow through the liver causes esophageal varices. Liver damage resulting from cirrhosis of the liver is one cause, but anything that reduces liver blood flow such as liver cancer or biliary atresia can have this result.

   Learning Outcome: 37-2

9. D

   Rationale: The liver is highly vascular so post-procedure it would be important to monitor for bleeding and apply pressure at the puncture site.

   Learning Outcome: 37-10

10. A

    Rationale: Ascites results in an increased abdominal girth. The remaining options would not alter abdominal girth in most instances and would not require daily measurements.

    Learning Outcome: 37-4

11. D

    Rationale: Inflammatory and infectious disorders often result in diarrhea so it would be important for the nurse to monitor for and treat crampy pain and diarrhea. Determining the cause of the inflammation and infection would be helpful in both treatment and reduction of reoccurrence. Electrolytes may become imbalanced due to loss of electrolytes in diarrhea.

    Learning Outcome: 37-6

12. D

    Rationale: GERD is most commonly diagnosed in Caucasians.

    Learning Outcome: 37-7

13. C

    Rationale: Clients should be instructed to eat more frequent, smaller meals to prevent over taxing the GI system following gastric surgery which will reduce the risk of dumping syndrome and loss of both nutrients and electrolytes. Increasing fluids will increase the risk of dumping by hyperextending the stomach. Clients should avoid lying down for 2–3 hours following meals. Foods high in carbohydrates are more easily metabolized and do not impact dumping syndrome as the client should eat well rounded meals.

    Learning Outcome: 37-10

14. A

    Rationale: Bowel function is improved with adequate intake of fluid and fiber (residue). A low residue diet would be incorrect as residue should be increased. While option 3 may be correct it would not contribute to improving bowel regularity. The foods in option 4 are flatus producing.

    Learning Outcome: 37-5

15. D

    Rationale: The stoma should be assessed and any complaint of discomfort, altered skin integrity, or edema should be reported.

    Learning Outcome: 37-8

Chapter 38 Clients with Endocrine System Disorders

Matching

1.	D	6.	B	11.	B	16.	D	21.	E
2.	C	7.	D	12.	F	17.	D	22.	B
3.	A	8.	A	13.	A	18.	F		
4.	E	9.	E	14.	E	19.	A		
5.	B	10.	C	15.	C	20.	C		

Learning Outcomes

1. See section entitled "Structure and Function of the Endocrine System."
   Learning Outcome: 38-1
2. See section entitled "Structure and Function of the Endocrine System."
   Learning Outcome: 38-2
3. See section entitled "Pituitary Disorders."
   Learning Outcome: 38-3
4. See sections entitled "Thyroid Disorders" and "Parathyroid Disorders."
   Learning Outcome: 38-4
5. See sections entitled "Thyroid Disorders" and "Parathyroid Disorders."
   Learning Outcome: 38-5
6. See section entitled "Diabetes Mellitus."
   Learning Outcome: 38-6
7. See section entitled "Diabetes Mellitus."
   Learning Outcome: 38-7
8. See section entitled "Diabetes Mellitus."
   Learning Outcome: 38-8
9. See section entitled "Adrenal Gland Disorders."
   Learning Outcome: 38-9

Apply What You Learned

1. Type 2 diabetes mellitus is also known as *non-insulin-dependent diabetes mellitus* (NIDDM). It affects 90% of the diabetic population and occurs more frequently in adults over 40. It develops more slowly than Type 1 diabetes mellitus, and heredity and obesity play a significant role. In Type 2 diabetes mellitus, the pancreas continues to make insulin but the body cells are affected by the increased weight and are unable to use the insulin. Symptoms may go undetected until a routine urinalysis reveals glucose in the urine. Type 2 diabetes mellitus is usually treated with oral hypoglycemics, although

insulin may also be required. Clients with a family history of diabetes are at higher risk for developing it.

2. The most common symptoms are known as the *three Ps:*

Polyuria—Excessive urination occurs as the body tries to eliminate the excess sugar in the blood.

Polydipsia—Excessive thirst occurs because the body is attempting to counteract the excessive loss of urine. Blood viscosity increases as the blood sugar level rises, so the body begins to draw fluid from the cells.

Polyphagia—Voracious hunger occurs as the body recognizes the need for energy and demands fuel. The person loses weight because the body is unable to utilize glucose for energy and starts to use the body's fat and protein stores. Hyperglycemia results from the lack of insulin production, and the person feels weak and lacks energy because of the ineffective glucose utilization.

3. Diabetes mellitus greatly increases the health risks in people with other disorders. Your client is an African American male with hypertension. The client's risk of stroke is two to four times higher than that of an adult without diabetes. Diabetes mellitus is the sixth leading cause of death among African Americans. It is not uncommon for these clients to view the disease as a death sentence. It will be important for the nurse to incorporate the client's preferences into his treatment plan to support compliance and promote healthy behaviors.

4. Diabetes is treated by balancing *diet, exercise,* and *medication.* The client with Type 2 diabetes is usually overweight, and losing weight becomes part of the treatment plan. Losing weight will lower the blood sugar, blood pressure, and cholesterol. It will also increase the sensitization of the insulin receptor sites, so the client will require less medication.

Diet—Diet management is the key to diabetic control. The dietitian is a vital member of the interdisciplinary team and works with the physician to determine an individualized diet plan for the client. Diets are based on creating a plan that allows the client to make modifications during times of exercise and illness.

The client may need to lose weight and will have caloric restriction. The timing of meals and snacks must coincide with medication action. The client is instructed to avoid skipping or delaying meals and snacks. A common diet seen in the clinical setting is an 1800-calorie American Diabetes Association diet.

Exercise—Exercise is the second important step in maintaining blood sugar control. For the Type 2 diabetic, exercise coupled with weight loss may be enough to control blood sugar levels. During exercise, body cells become more sensitive to insulin and glucose. The body then burns the sugar for energy and needs less insulin.

There are many benefits of exercise, including decreased blood pressure, decreased stress, and lowered heart rate. Clients with diabetes should discuss their exercise plan with their physician and be consistent in maintaining their exercise regimen.

Medication—The third cornerstone of diabetic control consists of two types of medication: insulin and oral hypoglycemics. Type 2 diabetics may need insulin during times of illness, increased stress, and trauma, but may return to the oral medications alone.

   Oral medications are not a form of insulin; instead, they stimulate the pancreas to produce insulin. Oral hypoglycemics also make the cell receptor sites more sensitive to the insulin produced. Most oral hypoglycemic medication is administered up to 30 minutes prior to a meal.

5. The LPN/LVN reinforces the dietary regimen and focuses education on helping the client and family make healthy food choices. The client needs to know that being diabetic does not mean he has to give up all the foods he likes, but he must pay attention to the foods he chooses to eat.

   Moreover, the LPN/LVN must ensure that the client understands the importance of maintaining an exercise routine and reinforces its benefits in controlling diabetes. Medication teaching is a critical nursing action that helps the client to understand what medication he or she is taking and why, its action, and its side effects or adverse reactions. If a client understands the need for the medication, he or she is more likely to take it as ordered.

Multiple Choice Questions

1. A

   Rationale: Luteinizing hormone is a tropic hormone secreted by the anterior pituitary. Insulin is secreted by the pancreas. Thymosin is secreted by the thyroid. Cortisol is treated by the anterior pituitary gland.
   Learning Outcome: 38-3

2. C

   Rationale: Melanin is secreted by the pineal gland.
   Learning Outcome: 38-2

3. B

   Rationale: Insulin is secreted by beta cells of the pancreas.
   Learning Outcome: 38-6

4. D

   Rationale: Diabetes insipidus is caused by a lack of ADH from the pituitary gland and is related to control of water and sodium, not sugar metabolism as in diabetes mellitus.
   Learning Outcome: 38-3

5. B

   Rationale: Primary hyperthyroidism is caused by an oversecretion of T_3 and T_4.
   Learning Outcome: 38-4

6. A

   Rationale: Hypocalcemia results in irritation of the muscles causing continuous muscle spasms and tremors because calcium is an important component to muscle contractility.
   Learning Outcome: 38-5

7. A

Rationale: Insulin is required for the cells to utilize glucose in the serum.

Learning Outcome: 38-6

8. B

Rationale: Peak time refers to the time when the medication is most effective or at its peak of activity.

Learning Outcome: 38-7

9. A

Rationale: Oral hypoglycemic agents should be administered 30 minutes before a meal so it begins to act at approximately the same time glucose from the meal begins to enter the bloodstream.

Learning Outcome: 38-6

10. A

Rationale: This client is displaying signs and symptoms of hypoglycemia which can only be confirmed by checking the serum blood sugar. A snack will be provided if hypoglycemia is confirmed.

Learning Outcome: 38-8

11. B

Rationale: Myxedema results from hyperthyroidism with hair loss as a common symptom.

Learning Outcome: 38-5

12. A

Rationale: While there are higher than necessary levels of calcium in the bloodstream (hypercalcemia), the increased secretion of parathormone results in inadequate uptake of calcium in the bones making them more fragile and subject to pathological fractures. The kidneys try to remove calcium from the blood stream to reduce the excessively high levels resulting in increased risk for calcium based calculi.

Learning Outcome: 38-5

13. C

Rationale: A profound effect of pheochromocytoma is elevation of blood pressure, often to extremely high levels so monitoring blood pressure is a priority nursing action.

Learning Outcome: 38-9

14. A

Rationale: Lack of corticosteroids results in Addison's disease which is one reason why it is important to teach clients taking corticosteroids like Prednisone to never discontinue them suddenly.

Learning Outcome: 38-9

15. C

Rationale: Cushing's disease often manifests with elevated serum glucose levels and resulting fatty tissue deposits.

Learning Outcome: 38-9

Matching

1. B	6. C	11. A	16. G	21. A	26. E
2. E	7. D	12. C	17. C	22. F	
3. F	8. E	13. F	18. D	23. G	
4. A	9. F	14. A	19. B	24. D	
5. D	10. B	15. E	20. C	25. B	

Learning Outcomes

1. See sections entitled "Structure and Function of the Urinary System" and "Factors Affecting Urinary Function."
   Learning Outcome: 39-1
2. See section entitled "Urine Characteristics."
   Learning Outcome: 39-2
3. See section entitled "Altered Urinary Elimination."
   Learning Outcome: 39-3
4. See section entitled "Basic Skills for Urinary Care."
   Learning Outcome: 39-4
5. See section entitled "Basic Skills for Urinary Care."
   Learning Outcome: 39-5
6. See section entitled "Kidney Disorders."
   Learning Outcome: 39-6
7. See section entitled "Renal Failure."
   Learning Outcome: 39-7
8. See section entitled "Ureteral, Bladder, And Urethral Disorders."
   Learning Outcome: 39-8

Apply What You Learned

1. In the older adult, an estimated 30% of nephrons are lost by age 80. Renal blood flow decreases because of vascular changes and a decrease in cardiac output. The ability to concentrate urine declines. Bladder muscle tone diminishes, causing increased frequency of urination and nocturia (awakening to urinate at night). Diminished bladder muscle tone and contractibility may lead to residual urine in the bladder after voiding, increasing the risk of bacterial growth and infection. Urinary incontinence may occur due to mobility problems or neurologic impairments. Urinary incontinence is *not* a normal part of aging, however.
2. Possible factors which may contribute to incontinence:
   - Bladder inflammation or other disease
   - Infection
   - Difficulties in independent toileting (mobility impairment)
   - Leakage when coughing, laughing, or sneezing
   - Cognitive impairment

3. Normal urine should be straw or light amber in color and transparent, with a faint aromatic odor. It should not be dark amber, cloudy, or thick, or have an offensive odor.

4. The client should drink at least six to eight 8-ounce glasses of water or fluid of choice per day. Careful perineal care should be provided after each episode of incontinence or defecation. Cleansing of the perineum must proceed from the cleanest area (meatus) to the most soiled area (anus) in order to prevent spreading of fecal material toward the urinary meatus. Providing foods or juices high in vitamin C will help to acidify the urine, decreasing the risk of bacterial growth.

5. Clients with incontinence or the inability to control elimination become much more susceptible to skin breakdown. Skin that is continually moist becomes macerated, or softened, by soaking in the urine. Urine that accumulates on the skin converts to ammonia, irritates skin further, and causes an offensive odor. The incontinent person requires meticulous skin care. Mild soap and water are used; the skin is dried gently but thoroughly; and clean, dry clothing or bed linen is provided. If the skin is irritated, the nurse may apply a barrier cream. The use of bed pads will help to absorb wetness and leaves a dry surface for contact with the skin.

6. Three appropriate nursing diagnoses are:
   - Altered urinary elimination
   - Risk for infection
   - Risk for impaired skin integrity

7. Nursing interventions/actions necessary for this client:
   - Develop and initiate a bladder training program.
   - Toilet regularly before and after meals and every 2 hours.
   - Cleanse skin thoroughly but gently after each incident of incontinence.
   - Cleanse the perineum from front to back.
   - Replace soiled clothing and bedding with clean, dry items.
   - Offer fluids such as water, orange juice, or cranberry juice every 15 minutes.
   - Monitor fluid intake.
   - Be respectful.
   - Provide privacy.
   - Maintain dignity.

Multiple Choice Questions

1. B

   Rationale: The bladder generally signals a need to void when 300 to 500 mL of urine stretch the bladder and trigger the stretch receptors. All other answers are incorrect.

   Learning Outcome: 39-1

2. A

   Rationale: Only sodium is an inorganic solute. Creatinine, ammonia, and uric acid are organic solutes.

   Learning Outcome: 39-2

3. C

Rationale: Normal intake is 1000 to 1500 mL so increasing fluid intake to 2000 to 3000 mL is required to reduce the risk of UTI or urinary calculi.

Learning Outcome: 39-3

4. B

Rationale: Normal urine pH is approximately 6.0 to 6.5

Learning Outcome: 39-4

5. B

Rationale: Ketone bodies are found in the urine when inadequate carbohydrates are consumed resulting in the breakdown of protein with byproducts of this catabolism found in the urine. Protein would be more likely found in urine if the client has kidney damage. A normal urinalysis does not include ketones and ketones are not normally found in the urine of pregnant women unless their carbohydrate intake is inadequate for energy production.

Learning Outcome: 39-5

6. A

Rationale: Pain in the flank is a common symptom as cysts grow on and around the kidney creating pressure. Pain on urination is a symptom of a urinary tract infection, reduced urine output indicates kidney damage, as does fluid and sodium retention.

Learning Outcome: 39-6

7. A

Rationale: Nephrosclerosis is a potential side effect of autoimmune damage to the kidney.

Learning Outcome: 39-7

8. A

Rationale: In order to prevent damage to the AV fistula it is important to avoid taking blood pressure readings in the involved arm. The other interventions may be indicated but are not the priority intervention.

Learning Outcome: 39-7

9. C

Rationale: Priority care requires assessment of the stoma and surrounding skin to prevent alterations in skin integrity. The other interventions would not be of greater importance when caring for this client as compared to any other client.

Learning Outcome: 39-8

10. A

Rationale: Escherichia coli are responsible for most urinary tract infections as pathogens are swept from the anus toward to the urethra, often secondary to improper wiping. While other bacteria can cause a UTI, they are not the most common agent.

Learning Outcome: 39-8

11. B

Rationale: Cholinergic medications are administered to stimulate improved bladder contraction for clients with urinary retention.

Learning Outcome: 39-8

12. D

Rationale: All of these strategies will help to reduce the risk of UTIs.

Learning Outcome: 39-8

13. D

Rationale: Bleeding should diminish and the urine should progress from bright red to pink to eventually a normal color over the first 24 to 48 hours following surgery.

Learning Outcome: 39-8

14. D

Rationale: A professional and sensitive approach by the nurse will reduce the client's discomfort and the nurse should avoid making embarrassing comments.

Learning Outcome: 39-8

15. D

Rationale: Bladder training can be highly effective and would be the first approach to reducing urinary incontinence. Intake of fluid would not be indicated and has the potential to be dangerous, resulting in dehydration. Adult diapers are often bulky and are not the first strategy to employ. Catheters increase the risk of urinary tract infection and are not recommended as treatment for incontinence.

Learning Outcome: 39-3

Chapter 40 Clients with Reproductive System Disorders

Matching

1. E	6. C	11. C	16. C	21. D
2. D	7. D	12. E	17. A	22. C
3. A	8. A	13. B	18. E	23. B
4. B	9. B	14. D	19. F	24. A
5. F	10. F	15. F	20. E	

Learning Outcomes

1. See section entitled "Reproductive Structure and Function."
   Learning Outcome: 40-1
2. See section entitled "Obtaining A Comprehensive Sexual History."
   Learning Outcome: 40-2
3. See section entitled "Female Reproductive Health Issues."
   Learning Outcome: 40-3
4. See section entitled "Breast Disorders."
   Learning Outcome: 40-4
5. See sections entitled "Uterine Disorders" and "Menopause."
   Learning Outcome: 40-5
6. See section entitled "Tumors and Ectopic Disorders."
   Learning Outcome: 40-6
7. See section entitled "Female Reproductive Health Issues."
   Learning Outcome: 40-7
8. See section entitled "Male Reproductive Health Issues."
   Learning Outcome: 40-8
9. See section entitled "Family Planning Issues."
   Learning Outcome: 40-9

10. See section entitled "Contraception."
    Learning Outcome: 40-10
11. See section entitled "Infertility Issues."
    Learning Outcome: 40-11

Apply What You Learned

Invasive carcinoma—condition in which cancer cells have spread to the surrounding tissues

Peau d'orange—dimpled skin condition seen in breast cancer

Nipple retraction—inversion of the nipple

Breast-conserving surgery—removing the tumor, surrounding tissue, and several lymph nodes; may be followed by radiation treatments

1. Decisional conflict: Treatment options
2. Discuss the disease process and options. Provide an opportunity for the client to ask questions. Make eye contact if culturally acceptable. Answer questions simply and honestly.
3. Reinforce preoperative teaching and routine postoperative care, including pain control, wound care, activity restrictions, diet, special equipment, such as a JP drain, and IV fluids.
4. Nurse's notes should contain all of your teaching points to include the client's acknowledgment of understanding and any questions that might arise during the session.

Multiple Choice Questions

1. C
   Rationale: The endometrium is an internal structure. It is the inner lining of the uterus. The remaining options are visible externally.
   Learning Outcome: 40-1
2. A, C, D
   Rationale: A nonjudgmental and nonthreatening environment along with respecting client privacy is essential to developing a relationship that fosters discussion of highly personal matters. It is important to consider the cultural needs of clients from other ethnicities because it may impact their willingness to share personal information.
   Learning Outcome: 40-2
3. A
   Rationale: Sexually transmitted infections and infections of the reproductive system can often be prevented by client teaching. Tumors, structural changes, and blockages are unlikely to be impacted by nursing interventions.
   Learning Outcome: 40-3
4. D
   Rationale: Chocolate and caffeine have been found to increase the occurrence of fibrotic lumps in the breast.
   Learning Outcome: 40-4

5. B

   Rationale: Excessive exercise can lead to amenorrhea. Menstruation will usually return when exercise is decreased.

   Learning Outcome: 40-5

6. C

   Rationale: The human papilloma virus (HPV) has been highly associated with cervical cancers.

   Learning Outcome: 40-6

7. A, D

   Rationale: Microscopic slides are used to collect specimens from the vagina and a large paper bag is used to collect all clothing worn by the rape victim, and all are sent to the lab to examine for microscopic evidence.

   Learning Outcome: 40-7

8. C

   Rationale: Alprostadil (prostaglandin E) is a medication, usually supplied as a urethral suppository, to treat erectile dysfunction.

   Learning Outcome: 40-8

9. D

   Rationale: The intrauterine device is more effective than a diaphragm, vaginal sponge or female condom. Effectiveness of a diaphragm or vaginal sponge is increased if used in conjunction with a spermicidal jelly.

   Learning Outcome: 40-10

10. C

    Rationale: 20% of infertility issues are shared with both the male and the female and require a shared approach to improve conception.

    Learning Outcome: 40-11

Chapter 41 Clients with Sexually Transmitted Infections

Matching

1. C	6. C
2. E	7. D
3. D	8. B
4. A	9. A
5. B	

Learning Outcomes

1. See section entitled "Prevention."

   Learning Outcome: 41-1

2. See section entitled "Prevention."

   Learning Outcome: 41-2

3. See section entitled "Diagnostic Tests for STIs."

   Learning Outcome: 41-3

4. See section entitled "Diagnostic Tests for STIs"
   Learning Outcome: 41-4
5. See section entitled "Nursing Care."
   Learning Outcome: 41-5
6. See section entitled "Nursing Care."
   Learning Outcome: 41-6

Apply What You Learned

1. Explanation focusing on transmission and treatment of HIV:
   - **Transmission:** Transmission of sexually transmitted diseases occurs when clients come in contact with infected body fluids or lesions. This transmission is likely to occur during unprotected oral, genital, or anal sexual contact. Heterosexual *and* homosexual male *and* female partners are *all* at risk of transmitting and contracting these infections.
   - **Treatment:** Currently, treatment for HIV and AIDS focuses on suppression of the virus and correction of the various diseases afflicting the client. New medications are being developed that do not cure the illness, but reduce symptomatology and support optimal functioning.
2. Pathophysiology of HIV and AIDS:
   - AIDS is a relatively new disease. It was not identified as a separate disorder until 1981. A short 2 years later, the retrovirus HIV was identified as the causative agent. Following exposure to infected body fluids, the antibody response occurs within 6 weeks to 6 months. During this period the client is typically asymptomatic. Development of AIDS may not occur for up to 10 years. Clinical manifestations vary but are generally neurologic and/or related to immunosuppression.
3. Four discharge considerations:
   - Ensure that the client understands the need to inform all sexual partners to prevent future transmission and avoid complications.
   - Ensure that the client understands the need to use latex condoms for sexual activity, and educate on proper use and disposal, including hand washing.
   - Explain to the client the importance of health care behaviors which will reduce the risk of transmission of sexually transmitted diseases: urinating and bathing following intercourse, abstinence or monogamy, and avoiding the abuse of intravenous drugs or sexual relations with those who engage in this practice.
   - Encourage the client to regularly contact the healthcare clinic and/or provider for ongoing evaluation and support.

Multiple Choice Questions

1. B
   Rationale: Only diagnoses of gonorrhea neisseria must be reported according to CDC guidelines.
   Learning Outcome: 41-5

2. C

   Rationale: While it is not uncommon for there to be no symptoms presented, if symptoms of secondary syphilis are presented they will be seen 6 weeks after appearance of initial chancre and the client will report flu-like symptoms.

   Learning Outcome: 41-4

3. C

   Rationale: Jarisch-Herxheimer reaction is characterized by fever, headache, myalgia, and significant chancre changes such as edema and bright coloring secondary to the rapid destruction of spirochetes during treatment with penicillin.

   Learning Outcome: 41-5

4. C

   Rationale: Dysuria, urinary frequency, and pelvic pain are often experienced by women after contact with *chlamydia trachomatis*.

   Learning Outcome: 41-4

5. A

   Rationale: *Candida albicans* is a common cause of yeast or fungal type infections.

   Learning Outcome: 41-4

6. D

   Rationale: Once contracted, herpes genitalis cannot be cured and must be managed in order to reduce exacerbations.

   Learning Outcome: 41-6

7. D

   Rationale: Improved antiretroviral medications have prolonged the time from HIV infection to conversion to AIDS to as long as 10 years or more.

   Learning Outcome: 41-4

8. B

   Rationale: A frequent first early symptom following exposure to gonorrhea is urethritis or inflammation of the urethra.

   Learning Outcome: 41-2

9. D

   Rationale: Frothy foul smelling vaginal discharge, pruritus, and lower abdominal pain are associated with trichomoniasis infection.

   Learning Outcome: 41-4

10. B

    Rationale: A gram stain is required to diagnose gonorrhea.

    Learning Outcome: 41-3

11. A

    Rationale: Acyclovir is an effective medication used for the treatment of herpes, but it is important to begin treatment as soon as the outbreak begins.

    Learning Outcome: 41-4

12. D

    Rationale: Metronidazole (Flagyl) is used to treat trichomoniasis.

    Learning Outcome: 41-4

13. C

   Rationale: Cryotherapy is used to freeze and remove warts resulting from human papillomavirus.

   Learning Outcome: 41-4

14. D

   Rationale: This client requires more information about the transmission of STIs as well as strategies for reducing the risk associated with unprotected sexual encounters.

   Learning Outcome: 41-5

15. D

   Rationale: Transmission, treatment, and length of time abstinence is recommended to allow time for recovery are all important factors to be included in the teaching plan.

   Learning Outcome: 41-6

Chapter 42 Health Promotion of Older Adults

Matching

1. B		5. C		9. F	
2. D		6. C		10. B	
3. E		7. D		11. E	
4. A		8. A			

Learning Outcomes

1. See section entitled "Gerontology."
   Learning Outcome: 42-1
2. See section entitled "Factors that Affect the Aging Process."
   Learning Outcome: 42-2
3. See sections entitled "Physiologic Changes of Older Adults" and "Sensory Changes in Older Adults."
   Learning Outcome: 42-3
4. See section entitled "Continence Training."
   Learning Outcome: 42-4
5. See section entitled "Psychosocial Changes and Adaptations."
   Learning Outcome: 42-5
6. See section entitled "Special Health Concerns of Older Adults."
   Learning Outcome: 42-6
7. See section entitled "Safety Issues for Older Adults."
   Learning Outcome: 42-7
8. See section entitled "Caregiver Stress."
   Learning Outcome: 42-8

Apply What You Learned

1. Culture influences the way we view aging, as well as our views about wellness and illness. Older adults may continue to follow their native health practices to prevent illness. They may use prayer, light candles, or wear an amulet. The nurse should find ways to reinforce clients' views as they teach and promote other methods of health maintenance and health promotion. It is important for the nurse to address these issues in a nonjudgmental manner, and recognize that many cultural practices and folk remedies actually work.

2. Both visual and hearing deficits may be present.

   Visual Considerations—The eyes incur many functional and structural changes with aging. The eyelids sag as they lose elasticity and thickness. Older adults often complain of dry, itchy, or burning eyes due to decreased tear production. The over-fifty population commonly experiences presbyopia. Members of this age group often hold reading materials at arm's length. Printed materials should be readable using a large font and contrasting color.

   Hearing Considerations—The tympanic membranes in the ear become thinner, as do other body tissues. The muscles that support the tympanic membrane show atrophic changes related to the aging process. The older adult's hearing becomes altered. This condition is called *presbycusis*. It affects an estimated 13% of persons over the age of 65, with men affected more than women. Do not shout, but instead speak clearly and slowly, enunciating the words carefully.

3. Three key points applicable to a diverse group of aging adults are:
   - Health conditions refer to the way a person has taken care of his or her body.
   - There are certain predictable changes that occur as the human body ages.
   - Most body systems are less efficient in the older adult due to the effects of aging.

Multiple Choice Questions

1. D
   Rationale: The psychosocial stage faced by older adults is ego integrity versus despair, when they review their life and determine if they have met their goals. Trust versus mistrust occurs in infancy, generativity versus stagnation occurs in middle aged adults, and role identify vs role confusion occurs in adolescence.
   Learning Outcome: 42-5

2. A
   Rationale: Only slowed immune response is a normal change that occurs with aging. All of the other options would be abnormal and represents a form of pathophysiology requiring intervention.
   Learning Outcome: 42-3

3. A

Rationale: Intermittent claudication is caused by insufficient blood supply to the tissues caused by arterial occlusive diseases. Coronary artery disease may promote arterial occlusive disorders but is not the direct cause of intermittent claudication. Varicose veins and venous stasis do not play a role in intermittent claudication.

Learning Outcome: 42-6

4. B

Rationale: Insulin resistance and reduced production of insulin increase the older adult's risk of diabetes mellitus. The other options are not common age-related problems in the older adult.

Learning Outcome: 42-6

5. B

Rationale: As the pH in the vaginal mucosa changes it allows for a more yeast accommodating environment that increases risk of yeast infection. The other options do not contribute to yeast infections.

Learning Outcome: 42-3

6. D

Rationale: Older adults are at increased risk for heat stroke or heat exhaustion because they have fewer and less active sweat glands so they perspire less, an important component to thermoregulation. As a result, they have fewer mechanisms to reduce internal temperature in hot weather. The other options are not true.

Learning Outcome: 42-6

7. B

Rationale: Older adults are more likely to have graying or white hair because of the loss of pigment cells in their hair bulbs. The other options are not true.

Learning Outcome: 42-3

8. B

Rationale: It is normal for older adults to lose muscle tone and flexibility, although participation in safe exercise programs can help to diminish this effect somewhat. The other options are indications of abnormal findings and indicate pathophysiology.

Learning Outcome: 42-3

9. A

Rationale: Sensation declines with age so the older adult is at increased risk of burns. The best instructions provided to the unlicensed assistive personnel is to test bathwater to avoid burns.

Learning Outcome: 42-7

10. D

Rationale: Older adults often report being cold because the body's temperature regulating mechanism decreases with age and the older adult's ability to adapt to changes in environmental temperature decreases as a result.

Learning Outcome: 42-7

11. C

Rationale: Kegal exercises are referred to as pelvic muscle exercises and can also help reduce episodes of incontinence.

Learning Outcome: 42-7

Chapter 43 Nursing Care of Ill Older Adults

Matching

1.	C	5.	A	9.	E
2.	D	6.	B	10.	A
3.	E	7.	C	11.	B
4.	F	8.	D		

Learning Outcomes

1. See section entitled "Role of LPNs/LVNs."
   Learning Outcome: 43-1
2. See section entitled "Abnormal Changes in Older Adults."
   Learning Outcome: 43-2
3. See section entitled "Special Concerns of the Hospitalized Older Adult."
   Learning Outcome: 43-3
4. See section entitled "Special Concerns of the Hospitalized Older Adult."
   Learning Outcome: 43-4

Apply What You Learned

Aging—Progressive changes related to the passage of time

Physical—Concerning or pertaining to the body

Psychosocial—Related to both psychologic and social factors

Behaviors—The actions or reactions of an individual under specific circumstances

Lifestyles—Pattern of living and behavior of an individual, society, or culture

1. Arthritis, hypertension, hearing and vision impairments, cardiovascular diseases, cataracts, sinusitis, orthopedic disorders, diabetes, and Alzheimer's disease.
2. Answers will vary.
3. Early detection of diseases, immunizations, injury prevention, self-management techniques. People who are physically active, eat a healthy diet, do not use tobacco, and practice other healthy behaviors reduce their risk for chronic illnesses and have half the rate of disability as those who do not.

Multiple Choice Questions

1. A, D, E
   Rationale: When caring for the older adult, it is important to balance the need for autonomy in the client with the time constraints of the nurse. Additional time may be required and the nurse will need to be patient.
   Learning Outcome: 43-1

2. C

   Rationale: Rosacea can cause swelling and enlargement of the nose, and may also cause conjunctivitis due to alterations in the chemical composition of the tears.

   Learning Outcome: 43-2

3. A

   Rationale: Gout is a form of arthritis caused by accumulation of uric acid crystals initially found in the big toe in most cases.

   Learning Outcome: 43-2

4. B

   Rationale: The older adult is at greater risk for pressure ulcers, and the nurse must provide care to reduce risks including careful transfers to prevent shearing.

   Learning Outcome: 43-3

5. D

   Rationale: Because many systems are involved (nausea – GI system, jaundice – liver, confusion – neurological system, elimination – kidney) polypharmacy would be the first consideration versus a problem with one specific system.

   Learning Outcome: 43-4

6. A

   Rationale: Alzheimer's disease has been associated with alterations in neurotransmitters, specifically norepinephrine and dopamine.

   Learning Outcome: 43-2

7. D

   Rationale: Cardiomegaly is enlargement of the heart, specifically the left ventricle, which must work harder and hypertrophies as a result.

   Learning Outcome: 43-2

8. C

   Rationale: Diplopia is associated with the eyes and is defined as double vision.

   Learning Outcome: 43-2

9. A

   Rationale: Dementia can occur at any age, although it is most commonly seen in older adults, and can result from drug overdosage, withdrawal, or polypharmacy.

   Learning Outcome: 43-2

10. C

    Rationale: Varicose veins may occur due to increased pressure caused by adequate arterial supply and reduced venous return secondary to inactivity of the muscles in the leg, which normally contract to promote blood return to the heart.

    Learning Outcome: 43-2

Matching

1.	B	5.	D	9.	A
2.	F	6.	C	10.	F
3.	A	7.	C	11.	B
4.	E	8.	D	12.	E

Learning Outcomes

1. See section entitled "Chronic Illness."
   Learning Outcome: 44-1
2. See sections entitled "Factors Associated with Chronic Illness" and "Prevention of Chronic Illness."
   Learning Outcome: 44-2
3. See section entitled "LPN/LVN Role in Care of Clients with Chronic Illness."
   Learning Outcome: 44-3
4. See section entitled "Terminal Illness."
   Learning Outcome: 44-4
5. See section entitled "LPN/LVN Role in Care of Clients with Terminal Illness."
   Learning Outcome: 44-5
6. See section entitled "Nursing Care."
   Learning Outcome: 44-6
7. See section entitled "Nursing Care."
   Learning Outcome: 44-7
8. See section entitled "Definitions and Signs of Death."
   Learning Outcome: 44-8
9. See section entitled "Legal Issues in Terminal Illness."
   Learning Outcome: 44-9
10. See section entitled "Definitions and Signs of Death."
    Learning Outcome: 44-10
11. See section entitled "Definitions and Signs of Death."
    Learning Outcome: 44-11
12. See section entitled "Care After Death."
    Learning Outcome: 44-12

Apply What You Learned

Suggested Answers

1. Signs of impending death can be found in Box 44-4 on page 1230 in your textbook.
2. It would be important to point out the signs you noted and inform Mrs. Montgomery that you believe her husband will be gone soon. This allows her to make the decision about whether or not she wants to go to the cafeteria. She may feel extremely guilty or bad if she is not with him when he dies.

3. The nurse should prepare a cot for Mrs. Montgomery and make her as comfortable as possible. The nurse may also ask her if she would like anyone called to keep her company.

Multiple Choice Questions

1. A, B, D
   Rationale: Age, culture, and genetics are all factors associated with chronic illness. Pain tolerance and education may impact how they cope with chronic illness, but are not associated with the development of chronic illness.
   Learning Outcome: 44-1

2. C
   Rationale: The client can adjust their lifestyle by making healthier choices to reduce the risk of chronic illness. Race and culture are not changeable, while increased income may not prevent the risk.
   Learning Outcome: 44-2

3. B
   Rationale: The nurse can best help the client by encouraging independence and providing only the assistance the client requires. Not every chronically ill client has decubitus ulcers.
   Learning Outcome: 44-3

4. D
   Rationale: With palliative care, interventions are provided to maintain the client's comfort and diagnostic, and other invasive procedures are not performed.
   Learning Outcome: 44-4

5. A
   Rationale: The goal of care for the client with a terminal illness is to meet as many needs and expectations as possible and provide a source of support for expression of fears and concerns. Clients may prefer to be alone with their families and avoid social situations. Flexibility may be required regarding visitation rules. The nurse can provide updates on client status.
   Learning Outcome: 44-5

6. B
   Rationale: The client's mentation will frequently change and they may become agitated, confused, or restless, or their level of consciousness may change. Reduced appetite, urine output, and temperature is anticipated.
   Learning Outcome: 44-6

7. A
   Rationale: The priority when caring for the dying client and their families is to meet their emotional needs, and help them to recognize and understand the significance of their loved one's changes in condition. Families should be allowed to respond as they see fit, the client should be positioned for comfort, and the expectation of decreased renal function is anticipated.
   Learning Outcome: 44-7

8. D
   Rationale: As cardiac output decreases, the client's pulse is anticipated to become weak and thready and may increase or decrease.
   Learning Outcome: 44-8

9. C

Rationale: The "comfort measures only" order indicates only palliative care is to be administered. DNRs indicate the client is not to be resuscitated but does not rule out restorative care while the client is alive. A living will discusses the client's preferences, but does not indicate only palliative care is to be delivered when it is written. Durable power of attorney directs who is to make decisions for the client if they are unable to make decisions for themselves.

Learning Outcome: 44-9

10. D

Rationale: If there is an absence of electrical current from the brain, the client is brain dead. Total lack of response indicates the client has an altered level of consciousness, but can indicate the client is in a coma without being brain dead. Destruction of the spinal cord creates paralysis, but doesn't indicate death. Lack of reflexes is not an indicator of death.

Learning Outcome: 44-10

Chapter 45 Caring for Clients with Cancer

Matching

1. D	1. D
2. E	2. A
3. B	3. E
4. C	4. C
5. A	5. B

Learning Outcomes

1. See chapter introduction.
   Learning Outcome: 45-1
2. See section entitled "Normal Cells versus Cancer Cells."
   Learning Outcome: 45-2
3. See section entitled "Cancer Prevention and Cancer Screening."
   Learning Outcome: 45-3
4. See section entitled "Factors Affecting Choice of Diagnostic Evaluation."
   Learning Outcome: 45-4
5. See section entitled "Nursing Implications in Diagnostic Evaluation."
   Learning Outcome: 45-5
6. See section entitled "Diagnostic Tests."
   Learning Outcome: 45-6
7. See section entitled "Treatment Planning."
   Learning Outcome: 45-7
8. See section entitled "Nursing Care."
   Learning Outcome: 45-8
9. See section entitled "Cancer Care for Special Populations."
   Learning Outcome: 45-9

Suggested Answers

The priority of care is to prevent complications by padding Matthew's crib in case he has another seizure and create a safe environment for him. Other priorities include providing support for his parents, and offering to phone family or friends, calling for their spiritual support person if desired, and encouraging them to share their thoughts and feelings.

Because Matthew's cancer is in the brain, chemotherapy will not cross the blood-brain barrier unless it is administered intrathecally. Children cannot have their brains irradiated; it causes significant damage because their brains are growing rapidly. The option of minimally invasive surgery or genetic therapy may be considered depending on where they live, because these options are generally only available in major centers.

Multiple Choice Questions

1. D
    Rationale: One of the reasons why cancer cells are so dangerous is the speed and continuity with which they grow. Unlike normal cells, cancer grows faster and never enters the resting phase in the cell cycle.
    Learning Outcome: 45-2
2. C
    Rationale: The genes in cancer cells are called oncogenes.
    Learning Outcome: 45-1
3. D
    Rationale: Thirty minutes of physical activity everyday helps to prevent cancer. Unprotected sex increases the risk of cancer, specifically HPV. Sunscreen should have a minimum SPF of at least 15.
    Learning Outcome: 45-3
4. A, B, D, E
    Rationale: All of these play a role in the client's choice of evaluation except those clients with a goal of palliative treatment who would most likely not choose any evaluation method.
    Learning Outcome: 45-4
5. B, D, E
    Rationale: Although concerns about getting too close to the client may lead to distancing, these certainly would not be the nurse's priorities of care for the client with cancer. However, exploring the needs of the family and providing proper referrals will be important, as will acting as a source of comfort for the client.
    Learning Outcome: 45-5
6. A
    Rationale: Duke's staging system is most often used to stage colorectal cancer.
    Learning Outcome: 45-6

7. A, B, D, E

   Rationale: The client's mental status will not factor into the decision regarding the appropriateness of surgical intervention to treat cancer.

   Learning Outcome: 45-7

8. A

   Rationale: A realistic goal is that the client will remain infection free until his immune system returns to normal function, which will likely take several weeks after the end of chemotherapy. The client should not eliminate activity, although he may not feel like being as active as he was before. He does not need to limit social activities, but should use care to avoid infected people.

   Learning Outcome: 45-8

9. A, C

   Rationale: Nutrition and family support play an important role in the client's recovery. Because cancer cells grow quickly, they consume a large amount of nutrients, so the client must increase the amount of calories and nutrients taken in to maintain a stable weight. Family support reduces the client's stress and anxiety, helping them to use their energy to fight the disease. The type of treatment will depend on the client, the location, and the type of cancer.

   Learning Outcome: 45-9

10. B, D

    Rationale: Radiation can cause temporary or permanent alterations in taste and fibrosis of lung tissue, depending on the area being irradiated. Hair loss is more likely than hair growth. Susceptibility to infection is more likely with chemotherapy, and there is no impact on blood coagulation.

    Learning Outcome: 45-7

Chapter 46 Long-Term Care and Rehabilitation Nursing

Matching

1.	E	6.	D
2.	F	7.	A
3.	G	8.	C
4.	B		
5.	H		

Learning Outcomes

1. See section entitled "Levels of Care."
   Learning Outcome: 46-1
2. See section entitled "Roles of the LPN/LVN in Long-Term Care Nursing."
   Learning Outcome: 46-2
3. See section entitled "Roles of the LPN/LVN in Long-Term Care Nursing."
   Learning Outcome: 46-3
4. See section entitled "Onsite Healthcare Team."
   Learning Outcome: 46-4

5. See sections entitled "Specialized Needs of Younger Clients in Long-Term Care" and "Rehabilitation Nursing"
   Learning Outcome: 46-5
6. See section entitled "Rehabilitation Nursing."
   Learning Outcome: 46-6
7. See section entitled "Legal and Ethical Concerns in Long-Term Care."
   Learning Outcome: 46-7
8. See section entitled "Reimbursement for Long-Term Care and Rehabilitation."
   Learning Outcome: 46-8

Apply What You Learned

Suggested Answers

1. You can provide teaching regarding the value and importance of rehabilitation in helping her to regain her independence. It may be helpful to have someone from the rehabilitation facility speak with her or send her pictures of the place where she'll be going. Her son may be able to visit the facility and learn more about it and share his findings with his mother.

2. Use of therapeutic communication, including open-ended questions, active listening, and reflecting back what the client says may help the nurse learn more about the client's feelings. In order to keep the client from closing down, it is important that the nurse not express an opinion over the best choice, but rather listen to what the client wants and attempt to broker a compromise between the client and family. Ultimately, the client has the right of self-determination no matter what the family thinks, but a compromise can make the situation more tolerable for all concerned.

3. Perhaps a bedroom can be created on the main floor if there is a bathroom on that floor. A home aide can be hired to come in once a week or once every other week to do laundry or a family member can assist with this chore to keep Mrs. King from having to go downstairs. If there is no bathroom on the main floor, a commode could be placed in a private spot for urination so Mrs. King need only climb the stairs at bedtime. The home can be assessed for other safety risks that can be resolved to make her home a safer place.

Multiple Choice Questions

1. C
   Rationale: Assisting clients with ADLs, such as bathing, would be considered custodial care. Occupational therapy, medication administration, or dressing changes are considered skilled nursing care.
   Learning Outcome: 46-1
2. B, D
   Rationale: The LPN supervises UAPs and delegates tasks with supervision. Setting up appointments is within the scope of practice for the LPN/LVN, although a unit clerk may or may not be available to assist with these types of tasks. In most states, the LPN/LVN does not administer IV push medications, and although they may contribute to the plan of care, they do not develop a

plan of care. Clients should never be allowed in the nurse's private vehicle, nor should the nurse drive a vehicle owned by the facility unless specific insurance and legal arrangements have been made due to the risk of liability if an untoward event occurred.

Learning Outcome: 46-2

3. B, D, E

Rationale: The nurse notifies the funeral home when a client dies, and should administer all tube feedings because of the level of skill involved. Other tasks can be delegated to the UAP when appropriate.

Learning Outcome: 46-3

4. B

Rationale: Occupational therapists help the client adapt to injury or illness in order to remain as independent as possible when performing ADLs, so it would be the occupational therapist who would determine the best type of adaptive device required to help the client perform specific activities.

Learning Outcome: 46-4

5. B

Rationale: The child must have school incorporated into the environment. The other options are important to all clients in the rehabilitation or long-term care facility.

Learning Outcome: 46-5

6. D

Rationale: The nurse's role is to observe, assess, and monitor for signs and symptoms of complications to allow for rapid treatment in order to prevent further loss of function. The nurse contributes to development of the rehab program, but is not responsible for developing it. Teachers are hired to meet pediatric clients' school needs. Clients in rehabilitation should be encouraged to be as autonomous as possible in preparation for discharge.

Learning Outcome: 46-6

7. A

Rationale: The nurse's responsibility is to report the event to the supervisor, who will perform a more thorough investigation to determine if further reporting is necessary.

Learning Outcome: 46-7

8. D

Rationale: Medicare covers the cost for the first 100 days if the need for skilled care can be demonstrated.

Learning Outcome: 46-8

9. B

Rationale: The Omnibus Budget Reconciliation Act was passed to improve care in nursing homes and extended care facilities.

Learning Outcome: 46-1

10. A, B, C, E

Rationale: All of these procedures may be performed by the LPN/LVN, depending on state nurse practice acts, except for pushing IV medications, which is not allowed in most locations. Of course, it must be permissible by facility policy as well as nurse practice acts.

Learning Outcome: 46-2

Matching

1.	E	6.	C
2.	D	7.	D
3.	B	8.	E
4.	C	9.	A
5.	A	10.	B

Learning Outcomes

1. See section entitled "Emergency Care and Urgent Care."
   Learning Outcome: 47-1
2. See section entitled "Initial Contact."
   Learning Outcome: 47-2
3. See section entitled "Admission to EC or UC."
   Learning Outcome: 47-3
4. See section entitled "Airway Management and CPR."
   Learning Outcome: 47-4
5. See section entitled "Shock."
   Learning Outcome: 47-5
6. See section entitled "Trauma in the Emergency Center."
   Learning Outcome: 47-6
7. See sections entitled "Near Drowning," "Poisoning and Bites," "Psychiatric Emergencies," and "Rape."
   Learning Outcome: 47-7
8. See section entitled "Bioterrorism and Terrorist Attacks."
   Learning Outcome: 47-8
9. See section entitled "Burns."
   Learning Outcome: 47-9
10. See section entitled "Death in the EC."
    Learning Outcome: 47-10
11. See procedures at end of chapter.
    Learning Outcome: 47-11

Apply What You Learned

Suggested Answers

1. This client has symptoms of shock and based on the report of earache, it may be septic shock, although that can only be confirmed by blood cultures.
2. The client should be placed in a Trendelenburg position and oxygen saturation should be measured. The nurse may prepare for IV insertion by collecting the necessary equipment, but it cannot be started until an order is received from the provider.
3. The nurse may anticipate orders to start an IV, draw blood cultures, administer antibiotics, and admit the client to the acute care facility.

Multiple Choice Questions

1. A, C, E
   Rationale: The LPN/LVN will perform interventions, administer IV piggy-back medications, and reinforce client teaching. The RN creates discharge plans, but the LPN/LVN helps to reinforce teaching. The LPN/LVN can input their own data into the ED information system without asking the RN to chart for them.
   Learning Outcome: 47-1

2. C
   Rationale: During incidents with mass casualties, an incident command center is created to control the response to the tragedy. It is usually manned by police, fire, and healthcare personnel.
   Learning Outcome: 47-2

3. B
   Rationale: Clients with an undiagnosed problem, especially if the problem is related to head trauma, will not receive analgesics until seen by the provider.
   Learning Outcome: 47-3

4. D
   Rationale: The venturi mask is considered a low-flow device.
   Learning Outcome: 47-4

5. A
   Rationale: This client is highly suspect for septic shock secondary to the diagnosis of infection several days ago.
   Learning Outcome: 47-5

6. B
   Rationale: RICE stands for rest, ice, compress, and elevate, and is the treatment protocol for soft tissue injuries such as sprains and strains.
   Learning Outcome: 47-6

7. C
   Rationale: *Bacillus anthracis* is anthrax, which would create serious concern regarding the possibility of bioterroism.
   Learning Outcome: 47-8

8. D
   Rationale: 9% for the right leg, 9% for the arms, and 18% for the anterior trunk totals 36%.
   Learning Outcome: 47-9

9. B
   Rationale: The nurse prepares the body for donation of organs if the client has signed an organ donor card and/or has family approval for donation. The family should not be notified of the client's death by phone. The nurse supports the family but does not counsel them. The care of the client is performed before they are taken to the morgue.
   Learning Outcome: 47-10

10. A
    Rationale: The nurse can apply a splint, but does not apply a cast. The client is measured while lying on the stretcher and is instructed to place weight on the arm, not the axilla, when crutch walking.
    Learning Outcome: 47-11

Matching

1. C
2. D
3. E
4. A
5. B

6. B
7. A
8. D
9. C

Learning Outcomes

1. See section entitled "Community Care Settings."
   Learning Outcome: 48-1
2. See section entitled "Community Care Settings."
   Learning Outcome: 48-2
3. See section entitled "School Health Office or Clinic."
   Learning Outcome: 48-3
4. See section entitled "Community Care Settings."
   Learning Outcome: 48-4
5. See procedures at end of chapter.
   Learning Outcome: 48-5
6. See procedures at end of chapter.
   Learning Outcome: 48-6
7. See procedures at end of chapter.
   Learning Outcome: 48-7

Apply What You Learned

Suggested Answers

1. The nurse should report acute physical problems to the physician because the client requires rapid intervention, and care will be slowed if the nurse reports to anyone other than the physician.
2. The nurse should clarify the request with the physician because oxygen is considered a medication and requires a doctor's order. Furthermore, nurses do not accept orders from medical assistants who do not have the authority to give these orders.
3. Questions related to benefits of employment should be directed to the office manager, who is responsible for the smooth running and staffing of the facility.

Multiple Choice Questions

1. D
   Rationale: Assisted living facilities require clients be able to meet most needs independently, but are able to assist with some degrees of personal

care, often providing communal dining in a cafeteria within the building and checking on clients to make sure they are okay.
Learning Outcome: 48-1

2. B, C, D
Rationale: The LPN/LVN admits new clients, performs lab tests, and can conduct electrocardiograms. However, they are responsible to the physician, not the office manager, unless the office manager is an RN. The LPN/LVN does not perform simple surgical procedures, but may assist the physician performing them.
Learning Outcome: 48-2

3. B, D
Rationale: The nurse administers basic first aid and provides client teaching. Providing aspirin is prescribing, which is outside the scope of practice. The nurse reports to the RN or physician, not to the principal of the school.
Learning Outcome: 48-3

4. C
Rationale: The nurse working in home care and hospice works far more autonomously than in many other settings. The nurse must have well-developed observational and critical thinking skills to succeed and this is not generally recommended for new graduates.
Learning Outcome: 48-4

5. A, C
Rationale: The nurse will require black and red pens for charting unless the facility is digital. Thank the client for their cooperation in order to foster a better nurse/client relationship. Medical terminology should be avoided when questioning the client. Sometimes, closed-ended questions are needed when specific data is required. The nurse should sit at eye level with the client while obtaining information.
Learning Outcome: 48-5

6. B, C, D, E
Rationale: Suturing the wound is outside the LPN/LVN's scope of practice. The other options are valid LPN/LVN responsibilities.
Learning Outcome: 48-6

7. B, C, D, E
Rationale: Sigmoidoscopy is performed by a physician, but all of the other options can be performed by the nurse autonomously.
Learning Outcome: 48-7

8. D
Rationale: Hepatitis B immunization may be initiated before the baby is discharged from the hospital after delivery or anytime thereafter.
Learning Outcome: 48-3

9. D
Rationale: When a client is in acute distress, they should never be left alone and should be monitored constantly.
Learning Outcome: 48-3

10. A
Rationale: The Ishihara exam measures near vision, whereas the Snellen chart measures distance vision; the Hardy-Rand-Rittler exam measures color perception.
Learning Outcome: 48-7

Matching

1. C	5. A	9. E	13. A
2. E	6. C	10. B	14. B
3. D	7. D	11. E	5. C
4. B	8. A	12. F	16. D

Learning Outcomes

1. See section entitled "Mental Health."
   Learning Outcome: 49-1
2. See section entitled "Mental Disorders."
   Learning Outcome: 49-2
3. See section entitled "Child and Adolescent Mental Health."
   Learning Outcome: 49-3
4. See section entitled "Treatment for Mental Health Disorders."
   Learning Outcome: 49-4
5. See section entitled "Nurses' Role in Mental Health Promotion."
   Learning Outcome: 49-5
6. See section entitled "Schizophrenia."
   Learning Outcome: 49-6
7. See section entitled "Mood Disorders."
   Learning Outcome: 49-7
8. See section entitled "Personality Disorders."
   Learning Outcome: 49-8

Apply What You Learned

Suggested Answers

1. This client is highly likely to be experiencing the mood disorder of major depression as characterized by his social withdrawal, disinterest in things around him, sleep disturbance, and sad affect.
2. The most important question to ask this client is, "Are you planning or thinking about hurting yourself or someone else?" Clients experiencing major depression are far more likely to hurt themselves and must be assessed to prevent self-harm.
3. The physician and/or nurse supervisor should be notified of the client's condition so appropriate treatment and referrals can be initiated.

Multiple Choice Questions

1. D
   Rationale: A mentally healthy person has a sense of the meaning of life, accurately evaluates reality, displays flexibility toward change and conflict, and does not attempt to control others.
   Learning Outcome: 49-1

2. C

   Rationale: 1 in 2 people have a psychiatric or substance abuse problem at some point in their lives, so it is of great importance that nurses learn to assess for these issues.

   Learning Outcome: 49-2

3. B

   Rationale: Half of all cases of mental illness begin at age 14 and failure to properly intervene will cause many of these children to develop more serious problems before diagnosis.

   Learning Outcome: 49-3

4. D

   Rationale: The aim of milieu therapy is to create a safe and structured environment, allowing the client to feel free to perform the work of improving mental health.

   Learning Outcome: 49-4

5. A

   Rationale: Tertiary care is aimed at rehabilitation and reducing complications of disease, so the nurse who reminds the client diagnosed with schizophrenia to attend group therapy is providing tertiary care. Option B is primary care. Options C and D are secondary care.

   Learning Outcome: 49-5

6. D

   Rationale: Anhedonia is the inability to feel pleasure, which would be a negative symptom. Other options are positive symptoms.

   Learning Outcome: 49-6

7. D

   Rationale: MAOIs are powerful and effective drugs, but interact with many substances, including foods containing the amino acid tyramine, so careful client teaching is required when these drugs are prescribed.

   Learning Outcome: 49-7

8. C

   Rationale: The client with histrionic personality disorder is very emotional and dramatic in an attempt to seek attention, but rarely is able to form a satisfying relationship because they always want to be the center of attention.

   Learning Outcome: 49-8

9. A, C, E

   Rationale: Appropriate and realistic outcomes for the client with a mood disorder include performing ADLs independently, agreeing not to harm themselves, and falling asleep within 30 minutes of going to bed. Everyone is different so it may not be possible to sleep for 5 to 6 hours, but the goal is to have the client awaken feeling rested. Feelings of anger should not be suppressed, but expressed in a healthy way that helps to resolve conflicts instead of inflaming them.

   Learning Outcome: 49-7

10. B, D, E

    Rationale: Schizophrenia is diagnosed more frequently in family members of schizophrenics, so there is a familial association. People born or raised in an urban area have a greater risk for having schizophrenia. Reduced immune

function and an increase in cytokines (interleukin-6), and abnormalities in leukocytes and immunoglobulins have been reported in people with schizophrenia, but it is hard to know if this is caused by the medications prescribed to treat the disease or the disease itself. People with schizophrenia are born more frequently in the winter and spring than in the summer or fall.
Learning Outcome: 49-6

Chapter 50 Substance Abuse and Eating Disorders

Matching

1.	F	6.	B	11.	C
2.	G	7.	E	12.	B
3.	D	8.	F	13.	A
4.	A	9.	E		
5.	C	10.	D		

Learning Outcomes

1. See section entitled "Substance Abuse and Dependency."
   Learning Outcome: 50-1
2. See sections entitled "Alcohol" and "Other CNS Depressants."
   Learning Outcome: 50-2
3. See section entitled "Substance Abuse."
   Learning Outcome: 50-3
4. See section entitled "Substance Abuse."
   Learning Outcome: 50-4
5. See section entitled "Collaborative Care."
   Learning Outcome: 50-5
6. See section entitled "Substance Dependency among Nurses."
   Learning Outcome: 50-6
7. See section entitled "Eating Disorders."
   Learning Outcome: 50-7
8. See section entitled "Eating Disorders."
   Learning Outcome: 50-8

Apply What You Learned

Suggested Answers

1. The nurse might tell the client that he has taken the first step in the act of sobriety and would then ask the client when he had his last drink, because this is important in determining the possible occurrence of DTs.
2. Arrangements should be made for the client to be admitted to a detoxification unit first until his system is cleared of alcohol and withdrawal symptoms are over. At that time, he may be admitted to an inpatient unit or treated by an outpatient center to help him overcome the psychological issues of addiction.

Multiple Choice Questions

1. A

    Rationale: Clients with a physical dependence on a substance will experience symptoms of withdrawal that may cause them to relapse and continue use of the substance in order to reduce the symptoms. Addiction involves the psychosocial components of abuse, tolerance is the amount of substance required to create the same effect, and lack of willpower is not a component of the issue of abuse and dependence.

    Learning Outcome: 50-1

2. D

    Rationale: Asians are unlikely to experience alcoholism because of the genetic variant found in people from this culture.

    Learning Outcome: 50-2

3. C

    Rationale: These symptoms are often found in clients using amphetamines that depress appetite and act as a stimulant.

    Learning Outcome: 50-3

4. B

    Rationale: As the client withdraws from a substance, they are unable to protect themselves and often require a low stimulation environment.

    Learning Outcome: 50-4

5. B

    Rationale: Alcoholics Anonymous was founded on the idea that a group of people sharing a common problem offers a sense of community that helps to provide strength and support to maintain sobriety.

    Learning Outcome: 50-5

6. D

    Rationale: To protect the privacy of the coworker, it is best to notify the supervisor as opposed to the staff nurse who happens to be in charge that day.

    Learning Outcome: 50-6

7. C

    Rationale: The client with bulimia nervosa follows binge eating with compensatory behavior resulting in purging of the excess intake.

    Learning Outcome: 50-7

8. D

    Rationale: Social support has been shown to be effective in all substance abuse issues, including food.

    Learning Outcome: 50-7

9. B

    Rationale: BMI is calculated by multiplying weight by 703 and dividing by the height (in inches) twice: $215 \times 703 = 151145 \div 71 = 2128.8 \div 71 = 29.98$

    Learning Outcome: 50-7

10. C

    Rationale: A street name of codeine is pancakes and syrup.

    Learning Outcome: 50-3

Matching

1. F	6. A	11. A	16. F	21. F
2. D	7. F	12. C	17. D	22. C
3. E	8. E	13. C	18. B	23. B
4. B	9. D	14. E	19. E	24. A
5. C	10. B	15. A	20. G	25. D

Learning Outcomes

1. See section entitled "Preconception."
   Learning Outcome: 51-1
2. See section entitled "Fertilization and Fetal Development."
   Learning Outcome: 51-2
3. See section entitled "Signs of Pregnancy."
   Learning Outcome: 51-3
4. See section entitled "Maternal Changes during Pregnancy."
   Learning Outcome: 51-4
5. See section entitled "Nursing Care."
   Learning Outcome: 51-5
6. See section entitled "Discomforts of Pregnancy."
   Learning Outcome: 55-6
7. See section entitled "Nursing Care."
   Learning Outcome: 55-7
8. See section entitled "Nursing Care."
   Learning Outcome: 55-8
9. See procedures at end of chapter.
   Learning Outcome: 55-9
10. See procedures at end of chapter.
    Learning Outcome: 55-10

Apply What You Learned

Suggested Answers

1. Topics to cover include: making healthy diet choices, use of prenatal vitamins, symptoms to report to the doctor, toxins to avoid, exercises to perform or avoid, importance of avoiding alcohol, clothing adaptations, hygiene, and importance of fluids. A complete list can be found in Box 51-4 on page 1427.
2. Teaching should be performed after she calls her boyfriend because she will be more able to hear what the nurse is saying versus sitting there waiting to get finished so she can make an important phone call.

Multiple Choice Questions

1. A, C, D
   Rationale: Foods high in folic acid include liver, milk, and kidney beans. A more complete list can be found in Box 51-1 on page 1411.
   Learning Outcome: 55-1

2. C
   Rationale: The villus secures the blastocyst to the uterus.
   Learning Outcome: 55-2

3. D
   Rationale: Amenorrhea is a presumptive sign because there can be other causes of a missed menstrual period other than pregnancy. Furthermore, it is possible to be pregnant and still have regular menstrual periods.
   Learning Outcome: 55-3

4. B
   Rationale: An increase in platelets, fibrin, fibrinogen, and other coagulation factors coupled with venous stasis can lead to thrombus formation, and is a risk faced by the women in the last half of pregnancy.
   Learning Outcome: 55-4

5. A
   Rationale: Heartburn can often be reduced by eating small amounts of food frequently and avoiding spicy foods. Risk for heartburn increases as fetal size increases, pushing contents of the stomach into the esophagus.
   Learning Outcome: 55-6

6. D
   Rationale: Generally the client should gain no more than 25 to 35 pounds throughout the pregnancy.
   Learning Outcome: 55-5

7. C
   Rationale: Fluid that leaks from the nipple should be rubbed into the skin of the nipple to lubricate and promote breast health.
   Learning Outcome: 55-7

8. A
   Rationale: The sudden occurrence of double vision is highly suspect for possible pregnancy-induced hypertension; the client should be seen to assess blood pressure.
   Learning Outcome: 55-8

9. D
   Rationale: D is correct and fetal heart rate should be assessed any time the mother accesses health care. Gel should be applied to the Doppler, not to the mother's abdomen. The diaphragm should be positioned midline of the woman's abdomen halfway between the umbilicus and symphysis pubis, not left of midline. When checking the fetal pulse against the mother's, if they are the same, the Doppler should be repositioned, not the mother.
   Learning Outcome: 55-9

10. C
   Rationale: The fetal ultrasound is performed by a trained ultrasound technician, not the nurse.
   Learning Outcome: 55-10

Chapter 52 Care of Women during High-Risk Pregnancy

Matching

1. D
2. C
3. B
4. E
5. A

6. E
7. D
8. A
9. B
10. C

Learning Outcomes

1. See section entitled "Risk Factors in Pregnancy."
   Learning Outcome: 52-1
2. See section entitled "Risks of Pregnancy to the Adolescent Mother."
   Learning Outcome: 52-2
3. See sections entitled "Tests Used to Assess Maternal Well-Being" and "Assessing Fetal Well-Being."
   Learning Outcome: 52-3
4. See section entitled "Complications of Pregnancy."
   Learning Outcome: 52-4
5. See section entitled "Medical Conditions Complicated by Pregnancy."
   Learning Outcome: 52-5
6. See section entitled "Nursing Care."
   Learning Outcome: 52-6

Apply What You Learned

Suggested Answers

1. Urine should be assessed for the presence of glucose and protein that could indicate signs of gestational diabetes or preeclampsia, blood pressure monitoring with vital signs and fetal heart tones should be performed every four hours to assess for early signs of preeclampsia, client should be assessed for contractions, rupture of membranes, pain, or any signs of problems.
2. Listening to three fetal heart tones can be quite challenging, but the nurse can increase the chances of hearing each of the different heart tones by knowing the placement of each of the fetus. Generally heart tones will be heard in three different locations on the mother's abdomen closest to the position of the heart in each fetus. These locations where fetal heart tones are best heard should be documented to make it easier for successive checks to be performed.

3. This client may require an IV for administration of medications to stop labor, should be repositioned on her side to prevent hypotension secondary to pressure of the babies on the maternal great vessels, and need skin care to prevent loss of skin integrity, assistance to reduce stress, and activities to reduce boredom. You may have thought of other needs as well.

Multiple Choice Questions

1. C
   Rationale: Although being unmarried does not place the client in a high-risk category, it is one factor that can increase risk and falls under the sociodemographic group of factors.
   Learning Outcome: 52-1

2. C
   Rationale: The client who smoked and drank alcohol during the early weeks of the pregnancy is at greatest risk because fetal organ development is completed by 6 to 8 weeks gestation.
   Learning Outcome: 52-2

3. D
   Rationale: The indirect Coombs' test looks for maternal antigens that attack the fetal blood cells if incompatibility exists.
   Learning Outcome: 52-3

4. A
   Rationale: Hyperemesis gravidarum presents with frequent vomiting that if not corrected can lead to dehydration, with reduced urine output, electrolyte imbalance, and elevated BUN. Treatment may include antiemetics and IV fluid to replace fluid volume.
   Learning Outcome: 52-4

5. D
   Rationale: Pyrimethamine is administered to treat clients with toxoplasmosis and may cause the symptoms described.
   Learning Outcome: 52-5

6. D
   Rationale: Fetal ultrasound requires a doctor's order, but the other assessments can be performed without an order and are nursing orders. Cervical examination is contraindicated in some cases, such as mothers with vaginal bleeding.
   Learning Outcome: 52-6

7. C
   Rationale: This client is displaying early signs of mild preeclampsia that require immediate intervention to prevent worsening symptoms.
   Learning Outcome: 52-7

8. A
   Rationale: Preeclampsia, unfortunately, is a commonly diagnosed disorder in women, especially primiparas under 20 or over 35.
   Learning Outcome: 52-4

9. B
   Rationale: If the mother has a herpes lesion on the genitals, a C-section will be performed to prevent transmission to the baby.
   Learning Outcome: 52-5
10. B
   Rationale: Low alpha-fetoprotein findings are an indication of a possible (not definite) diagnosis of Down's syndrome.
   Learning Outcome: 52-3

Chapter 53 Care of Women during Labor and Birth

Matching

1.	C	6.	A	11.	C	16.	F
2.	F	7.	D	12.	B	17.	B
3.	B	8.	E	13.	E	18.	C
4.	E	9.	A	14.	D		
5.	D	10.	F	15.	A		

Learning Outcomes

1. See sections entitled "Beginning of Labor," "Signs of Impending Labor," and "Variables Affecting Labor."
   Learning Outcome: 53-1
2. See section entitled "Stages of Labor."
   Learning Outcome: 53-2
3. See section entitled "Nursing Care."
   Learning Outcome: 53-3
4. See sections entitled "Birth" and "Recovery."
   Learning Outcome: 53-4
5. See section entitled "High-Risk Labor and Birth."
   Learning Outcome: 53-5

Apply What You Learned

Suggested Answers

1. When a woman delivers via Cesarean section, the risk to the baby is greater because the fetus does not squeeze through the vaginal canal, may not be exposed to the stress of labor if the C-section is planned in advance as opposed to performing it emergently, and the fetus is exposed to any anesthesia administered to the mother. The mother must undergo surgery, with an incision that has the potential for infection and the risks that accompany any surgery. Although C-section outcomes are generally good, they are not the best or safest option for the mother or the fetus, so should not be allowed as a choice.

2. Lamaze is based on the idea that pain is a learned reflex and through proper breathing and relaxation exercises, the pregnant woman can reduce the pain of labor. The woman and her partner attend classes prior to beginning labor to learn the various techniques in preparation for labor and delivery.

3. The Leboyer method of delivery has the fetus immersed into water during or shortly after birth. The idea is that it allows the baby to be born with less trauma and makes the process more gentle. However, the baby's first cry after birth is essential to alveoli expansion and delivery into water can make it harder to assess possible complications, such as meconium or bleeding.

Multiple Choice Questions

1. D
   Rationale: Passage of the mucus plug generally precedes labor by 24 to 48 hours and indicates the onset is impending.
   Learning Outcome: 53-1

2. A
   Rationale: The ideal presentation is occiput ROA because the baby presents with the top back of the head.
   Learning Outcome: 53-1

3. B
   Rationale: Engagement is when the fetal head (or presenting part) falls into the true pelvis. This may occur as early as 2 weeks prior to the onset of labor and is sometimes called "lightening" because the mother feels lighter and can breathe more easily as the fetus moves down and away from the diaphragm.
   Learning Outcome: 53-2

4. D
   Rationale: Breathing techniques can help the mother to relieve muscle tension that interferes with labor progression and increases pain. The mother is often assisted by squatting or walking as opposed to lying supine. The mother in labor is often NPO except for ice chips. The woman does not push until full dilation occurs and then pushes with contractions, not between contractions.
   Learning Outcome: 53-3

5. A, B, D
   Rationale: The LPN/LVN checks functioning of equipment, provides assistance, and arranges the sterile instruments in the birthing room. IV push medications and assessment are the role of the RN.
   Learning Outcome: 53-4

6. A
   Rationale: The priority is to remain with the woman while having someone call EMS. The nurse should have the mother pant to avoid pushing, and should not touch the infant's head or the umbilical cord. If the baby is born before EMS arrives, an intact umbilical cord allows for oxygen exchange between the mother and fetus until help arrives. The baby should be wrapped in blankets and placed on the woman's abdomen.
   Learning Outcome: 53-5

7. B, C

Rationale: Dystocia is often the result of cephalopelvic disproportion and the risk of fetal harm increases after approximately 24 hours of labor, so this would be an indicator of need for C-section. If the cord prolapses, the woman is positioned to relieve pressure on the cord and the woman is rushed to C-section. Precipitous birth is rapid vaginal delivery and some malpresentations do not require C-section, but must be assessed on a case-by-case basis. The mother's preference is not a good reason to perform a C-section and would not indicate need for an immediate C-section.

Learning Outcome: 53-5

8. A

Rationale: A soft fundus below the umbilicus would increase the risk of abnormal bleeding, and the client should be assessed for a full bladder.

Learning Outcome: 53-2

9. B

Rationale: Contractions felt in the back or abdomen could be Braxton-Hicks contractions. Progressive dilation of the cervix in the increasing anterior position that increases with walking indicates true labor.

Learning Outcome: 53-1

10. D

Rationale: The release of oxytocin initiates labor contractions.

Learning Outcome: 53-2

Chapter 54 Care of Postpartum Women

Matching

1. E		6. A
2. C		7. H
3. F		8. D
4. B		
5. G		

Learning Outcomes

1. See section entitled "Body Systems Adaptations."
   Learning Outcome: 54-1
2. See section entitled "Psychological Changes."
   Learning Outcome: 54-2
3. See section entitled "Fathers, Siblings, and Others."
   Learning Outcome: 54-3
4. See section entitled "Nursing Care."
   Learning Outcome: 54-4
5. See section entitled "Nursing Care."
   Learning Outcome: 54-5
6. See section entitled "Nursing Care."
   Learning Outcome: 54-6

7. See section entitled "Nursing Care."
   Learning Outcome: 54-7
8. See section entitled "Postpartum Care after Cesarean Section."
   Learning Outcome: 54-8
9. See section entitled "Postpartum Care after Cesarean Section."
   Learning Outcome: 54-9
10. See section entitled "New Family."
    Learning Outcome: 54-10
11. See section entitled "Breastfeeding."
    Learning Outcome: 54-11

Apply What You Learned

Suggested Answers

1. The nurse might say something such as, "It's very frustrating when you first start to breast feed. Most women encounter problems at first and then things fall into place." This will show the mother that you understand the frustration involved and also reassure her that it's a common problem that will resolve with time.
2. The nurse can help the mother by showing her how to hold the infant, how to improve latching on, and how to encourage the let-down reflex. The nurse should talk about treating discomfort that may occur with engorgement, cracked nipples, and uterine cramping during breast feeding. Finally, the nurse can provide a referral to the La Leche League if needed.

Multiple Choice Questions

1. C
   Rationale: Lochia alba is a whitish vaginal discharge that can continue until the fourth to sixth week postpartum and gradually subsides.
   Learning Outcome: 54-1
2. D
   Rationale: During the letting-go stage, parents have adequately processed the birth and are ready to return to a normal life after having a baby. Social interactions become increasingly more important.
   Learning Outcome: 54-2
3. A, B, C, D
   Rationale: The nurse helps the mother create a support network by helping her to examine the friends and family in her life that she can depend on. Many people are happy to help a new mother, so this is an optimal time to request their help. The mother should consider things someone could do for her that would be helpful.
   Learning Outcome: 54-3
4. B
   Rationale: The nurse may use the mnemonic of BUBBLE to help remember important areas of the assessment: B — Breast, U — uterus, B — bowel, B — bladder, L — lochia, E — episiotomy/incision.
   Learning Outcome: 54-4

5. C
   Rationale: Pain of 7 in a newly postoperative client should be treated with morphine to allow the client to rest comfortably.
   Learning Outcome: 54-5

6. A
   Rationale: The new mother should drink at least 1000 mL of fluid per day in order to maintain homeostasis.
   Learning Outcome: 54-6

7. A
   Rationale: The client should be told to listen to her body and rest whenever she feels tired or when the opportunity arises. Telling new mothers to sleep when the baby sleeps is often effective. Eating whenever she is hungry could result in weight gain. Normal maintenance doesn't occur for 4 to 6 weeks in most cases. Postpartum exercises begin with simple exercises and are advanced according to the woman's response.
   Learning Outcome: 54-7

8. B
   Rationale: If the baby doesn't eat for 8 hours, the mother should notify the pediatrician.
   Learning Outcome: 54-8

9. B
   Rationale: A few women may feel very little pain and decline pain mediation following C-section. Food and fluid should he held until bowel sounds return. This client will have the same lochia as a woman who delivered vaginally. An indwelling catheter is not routinely placed and is often removed once full sensation returns, if required.
   Learning Outcome: 54-9

10. D
    Rationale: The difference between breast milk and formula is not great but breast milk is more easily digested and contains natural immunities. Breast feeding is best, but women who choose not to breast feed should not be made to feel guilty for their choice.
    Learning Outcome: 54-11

Chapter 55 Care of High-Risk Postpartum Women

Matching

1.	D	4.	F
2.	E	5.	B
3.	A	6.	C

Learning Outcomes

1. See entire chapter.
   Learning Outcome: 55-1
2. See section entitled "Preeclampsia."
   Learning Outcome: 55-2

3. See sections entitled "Postpartum Hemorrhage" and "Postpartum Thromboembolic Disease."
    Learning Outcome: 55-3
4. See section entitled "Postpartum Infections."
    Learning Outcome: 55-4
5. See section entitled "Postpartum Blues, Postpartum Depression, and Postpartum Psychosis."
    Learning Outcome: 55-5
6. See section entitled "Maternal Death."
    Learning Outcome: 55-6

Apply What You Learned

Suggested Answers

1. The nurse will assess the perineum, lochia, uterus, and breasts. The client should be questioned to assess pain and should be medicated for pain as needed. Encourage fluid intake and review documentation to determine when the client last voided. Assess for full bladder if she has not voided recently.
2. If the mother chooses to breast feed, she should assign one breast to each infant to prevent cross-contamination. She can be taught how to breast feed both infants at the same time or one at a time. She should be encouraged to feed them individually a few times a day as able in order to spend quality time with each of them.

Multiple Choice Questions

1. D
    Rationale: A classic sign of preeclampsia is protein in the urine, so the postpartum client's urine should be monitored and the amount of protein should decline and eventually stop.
    Learning Outcome: 55-1
2. B
    Rationale: Blood pressure should be rechecked every hour or more often, depending on how high the blood pressure is. Reflexes should also be checked because hypertension may be an indication of preeclampsia.
    Learning Outcome: 55-2
3. C
    Rationale: Uterine atony can occur as a result of prolonged third-stage labor, intrauterine infections, and/or oxytocin administration, and will lead to hemorrhage because the uterus does not adequately clamp down to stop bleeding.
    Learning Outcome: 55-3
4. B
    Rationale: These symptoms would indicate a systemic infection known as puerperal infection. Indications of a laceration or episiotomy infection would be more localized.
    Learning Outcome: 55-4

5. A

Rationale: Generally, a score of 13 or higher indicates a need for further assessment due to concern for a more serious postpartum depression or psychosis.

Learning Outcome: 55-5

6. B, C

Rationale: It is important to provide referrals to help support the family during this difficult time. A debriefing can help the nurse deal with feelings of grief and sadness and share feelings with others involved. The family is often in shock and is unable to understand detailed explanations that should be provided by the provider when the time comes. The nurse does not need to offer to babysit, and the decision to attend the funeral is up to each nurse to determine, but is not required.

Learning Outcome: 55-6

7. A

Rationale: These are classic signs of mastitis, which can be caused by a transfer of bacteria from the baby's mouth, or from milk stasis, which allows for the growth of pathogens.

Learning Outcome: 55-4

8. B

Rationale: Red discharge that continues beyond 2 weeks could indicate subinvolution, or delayed postpartum hemorrhage.

Learning Outcome: 55-3

9. C

Rationale: A pelvic hematoma is considered most dangerous because it develops rapidly, contains 250mL to 500mL of blood, and has few symptoms

Learning Outcome: 55-3

10. D

Rationale: Postpartum blues are anticipated and most women will experience them 2 to 3 days after birth as a result in changes in hormone levels. Some women will experience more serious symptoms consistent with postpartum depression or psychosis.

Learning Outcome: 55-5

Chapter 56 Care of Normal Neonates

Matching

1.	E	6.	C	11.	B	16.	B
2.	A	7.	D	12.	C	17.	A
3.	F	8.	A	13.	F	18.	C
4.	B	9.	F	14.	E		
5.	D	10.	E	15.	D		

Learning Outcomes

1. See section entitled "Physiologic Adaptations to Life."
   Learning Outcome: 56-1

2. See section entitled "Delivery Room Care."
   Learning Outcome: 56-2
3. See section entitled "Delivery Room Care."
   Learning Outcome: 56-3
4. See section entitled "Nursery Care."
   Learning Outcome: 56-4
5. See section entitled "Gestational Age."
   Learning Outcome: 56-5
6. See section entitled "Characteristics of the Newborn."
   Learning Outcome: 56-6
7. See section entitled "Hygiene Care."
   Learning Outcome: 56-7
8. See section entitled "Vitamin K Administration Nutrition."
   Learning Outcome: 56-8
9. See section entitled "Common Procedures."
   Learning Outcome: 56-9
10. See section entitled "Discharge Teaching about Neonatal Care."
    Learning Outcome: 56-10

Apply What You Learned

Suggested Answers

Mrs. Snyder may want to include her husband in the teaching about care of the neonate. Ms. Timberlake should be asked who, if anyone, she would like to include. Mrs. Snyder has other children so the nurse needs to determine what she knows, what questions she has, and what information she may need. Although she has other children, it doesn't indicate that she knows everything or doesn't have misconceptions that need to be corrected. She may be overwhelmed by four children under age 6, so determining sources of support is important.

Ms. Timberlake, on the other hand, is a new mother and will most likely require more instructions regarding how to provide baby care, including routine care, bathing, feedings, and safety needs. Sources of support should be explored because caring for an infant independently can be very overwhelming.

Multiple Choice Questions

1. C
   Rationale: Often one of the first signs of respiratory distress is flaring of the nostrils that will then be followed by other more obvious symptoms.
   Learning Outcome: 56-1
2. C
   Rationale: An infant with an Apgar score of 2 to 3 is not meeting the most basic requirements for life and requires resuscitation.
   Learning Outcome: 56-2

3. B

Rationale: Identification of the newborn and mother is always performed in the delivery room to ensure the right baby is identified with the right mother before they are separated for the first time. Other options are generally performed in the newborn nursery.

Learning Outcome: 56-3

4. A, B, D

Rationale: To avoid baby snatching, access to the nursery and the OB unit is limited, a band is placed on the baby that will alarm if the baby is removed from the unit, and the parents are taught not to give the infant to anyone – no matter what they are told – if the person doesn't have proper facility identification. Infants are transported in the bassinet and are not carried from nursery to mother's room. Most routine procedures can be performed with the infant in the bassinet.

Learning Outcome: 56-4

5. D

Rationale: This method of gestational age determination is only 75 to 85% accurate because conception can occur during any period of time after menstruation begins and is based on women who conceive 10 to 14 days after the first day of the menstrual cycle begins. Furthermore, women may not remember the exact date their menstrual period begins, so the date could be off. The best means of determining gestation is by exam.

Learning Outcome: 56-5

6. B, D, E

Rationale: Telangiectatic nevi, or stork bites, are considered normal findings and are usually located on the back of the neck. Epstein's pearls look like teeth just erupting through the gums, but are actually white spots that will go away. Milia are the white spots that look like little whiteheads on the baby's nose that will subside within a few weeks of birth. Lanugo is found on premature infants. Strabismus is an abnormal ophthalmic finding.

Learning Outcome: 56-6

7. C

Rationale: The infant cannot be placed in a tub of water until after the umbilical cord falls off because the cord must dry in order to fall off.

Learning Outcome: 56-7

8. B

Rationale: Colostrum, the initial milk produced by the breast feeding mother, is very concentrated and is not high in fluid content, but it is high in calories, protein, and immunity, and is extremely valuable to the neonate's immunity.

Learning Outcome: 8

9. C

Rationale: All newborns in the United States are required to undergo newborn screening 24 hours after first feeding and again 7 days after feeding. Different states include different tests they screen for, and may require screening be done at different times (some states say 3 days and 14 days after first feeding) but all test for phenylketonuria (PKU) and maple syrup urine disease.

Learning Outcome: 56-9

10. B, C

Rationale: The nurse teaches umbilical cord care and how to diaper. Infants should be placed on their back to sleep. Children should never be left unattended on high surfaces in or out of an infant carrier. The baby does not need to be awakened at night to eat and should be allowed to sleep.
Learning Outcome: 56-10

Chapter 57 Care of the High-Risk Neonate

Matching

1.	E	6.	C
2.	G	7.	A
3.	J	8.	D
4.	H	9.	F
5.	I	10.	B

Learning Outcomes

1. See the introductory section.
   Learning Outcome: 57-1
2. See section entitled "General Care of the High-Risk Newborn."
   Learning Outcome: 57-2
3. See section entitled "Physiological Characteristics of Preterm and Postterm Newborns."
   Learning Outcome: 57-3
4. See section entitled "Newborns with Alterations in Growth."
   Learning Outcome: 57-4
5. See section entitled "Respiratory Conditions."
   Learning Outcome: 57-5
6. See section entitled "Congenital Heart Defects."
   Learning Outcome: 57-6
7. See section entitled "Congenital Nervous System Defects."
   Learning Outcome: 57-7
8. See section entitled "Gastrointestinal Conditions."
   Learning Outcome: 57-8
9. See section entitled "Metabolic Disorders."
   Learning Outcome: 57-9
10. See sections entitled "Congenital Genitourinary Defects" and "Musculoskeletal Defects."
    Learning Outcome: 57-10
11. See section entitled "Infants of Drug-Abusing Mothers."
    Learning Outcome: 57-11
12. See section entitled "Neonatal Infections and Sepsis."
    Learning Outcome: 57-12

Apply What You Learned

1. Specific strategies include hand hygiene, maintaining and protecting intact skin, following aseptic technique when performing invasive procedures, teaching parents to wash their hands, teaching siblings to kiss baby on top of the head and avoid kissing hands and face, encouraging parents to avoid exposing baby to large groups (i.e., grocery stores, church nurseries) until immune system matures.

2. Parents will need to be shown how to meet nutritional needs, safety needs, hygiene needs, follow-up medical care and well-baby needs, and medication administration, and all parents should learn CPR, but particularly those whose newborn is being discharged on a cardiorespiratory monitor and home oxygen therapy.

3. This mother is taking responsibility for the premature birth, which in many cases is not accurate. The nurse should sit with the mother and explore her feelings of guilt and provide information to explain that mothers can do everything right (prenatal care, avoiding teratogens, etc) and still deliver prematurely.

Multiple Choice Questions

1. B
    Rationale: These are classic symptoms of galactosemia and should be reported to the physician. Galactosemia is a condition normally screened for in the newborn screen.
    Learning Outcome: 57-9

2. D
    Rationale: Multiple births are classified as high risk and the delivery will be attended by a neonatology nurse in case the newborn requires resuscitation. Many multiple births turn out to be normal deliveries, but are considered high risk because they carry a higher than average risk.
    Learning Outcome: 57-1

3. D
    Rationale: Large-for-gestational-age newborns are at great risk for glucose instability and must be closely monitored for blood sugar levels for several days after birth.
    Learning Outcome: 57-4

4. A, B, C
    Rationale: Routine care includes feeding (even if feedings are administered via feeding tube), bathing, and activity. Suctioning and wound care are not routine or general care.
    Learning Outcome: 57-2

5. A
    Rationale: High percentage oxygen and mechanical ventilation places the infant at increased risk for the development of bronchopulmonary dysplasia (BPD) because of the damage done to the small alveoli. It also increases the risk of retinopathy of the newborn.
    Learning Outcome: 57-5

6. B

Rationale: The nurse would suspect this baby may be experiencing drug withdrawal, which would be confirmed by drug screening that can be conducted with a blood, urine, or saliva specimen.

Learning Outcome: 57-11

7. A

Rationale: Newborns do not demonstrate sepsis in the same way an adult would. Frequently symptoms of infection are vague and can include decreased temperature, apneic episodes, and lethargy demonstrated by poor feeding or failing to wake to feed.

Learning Outcome: 57-12

8. B

Rationale: When caring for a newborn with a congenital heart defect, assessment of capillary refill time can be a valuable indicator of cardiac output. Capillary refill time is tested by pressing on the center of the chest *gently*, letting go, and counting the seconds required for blanching to subside and tissue to become pink again.

Learning Outcome: 57-6

9. A

Rationale: Infants with cleft lip and/or palate can be very challenging to feed because they are unable to form suction and are at risk for formula entering the nasal area, resulting in aspiration. Teaching parents how to feed their infant and how to respond if they choke are important teaching points.

Learning Outcome: 57-8

10. C

Rationale: The assessment findings indicate the neonate is most likely premature. Characteristics of the premature infants include increased flexibility due to immature development of the musculoskeletal system, reduced creases in the footprint, and floppy muscle tone.

Learning Outcome: 57-3

Chapter 58 Pediatric-Focused Nursing Care

Matching

1. D
2. C
3. A
4. E
5. B

6. D
7. C
8. B
9. A

Learning Outcomes

1. See section entitled "Pediatric Anatomy and Physiology."
   Learning Outcome: 58-1
2. See section entitled "Collecting Data for Pediatric Assessment."
   Learning Outcome: 58-2

3. See section entitled "Collecting Data for Pediatric Assessment."
   Learning Outcome: 58-3
4. See section entitled "Adapting Nursing Care for the Pediatric Client."
   Learning Outcome: 58-4
5. See section entitled "Hospitalized Child."
   Learning Outcome: 58-5
6. See section entitled "Teaching Strategies with Pediatric Clients."
   Learning Outcome: 58-6
7. See section entitled "Terminally Ill Pediatric Clients."
   Learning Outcome: 58-7
8. See section entitled "Chronically Ill Pediatric Clients."
   Learning Outcome: 58-8
9. See section entitled "Pediatric Clients with Developmental and Cognitive Issues."
   Learning Outcome: 58-9
10. See section entitled "Identifying Disorders of Pediatric Clients by Age."
    Learning Outcome: 58-10

Apply What You Learned

Suggested Answer

Determine whether additional support may be helpful (counselor, spiritual leader, primary nurses who have cared for Jay throughout his extended hospitalization) and arrange for them to be called. Provide the family with a quiet, private place to gather and arrange for pillows if they need to stay overnight. Consult with family members to determine if any special needs or issues can be met. Be supportive, understanding, and a good listener if they want to talk.

Multiple Choice Questions

1. C
   Rationale: The airways of infants of small children are much narrower than an adults and even a small partial occlusion can reduce air exchange significantly, making them more likely to choke than an adult.
   Learning Outcome: 58-1
2. B
   Rationale: The preschooler truly wants to please and responds to positive reinforcement particularly well.
   Learning Outcome: 58-2
3. C
   Rationale: Because infants have such short, fat necks, it can be virtually impossible to adequately assess the carotid pulse.
   Learning Outcome: 58-3
4. D
   Rationale: The school-age child can begin to take increasing responsibility for self-administration of their own medications, and can be taught how to control chronic diseases such as diabetes or asthma.
   Learning Outcome: 58-4

5. **A**

    Rationale: The toddler wants to do things himself, showing that he is a big boy or girl, so the nurse must make allowances for this need as appropriate when planning care.

    Learning Outcome: 58-5

6. **B**

    Rationale: Puppets help to maintain the attention of preschoolers when providing health teaching.

    Learning Outcome: 58-6

7. **D**

    Rationale: Listening is often the most powerful tool for determining psychosocial needs of the terminal child. Listening includes not only hearing what they are saying but also what they aren't saying.

    Learning Outcome: 58-7

8. **A, B, C, E**

    Rationale: When caring for a child with a chronic illness it is important to answer their questions as honestly as possible, even when their questions are difficult to answer. Provide the information they need to know in a way that is appropriate for their development, making sure they understand what they have been told. Explore the child's understanding of what is occurring because they may interpret actions far differently than anticipated. As children develop, encourage them to participate in their own care in a developmentally appropriate way. The preschooler can go get the bottle with his medication in it, the school-age child can take his medication appropriately, and the adolescent can manage his disease with supervision from parents.

    Learning Outcome: 58-8

9. **D**

    Rationale: The Early Screening Inventory tests the child to determine whether they are capable of learning rather than testing their current knowledge or achieved development.

    Learning Outcome: 58-9

10. **B, C, D**

    Rationale: Normalization is helping the child with special needs meet their full capability by encouraging them to be self-sufficient, expecting normal behavior, and managing behavior, much as would be done with a normal child. The parents should not encourage handicapped behavior, but rather adaptive behavior to the handicap, and should not provide the child with excuses when frustrations occur, but encourage them to try again or try a different approach.

    Learning Outcome: 58-10

Matching

1.	D	5.	B	9.	E
2.	E	6.	C	10.	B
3.	F	7.	D	11.	C
4.	A	8.	F	12.	A

Learning Outcomes

1. See section entitled "Nutrition for the Infant and Toddler."
   Learning Outcome: 59-1
2. See section entitled "Vital Signs in Infants and Toddlers."
   Learning Outcome: 59-2
3. See section entitled "Well-Child Checkups for Infants and Toddlers."
   Learning Outcome: 59-3
4. See section entitled "Illnesses And Disorders."
   Learning Outcome: 59-4
5. See section entitled "Illnesses and Disorders."
   Learning Outcome: 59-5
6. See section entitled "Illnesses and Disorders."
   Learning Outcome: 59-6
7. See section entitled "Illnesses and Disorders."
   Learning Outcome: 59-7
8. See section entitled "Integumentary Disorders."
   Learning Outcome: 59-8
9. See section entitled "Psychosocial Disorders."
   Learning Outcome: 59-9

Apply What You Learned

Suggested Answers

Infrequent diaper changing, exacerbated by thin or inexpensive diapers that do not adequately absorb moisture, may be the cause of the infant's severe diaper dermatitis. The nurse needs to explore if the rationale for changing diapers infrequently is cost or if there is an element of neglect related to this situation. Concerns should be reported so that adequate follow-up can be provided after the mother leaves the clinic. Other clues, such as cleanliness, weight gain, response to stimuli, and shape of the head can all be indicators of the mother's care of the infant. The mother needs to be taught to change the diaper regularly before every feeding and more often if the child experiences diarrhea. The mother will also need to be taught how to treat the diaper dermatitis and when to notify the physician if the rash does not respond to prescribed treatment.

Multiple Choice Questions

1. C

   Rationale: Usually by 6 to 8 months, the infant can begin to pick up cheerios or other small objects as the pincer grasp improves. It is important to remember that these are suggested ranges for development and some children may develop sooner, while others will develop later.
   Learning Outcome: 59-1

2. D

   Rationale: A respiration of 24 in the newborn is a bit slow. It may be acceptable if the infant is in a deep sleep, but further assessment is required to determine if adequate oxygenation is occurring.
   Learning Outcome: 59-2

3. C

   Rationale: Hepatitis B is generally given at birth, again at 2 months, and the final immunization is given at 6 months. Boosters may be necessary as indicated by periodic titers to determine adequate immunity.
   Learning Outcome: 59-3

4. B

   Rationale: Cystic fibrosis is diagnosed by a positive sweat test. Bronchopulmonary dysplasia is diagnosed by x-rays, RSV is diagnosed by culture, and whooping cough is often diagnosed by symptoms.
   Learning Outcome: 59-4

5. A

   Rationale: Cerebral palsy is often seen in premature babies and may be related to insufficient oxygenation, causing damage to neurons. Down syndrome is a chromosomal disorder, Reye's syndrome is an acute encephalopathy believed to be related to administration of aspirin during a viral infection, and mental retardation may or may not accompany cerebral palsy and can be caused by any number of conditions.
   Learning Outcome: 59-5

6. A

   Rationale: A Logan clamp may be used after surgery, especially if the defect is large, to provide support for the lip and prevent separation of sutures.
   Learning Outcome: 59-6

7. B

   Rationale: Phimosis is the inability to retract the foreskin. Complications can include balanoposthitis (infection of the glans penis) and/or paraphimosis (inability to replace the foreskin over the glans).
   Learning Outcome: 59-7

8. C

   Rationale: Diaper rash is often dismissed as a minor problem, but it can actually be quite serious and can lead to systemic infection if not properly treated. It can range from mild in a small area to severe, covering the entire skin area under the diaper.
   Learning Outcome: 59-8

9. B, C

Rationale: After 6 months of age, infants will demonstrate stranger anxiety or fear of people they do not know, such as the nurse. This is compounded by separation anxiety caused by removing the child from the mother. This can be avoided by having the mother place the child on the scale and assist with measurements.

Learning Outcome: 59-9

10. A

Rationale: Members of the group described in this question are all at increased risk for sudden infant death syndrome (SIDS) and mothers should be taught how to reduce risk by placing infants on their backs to sleep, avoiding use of bumper pads, pillows, and blankets.

Learning Outcome: 59-4

Chapter 60 Care and Illnesses of Preschoolers (3 to 6 Years)

Matching

1.	C	6.	E
2.	E	7.	D
3.	B	8.	A
4.	A	9.	B
5.	D	10.	C

Learning Outcomes

1. See introduction to chapter.
   Learning Outcome: 60-1
2. See sections entitled "Nutrition for the Preschooler" and "Vital Signs in Preschoolers."
   Learning Outcome: 60-2
3. See section entitled "Respiratory Disorders."
   Learning Outcome: 60-3
4. See section entitled "Illnesses and Disorders."
   Learning Outcome: 60-4
5. See sections entitled "Nervous System Disorders" and "Sensory Disorders."
   Learning Outcome: 60-5
6. See section entitled "Illnesses and Disorders."
   Learning Outcome: 60-6
7. See section entitled "Integumentary Disorders."
   Learning Outcome: 60-7
8. See section entitled "Psychosocial Disorders."
   Learning Outcome: 60-8

Apply What You Learned

Suggested Answers

Wait approximately 30 to 60 minutes after he last vomited and then begin by giving him small amounts of plain water – approximately 1 teaspoon every 5 to 10 minutes. If tolerated, after 30 minutes amounts offered can be doubled. If he complains of nausea or vomits, stop offering fluid and begin again with one teaspoon an hour later. When oral fluids are tolerated, encourage fluids to replace those lost to diarrhea. When food is reintroduced into the diet the best foods are those that are easily digested such as the BRATT diet (Bananas, Rice, Applesauce, Tea, and Toast). If diarrhea continues for longer than 24 hours or vomiting continues for 12 hours and child cannot keep fluids down, the mother should call for an appointment so the child can be seen.

Multiple Choice Questions

1. D
   Rationale: Preschoolers can use a knife, fork, and spoon. They can generally draw a person with 6 parts, have opinions about good choices but cannot prepare food alone, and gain 1.5 to 5 kg per year.
   Learning Outcome: 60-1

2. B
   Rationale: Although calcium is required for growing bones, if taken in excess it can interrupt the normal absorption of iron.
   Learning Outcome: 60-2

3. C
   Rationale: Measles often causes skin sloughing and special skin care is needed to maintain comfort. Measles can create light sensitivity and environmental lighting must be limited, including light from television sets or computers.
   Learning Outcome: 60-3

4. C
   Rationale: Jehovah's Witnesses do not have an issue with transplantation of the organ, only with the blood contained within the organ. By draining all blood, the Jehovah's Witness can accept an organ transplantation without disturbing the beliefs of their religion.
   Learning Outcome: 60-4

5. A
   Rationale: Astrocytomas impact vision and grow quickly, causing increased intracranial pressure and seizures.
   Learning Outcome: 60-5

6. C
   Rationale: Osteomyelitis, if not treated aggressively and as early as possible, can be very difficult to contain and may lead to amputation of the affected bone.
   Learning Outcome: 60-6

7. D
   Rationale: Dermatophytes are fungi leading to fungal infections.
   Learning Outcome: 60-7
8. B
   Rationale: Children diagnosed with autism will frequently perform the same behavior over and over in an attempt at self-comforting. Thought processes are disturbed, leading to these types of behaviors.
   Learning Outcome: 60-8
9. B
   Rationale: Scurvy is caused by lack of vitamin C in the diet. Intake of vitamin C must occur daily because it is not stored in the body. Excess intake is lost through urine as it is removed by the kidney.
   Learning Outcome: 60-6
10. D
    Rationale: Compartment syndrome occurs when increased pressure in a limited space compromises circulation and nerve innervation, leading to possible necrosis.
    Learning Outcome: 60-6

Chapter 61 Care and Illnesses of School-Age Children (6 to 12 Years)

Matching

1. D
2. G
3. B
4. F
5. A
6. E
7. C

Learning Outcomes

1. See sections entitled "Nutrition for School-Age Children" and "Vital Signs in School-Age Children."
   Learning Outcome: 61-1
2. See section entitled "Illnesses and Disorders."
   Learning Outcome: 61-2
3. See sections entitled "Nervous System Disorders" and "Musculoskeletal Disorders."
   Learning Outcome: 61-3
4. See sections entitled "Gastrointestinal Disorders" and "Endocrine Disorders."
   Learning Outcome: 61-4
5. See section entitled "Urinary Disorders" and "Reproductive Disorders."
   Learning Outcome: 61-5
6. See section entitled "Integumentary Disorders."
   Learning Outcome: 61-6
7. See section entitled "Psychosocial Disorders."
   Learning Outcome: 61-7

Apply What You Learned

Suggested Answers

1. Michael's mother may be feeling guilty because she delayed bringing Michael to the doctor to find out what was wrong with his leg. The nurse can ask the mother what she is sorry for and explain that a delay of 1 to 2 weeks does not make a significant difference in the outcome or treatment, and that the tumor may have begun growing long before the symptom of pain began.

2. Michael is approaching adolescence when fitting in and keeping up with his peers is so important. It is important to help Michael realize that realistic prosthetic legs will make him look normal and some of the more advanced prostheses can keep him active in sports. He will need to be taught how to tell people about his prosthesis in a way that makes it cool rather than frightening, but the time to begin this discussion is not when he first gets news of his need for an amputation.

3. Initially the family is in shock and is trying to come to terms with the required surgery, so it is pointless to provide teaching because the family will not be able to take it in right now. It is best to answer questions simply and be there to provide support and show concern.

Multiple Choice Questions

1. C
   Rationale: This blood pressure is on the high side for an 8-year-old and would require further assessment to determine the reason for the elevation.
   Learning Outcome: 61-1

2. B
   Rationale: Chorea is the involuntary spasmodic movement of the extremities that may accompany rheumatic fever.
   Learning Outcome: 61-2

3. A
   Rationale: Kyphosis is the convex curvature of the spine, whereas lordosis is a concave curvature, scoliosis is a lateral S or C shaped curvature, and amblyopia is reduction in vision with no damage to the eye.
   Learning Outcome: 61-3

4. B
   Rationale: Polydipsia is one of the three P's of diabetes mellitus (polydipsia, polyphagia, and polyuria). Diabetics often have poor wound healing because of the elevated blood glucose that slows the healing process, and weight loss is secondary to inadequate metabolism of glucose.
   Learning Outcome: 61-4

5. D
   Rationale: Edema results from insufficient epoetin secretion, resulting in pale skin and tachycardia. Hypertension results because of the important role the kidney plays in maintaining normal pressure both through fluid regulation and control of renin-angiotensin production.
   Learning Outcome: 61-5

6. C
Rationale: MRSA is an infection that requires an intact chain of infection and any break in the link will prevent the spread of the pathogen.
Learning Outcome: 61-6

7. A
Rationale: Attention deficit-hyperactivity disorder (ADHD) is only diagnosed when other causes are ruled out.
Learning Outcome: 61-7

8. B
Rationale: Ewing's sarcoma is most frequently diagnosed in children, usually boys of Caucasian or Hispanic origins.
Learning Outcome: 61-3

9. C
Rationale: Hyperopia is diagnosed when light focuses behind the retina.
Learning Outcome: 61-3

10. D
Rationale: Five to 6 ounces is recommended, divided into 3 servings a day or approximately 2 ounces per meal.
Learning Outcome: 61-1

Chapter 62 Care and Illnesses of Adolescents

Matching

1.	E	4.	B
2.	D	5.	C
3.	F	6.	A

Learning Outcomes

1. See introduction to chapter.
Learning Outcome: 62-1
2. See sections entitled "Nutrition" and "Vital Signs in Adolescents."
Learning Outcome: 62-2
3. See section entitled "Special Concerns."
Learning Outcome: 62-3
4. See section entitled "Special Concerns."
Learning Outcome: 62-4
5. See section entitled "Illnesses and Disorders."
Learning Outcome: 62-5
6. See sections entitled "Nervous System Disorders" and "Musculoskeletal Disorders."
Learning Outcome: 62-6
7. See sections entitled "Gastrointestinal Disorders" and "Endocrine Disorders."
Learning Outcome: 62-7

8. See sections entitled "Urinary Disorders" and "Reproductive Disorders."
   Learning Outcome: 62-8
9. See section entitled "Integumentary Disorders."
   Learning Outcome: 62-9
10. See section entitled "Psychosocial Disorders."
    Learning Outcome: 62-10

Apply What You Learned

Suggested Answers

1. Brittany must deal with the fact that she was driving and caused the accident that resulted in her friend's death. This is compounded by her not requiring everyone to wear their seat belts. In addition to guilt and sorrow over her friends, she must also cope with paraplegia and the alteration to her body image caused by facial trauma. The nurse can best help her by encouraging her to share her feelings and thoughts, and help her learn positive coping strategies. She may require a referral to a counselor because her needs may be greater and last longer than the nurse can provide help for Brittany's family will also need help coping with the change in their daughter's life.
2. Brittany will have a need to talk with the other girls in the car with her. Peers are very important to the adolescent so she will need a care plan that encourages social interaction through use of computers, telephone, and face-to-face visits. She also must be helped to cope with alteration in body image secondary to the facial wounds. Teens do not like to feel 'different' and she will most likely want to avoid social interaction until her facial wounds heal.
3. She will require surgery to stabilize the spine and plastic surgery to repair the facial wounds. After her physical condition is stabilized, she will require rehabilitation to cover physical therapy and occupational therapy. Nursing care will be focused on preventing infection, promoting healing of wounds and fractures, cast care for her fractured arm, and stabilization of the fractured vertebra. She must be repositioned frequently to avoid loss of skin integrity. Bowel and bladder training is likely to be needed due to the location of the lumbar spine injury. Preparing Brittany for rehabilitation will be an important nursing function in the acute care setting.

Multiple Choice Questions

1. C
   Rationale: When the body begins to increase production of estrogens in the girl or androgens in the boy, the body responds with development of secondary sex characteristics and puberty begins.
   Learning Outcome: 62-1
2. A
   Rationale: The pulse rate is usually lower in an adolescent than an adult. Other vital signs are usually similar to that of an adult.
   Learning Outcome: 62-2

3. B

Rationale: The adolescent deserves the same level of confidentiality as an adult on these topics.

Learning Outcome: 62-3

4. D

Rationale: Accidents and injuries are the major cause of adolescent death, so it is of utmost importance that the nurse address issues such as driving safety to reduce the risk of death.

Learning Outcome: 62-4

5. A

Rationale: Treatment and prognosis for Hodgkin's lymphoma is based on the outcome of staging, which determines the number and location of lymph nodes involved.

Learning Outcome: 62-5

6. D

Rationale: An involuntary flex of the knees or hips is a positive Brudzinski sign, indicative of possible meningitis.

Learning Outcome: 62-6

7. C

Rationale: Recurrent abdominal pain with diarrhea that may be bloody is indicative of possible inflammatory bowel disease, which is diagnosed more frequently in clients of Jewish descent. Metabolic syndrome is associated with obese diabetics, meningitis presents with neurological symptoms such as headache, and hepatitis usually manifests with jaundice.

Learning Outcome: 62-7

8. A

Rationale: A radical orchectomy is used to treat testicular cancer. Testicular torsion is treated with orchiopexy and does not result in loss of the testes if surgical intervention is initiated within 4 to 6 hours.

Learning Outcome: 62-8

9. C

Rationale: Comedo is the medical terminology for an acne lesion.

Learning Outcome: 62-9

10. B

Rationale: This client is demonstrating signs and symptoms of depression and may be considering suicide, so the nurse must address the issue directly.

Learning Outcome: 62-10

Chapter 63 Leadership and Professional Development

Matching

1.	D	6.	E
2.	E	7.	D
3.	B	8.	B
4.	A	9.	A
5.	C	10.	C

Learning Outcomes

1. See section entitled "Licensure."
   Learning Outcome: 63-1
2. See section entitled "Licensure."
   Learning Outcome: 63-2
3. See section entitled "Nurse Practice Acts."
   Learning Outcome: 63-3
4. See section entitled "Leadership Styles."
   Learning Outcome: 63-4
5. See section entitled "Team Leading."
   Learning Outcome: 63-5
6. See section entitled "Delegation."
   Learning Outcome: 63-6
7. See section entitled "Reporting Techniques."
   Learning Outcome: 63-7
8. See section entitled "Handoff Procedure."
   Learning Outcome: 63-8
9. See section entitled "Paperwork."
   Learning Outcome: 63-9
10. See section entitled "Conflict Resolution."
    Learning Outcome: 63-10
11. See section entitled "Nursing Care Delivery Trends."
    Learning Outcome: 63-11
12. See section entitled "National Patient Safety Goals."
    Learning Outcome: 63-12

Apply What You Learned

Suggested Answers

1. The charge nurse needs to look at the assignments made at the beginning of the shift and consider whether this nurse may have had a heavier assignment than others on the unit. Did this nurse get away for a dinner break, or is this the nurse's dinner break because they couldn't get away earlier when they were assigned to dinner? It is important not to jump to conclusions and allow emotions to take over. First, thoroughly assess the situation to determine what is really going on.
2. The charge nurse needs to deal with this situation immediately because the unit needs this nurse's help and the assigned clients need care. After assessing the situation, the charge nurse needs to explain that the nurse must either care for their assigned clients or find another team member who can look after their clients while they take a break, if they are taking a dinner break. The charge nurse should explain the importance of always having someone covering each client and that it is the nurse's responsibility to find coverage.
3. The situation should be reported to the unit manager and it should be done in written form. The charge nurse should write what happened, how it was

handled, and the nurse's response as objectively as possible. If this nurse has a habit of disappearing like this, it is important for the nurse manager to be made aware of the situation, and that can only happen if there is open communication between charge nurses and nurse managers.

Multiple Choice Questions

1. A, B, C
   Rationale: To take the NCLEX-PN, the individual must be a high school graduate or hold an equivalency diploma. They must complete a nursing program that was approved by the state where the program is located. They also must either have a visa or be a U.S. citizen. Established residence is not required and it can be taken in any state, although licensure must be held in the state of residence if it is a compact state or the state where the nurse will work if it is not a compact state. It is not necessary to pass the NCLEX to apply to take the examination.
   Learning Outcome: 63-1

2. D
   Rationale: When the RN asks the LPN/LVN to perform an action this is a delegated nursing act.
   Learning Outcome: 63-2

3. B
   Rationale: This nurse has demonstrated the Nursing Code of Ethics that includes always putting the client first and collaborating with other members of the healthcare team. The nurse is not acting as a team leader and has not exceeded the scope of practice, because the nurse did not initiate the treatment, but discussed it with the physician, who can order the treatment if they believe it will benefit the client. The nurse has not delegated any action.
   Learning Outcome: 63-3

4. A
   Rationale: The autocratic leader makes unilateral decisions while dominating the team members, as demonstrated by this charge nurse.
   Learning Outcome: 63-4

5. C
   Rationale: One of the reasons for delegation is to ensure timely delivery of care for the client. If the nurse's client assignment requires more than the nurse can deliver independently, asking another to help can improve client care if delegation is performed properly, following the five rights of delegation.
   Learning Outcome: 63-6

6. D
   Rationale: These obligations are performed by the team leader, who is responsible for the smooth functioning of a unit on a given shift. The unit manager has 24-hour responsibility for the unit and has responsibilities such as budget management, staff management, and developing policies and procedures for the unit.
   Learning Outcome: 63-5

7. B

   Rationale: Taped report is listened to by the oncoming shift, while those about to go off shift provide client care and wait for report to be over so they can go home. Any questions that arise from the taped report must be tabled until the report is over, when the nurse can find the person on the previous shift who was responsible for the client's care to answer the question.
   Learning Outcome: 63-7

8. C

   Rationale: Incident reports are filed with risk management after review by the unit manager. Risk management compiles statistics to help the facility track when and why incidents occur and then make recommendations to change policies and procedures to reduce the risk of future incidents.
   Learning Outcome: 63-9

9. A

   Rationale: These nurses have reached a compromise to allow both to take off desired days while working a different day.
   Learning Outcome: 63-10

10. C

    Rationale: Functional nursing puts tasks at the center of work assignments with each member performing tasks at their level of education and experience.
    Learning Outcome: 63-11

Chapter 64 Preparing to Take the Licensure Exam

Matching

1. E
2. D
3. B
4. A
5. C

Learning Outcomes

1. See introduction to chapter.
   Learning Outcome: 64-1
2. See section entitled "Development of the NCLEX-PN."
   Learning Outcome: 64-2
3. See section entitled "Understanding the NCLEX-PN Plan."
   Learning Outcome: 64-3
4. See section entitled "Client Needs."
   Learning Outcome: 64-4
5. See section entitled "Computer Adaptive Testing."
   Learning Outcome: 64-5
6. See section entitled "Preparing and Reviewing for the Exam."
   Learning Outcome: 64-6
7. See section entitled "Evaluating Your Readiness to Take the Examination."
   Learning Outcome: 64-7

8. See section entitled "Applying to Take the NCLEX-PN."
   Learning Outcome: 64-8
9. See section entitled "Coping with Test Anxiety."
   Learning Outcome: 64-9
10. See section entitled "Taking the Examination."
    Learning Outcome: 64-10
11. See section entitled "Waiting for Your Results."
    Learning Outcome: 64-11

Apply What You Learned

Suggested Answer

ABCs help to prioritize, with airway considerations always chosen before other considerations. The nursing process guides choices, so if you have answers that represent assessments you can make, planning you can consider, interventions you can perform, or evaluations, you will always choose the answer that would be the next step in the nursing process. For example, if you find a client in a specific situation, you must assess them before you intervene. Another approach is to "remove the boulder first." For example, if the client is complaining of pain caused by wrinkles in the sheet, remove the wrinkles causing the problem before medicating for pain.

Multiple Choice Questions

1. D
   Rationale: The NCSBN conducts a vocational nursing job analysis every three years. If the analysis indicates the role or responsibilities of the nurse have changed significantly, they will adapt the test plan to accommodate the change.
   Learning Outcome: 64-2
2. C
   Rationale: Although you may encounter a few knowledge or comprehension questions, most of the test questions will be written at the application level or higher to see if you are able to take the information you learned throughout the program and apply it to actual nursing situations. Remember, you are tested on the academic level and not the "real world" level where you may see things that are not done correctly.
   Learning Outcome: 64-3
3. B
   Rationale: Pharmacological therapies are a subcategory of physiological integrity because medications are administered to help a client with a physiological or psychological problem resolve the issue.
   Learning Outcome: 64-4
4. A
   Rationale: You have up to 5 hours to answer a maximum of 205 questions, at which point the computer will end your examination. However, the test will

end when the computer calculates you have answered enough questions to demonstrate competence, which can come as soon as 75 questions. Be prepared – when the test is over there is no warning and the screen just suddenly goes blank.

Learning Outcome: 64-5

5. B

Rationale: Mock examinations are often offered with NCLEX-PN review books and are important to look for when deciding on the best book to buy. These mock exams may also be offered through standardized testing organizations or your nursing school and help you to practice taking an NCLEX-type test.

Learning Outcome: 64-6

6. B, D

Rationale: NCLEX review classes are offered by a variety of different organizations and may also be provided by your school to help graduates learn and prepare for their examination. Each student must evaluate their progress and readiness to determine if this would be helpful for you.

Learning Outcome: 64-7

7. B

Rationale: The test administering agency, currently Pearson Vue, will provide you with an authorization to test document that will arrive through the mail. Without this authorization, you will not be allowed into the testing center. When you receive your authorization to test, you must call to schedule an appointment time. When scheduling your appointment, consider your own preferences as to whether you are a morning person or an afternoon person.

Learning Outcome: 64-8

8. C

Rationale: Test anxiety

Learning Outcome: 64-9

9. B, C, E

Rationale: When preparing to take the exam tomorrow it is important to put both your mind and body in the best possible condition for the exam. Avoid studying the night before. Avoid stimulants like coffee, chocolate, or caffeinated soda and depressants such as alcohol. Stay active the day before the exam so you can sleep well and get a good night's sleep, so you aren't drowsy during the examination. Avoid heavy meals before the examination and do not drink excessive amounts of fluids, especially those that can act as a diuretic, for the hour before the exam because time spent going to the bathroom reduces the time you have to take the examination. The night before the exam, do something fun and relaxing but avoid movies, because recent research indicates they are overstimulating and will work against you.

Learning Outcome: 64-10

10. A, B, D

Rationale: Not everyone passes the test, but most do. If you should have a bad day and fail the test, use the results provided by the board of nursing to help you plan your study approach to take the exam again. The diagnostic profile will help you to determine areas of strength and weakness, pointing out what areas you did well on and which ones you missed most often. Getting a tutor, studying with others, or taking remediation programs can help

you strengthen areas of weakness. Talk to the director of your nursing program as they may be able to help you find resources in your community so the next time you take the test you do well.
Learning Outcome: 64-11

Chapter 65 Finding That First Job

Matching

1. C
2. F
3. A
4. E

5. D
6. B
7. D
8. E

9. A
10. C
11. B

Learning Outcomes

1. See section entitled "Portfolio."
   Learning Outcome: 65-1
2. See section entitled "Cover Letter."
   Learning Outcome: 65-2
3. See section entitled "Résumé."
   Learning Outcome: 65-3
4. See section entitled "Interviews."
   Learning Outcome: 65-4
5. See section entitled "Job Search."
   Learning Outcome: 65-5
6. See section entitled "Hiring Process."
   Learning Outcome: 65-6
7. See section entitled "Hiring Process."
   Learning Outcome: 65-7
8. See section entitled "Hiring Process."
   Learning Outcome: 65-8

Apply What You Learned

See Chapter 65 of main text for correct samples.

Multiple Choice Questions

1. C
   Rationale: The student should begin collecting material as soon as the quality of work reaches a caliber that will impress future employers, which generally begins at about the midpoint of your nursing program. Waiting until after graduation is too late to begin the process, because you will have lost some of the work you did throughout the program.
   Learning Outcome: 65-1

2. B

Rationale: The opening paragraph introduces yourself, explains what position you are applying for, and tells the reader where you heard about the job opening. It is in the second paragraph that you share your enthusiasm for the position. The closing paragraph thanks the reader for their consideration of your application and discusses how they can reach you. Nothing is written after the signature section.

Learning Outcome: 65-2

3. A

Rationale: The curriculum vitae is used by professionals with advanced education and experience to share information, such as published work or special research interest.

Learning Outcome: 65-3

4. D

Rationale: It is important to learn a little about the facility before arriving for the interview so you can explain what aspects of the organization appealed to you.

Learning Outcome: 65-4

5. B

Rationale: When you prepare to leave an organization to take a job elsewhere, it is customary to submit a letter or resignation providing at least 2 weeks' notice. It is highly unprofessional to leave an organization without providing adequate notice in writing.

Learning Outcome: 65-5

6. D

Rationale: Facilities may offer a small salary increase after the probationary period. Orientation is usually completed before the end of the probationary period because the facility needs time to evaluate your work while you are functioning independently. Most orientation and probationary periods last longer than 6 weeks.

Learning Outcome: 65-6

7. C

Rationale: Learning how to manage, and not just tolerate, stress is a very important skill in nursing. The amount of responsibility and the frequency of changing conditions make stress an expected part of the job. Always pointing out errors or things that can be done differently or showing other experienced nurses how to do their jobs will not lead to success. It is important to work as a member of the team and not as a single individual in order to provide the best client care.

Learning Outcome: 65-7

8. A

Rationale: Collaborative practice is indicated when the nurse works with others–both nursing and those from other professions. It allows input from all areas of the healthcare team, resulting in improved client care.

Learning Outcome: 65-8

9. B

Rationale: The purpose of the Federal Civil Rights Act was to stop employers from making hiring decisions based on anything that was not related to the skills and ability of the potential employee and limiting the personal information they can discuss in the interview process. This is true of all interviews, not just those in nursing.

Learning Outcome: 65-4

10. D

Rationale: Your portfolio is designed to help the interviewer see your specific skills and interests, so the portfolio should not include your hobbies and interests, especially if they do not relate to an area of the nursing profession.

Learning Outcome: 65-1